The Principles
and Practice of
Nurse Education

The Principles
and Practice of
Nurse Education

Third edition

Francis M. Quinn
University of Greenwich, London, UK

Stanley Thornes (Publishers) Ltd

First published in 1980 by Chapman & Hall
Second edition 1988
Third edition 1995 (ISBN 0-412-43550-0)

Reprinted in 1997 by
Stanley Thornes (Publishers) Ltd
Ellenborough House
Wellington Street
CHELTENHAM
GL50 1YW
United Kingdom

97 98 99 00 01 / 10 9 8 7 6 5 4 3 2

A catalogue record for this book is available from the British Library.

Library of Congress Cataloguing-in-Publication Data available

ISBN 0-7487-3170-9   1-56593-295-1 (USA)

Typeset by Photoprint, Torquay, Devon
Printed and bound in Great Britain by Scotprint, Musselburgh

Contents

Preface

The six years that have elapsed since publication of the second edition of this book have seen continuous and unprecedented changes within nurse education and health care. Mergers of Schools of Nursing and Midwifery, combined with moves into the higher education sector, have resulted in a significant reduction in the number of education providers nationally. Many nurse educators are re-appraising their academic qualifications in the light of their links with higher education, and undertaking further studies at undergraduate or postgraduate level.

The implementation of educational contracting with service providers has exposed nurse educators to market forces in education, which in turn has profound implications for existing curricula and resources. Within this climate of constant and major change, nurse educators have also had to plan and implement Project 2000 courses, develop post-registration frameworks at diploma and degree level and implement major quality assurance initiatives. The fact that change on such a scale is being implemented successfully is a tribute to the professional and personal commitment of nurse educators.

In this third edition I have addressed these major changes by including new chapters on Planning for teaching, Educational delivery systems, Course and pathway management, and Educational quality assurance, and by extensively revising and updating the other chapters. I have tried to maintain the book's emphasis on the practical application of educational principles to nursing, midwifery and health visiting education, supported by relevant theoretical perspectives; this is the formula that has proved so successful in previous editions.

In gathering experiences for this book I have received help, and not infrequently inspiration, from colleagues and students too numerous to mention individually; I hope they will accept this general acknowledgement of my deep gratitude for their contribution.

Finally, I would like to express my heartfelt thanks to my wife Carole and my children Hamnet and Tara for their patience and encouragement during the writing of this third edition.

Francis M. Quinn
Fleet
Hampshire, UK

Introduction: the changing context of nursing and midwifery education

1

The structure of nursing and midwifery education is undergoing fundamental changes of a near-revolutionary nature, both internal and external. The former includes the UKCC Post Registration Education and Practice (PREP) final proposals, and also the ENB Framework and Higher Award for Continuing Professional Education for Nurses, Midwives and Health Visitors. These internal changes are discussed in Chapter 12 (p. 305). The external changes include the links with higher education, Working Paper 10 (HMSO, 1989), and NVQs and of all these, perhaps the most significant is the development of partnerships with higher education (HE) institutions. Healthcare education is no stranger to HE; health visiting and district nursing has long been established in HE, as is the case for professions supplementary to medicine such as physiotherapy and radiography. Coping with changes in curriculum or with internal management arrangements can be stressful for teaching staff, but seem relatively minor upsets when compared with cultural upheaval consequent upon a merger with a university. Many Colleges of Nursing and Midwifery have now made this transition into the HE sector, whilst other have yet to make the step. Like most aspects of change, there are gains and losses in this move into HE; on the positive side there is the opportunity to utilize the facilities and expertise available in a university, and also the opportunity of becoming part of a much wider academic community. There is also the tremendous advantage of the management structure of HE which, unlike nursing and midwifery education, is very flat and non-hierarchical. For example, in a typical university department or school, there is one head or professor and the rest of the staff; even though there are different grades of lecturer e.g. lecturer and senior lecturer, this does not usually relate to line-management functions. Unlike nurse education, where management roles are reflected in seniority and salary, it is commonly found in universities that any member of the teaching staff might be given a major management responsibility such as a course directorship. It is also common for such roles to be rotate to another member of staff after a period of three or four years, so that he or she can bring in fresh ideas and approaches. It is probably true to say that there is much more academic freedom in HE compared with nurse education; for a start, there are limits to the amount of teaching that staff undertake, and there is more autonomy in the lecturer role. On the negative side, it is likely that accommodation, resources, and secretarial and administrative support are less satisfactory than those found in Colleges of Nursing and Midwifery, and there is the danger that nursing and midwifery education will become remote from the practice areas that it serves.

THE HIGHER EDUCATION (HE) SECTOR

The Further and Higher Education Act 1992 made major changes to further and higher education, including the establishment of the Funding Councils for England, Scotland and Wales. These replaced the Universities Funding Council (UFC) and the Polytechnics and Colleges Funding Council (PCFC) which were responsible for funding their relevant sectors before the end of the binary divide between universities and polytechnics. The HE sector includes existing and 'new' universities (ex-polytechnics) and also higher education colleges. The funding body for England is the Higher Education Funding Council for England (HEFCE) and its mission is to promote the quality and quantity of learning and research in higher education institutions, cost-effectively and with regard to national needs.

HE comes under the Department For Education (DFE), and the department has recently published *The Charter for Higher Education* (DFE, 1993) which explains the standards of service that students, employers, and the general public can expect from universities and colleges and other bodies involved in higher education in England. The standards cover areas such as prior information, applications, financial assistance, course aims and structure, equal opportunities, and information for employers.

Within the higher education sector there are a number of organizations concerned with issues of quality. The Higher Education Quality Council (HEQC) consists of three divisions: the Division of Quality Audit (DQA), which is responsible for undertaking quality audit of HE institutions throughout the UK; the Division of Credit and Access (DCA), which is responsible for quality assurance of credit ratings; and the Division of Quality Enhancement (DQE), which is responsible for gathering and disseminating information. HEQC works closely with the Quality Assessment Committees of the three Higher Education Funding Councils. The Quality Support Centre (QSC) was created out of the now-defunct CNAA research, development and information services, by the Open University, and provides information on quality issues to staff working in HE.

WORKING AS A LECTURER IN HIGHER EDUCATION (HE)

Nurse teachers may have mixed feelings about the move into HE, particularly as there is a significant salary differential between the NHS and HE sectors, with the advantage for the former. In HE, the 'career grade' is senior lecturer, i.e. this is as far as most academic staff will progress; the salary scale for this grade, however, equates with relatively low-seniority grades in nurse education, which raises interesting questions.

Academic staff in the ex-polytechnic universities have accepted what is known as the 'new contract' which, although subject to local variations, does have common elements across institutions.

The 'new' contract in HE

Typical statistics

1. Teaching hours per week: normally 18 hours teaching per week, which is 550 hours teaching per year.
2. Teaching weeks per year: normally 38 weeks per year, two of which are administration weeks.
3. Consecutive weeks of teaching: normally not more than 14 consecutive weeks teaching.
4. Annual leave: normally 35 working days paid holiday per year excluding bank holidays and statutory holidays.
5. Period of continuous leave: normally up to six weeks of continuous leave.

Typical duties

These include

1. teaching and tutorial guidance;
2. examining;
3. curriculum development;
4. administration;
5. being expected to work flexibly and efficiently and to maintain the highest professional standards;
6. being expected to participate in an appraisal scheme;
7. agreeing to exclusivity, i.e. obtaining permission to undertake certain external work; and
8. research and scholarly activity.

Research and scholarly activity (RSA)

As part of their normal duties academic staff are expected to engage in RSA, which includes writing books, articles and conference papers. RSA takes place throughout the year, but the weeks outside normal teaching and holiday entitlement are primarily devoted to RSA, which is principally self-managed and will be considered as part of the staff appraisal.

Research assessment exercises

These take place at intervals of four years or so and involve peer review of submissions from HE institutions. The exercise provides information about academic staff who are Active Researchers, and certain criteria have to be met by academic staff in order to be rated as an Active Researcher. From the first assessment exercise is seems that, to be considered an Active Researcher, a member of academic staff must have had a minimum of four papers published in refereed journals within the four years preceding the next assessment exercise. Departments and Schools in institutions of HE are awarded a research rating according to the number and quality of Active Researchers they have, and high ratings attract significant amounts of research funding.

WORKING FOR PATIENTS: WORKING PAPER 10

The Government White Paper *Working for Patients: Education and Training Working Paper 10* (HMSO, 1989) has ushered in a new approach to educational provision. Colleges of Nursing now have corporate status, and a competitive training environment has been introduced through a system of contracting for education. Colleges are no longer automatically funded to provide pre- and post-registration courses, but are required to bid through Regional Health Authorities for educational contracts with NHS Trusts/District Health Authorities. These service providers have become clients of the Colleges of Nursing, and as such will require them to provide education and training that meet identified staff development needs. This has necessitated a shift in orientation from a teacher-led to a client-centred approach to education, and if colleges cannot meet the requirements of the service providers, contracts will go elsewhere. Contracting for education is a means of ensuring that service providers obtain the education and training that best suits their staff development needs. As an alternative to sending staff on existing college courses, the service providers will be able to state precisely their specific education and training requirements. They will also be able to monitor the quality of the educational provision and give feedback to the college.

In turn, the colleges will have to adopt a client-centred approach to curriculum design and delivery, and teaching staff may have difficulty, initially, in accepting the shift of control from themselves to the service providers. They may also be anxious about the competitive contracting process, and what might happen if they fail to win contracts. However, it is not only hospitals that have trust status. General practitioners in a GP practice can opt to become a self-governing trust and this means that they would take responsibility for all aspects of their practice, including funding and staffing of community nursing services.

These changes have profound implications for nurse education, in both hospital and community. In the existing Project 2000 system of nurse education, the students spend half of their three-year programme in the

College of Nursing, and the other half on placements within the hospital and the community. During these placements the mentoring/supervision of students is carried out by the nursing staff, with little or no involvement of the nurse teachers from the college. In the past, this mentoring/supervision role was part of the job description of qualified nurses, but with the advent of the new trust contracts it is unlikely that this will be the case. If we look at this from the trusts' point of view, they may quite rightly ask why it is taken for granted that they provide mentorship/supervision of student nurses. Trusts may well feel that time spent by practitioners looking after students is time taken away from patient/client care, and that if mentorship/supervision is to be done, then it must be paid for.

Their point of view is made even more legitimate if we look at the educational contract between trust and college. The college contracts to provide nurse education to the trust, and the trust pays for this service. However, the trust itself (by its mentorship/supervision) is actually providing 50% of the educational activity that it is being charged for! This is clearly an anomalous situation, and it is almost certain to result in charges being levied for supervision/mentorship of student nurses in the future.

Another key issue here is the question of staff development for qualified nurses. In a GP trust, it is the GPs who would have to finance the staff development of health visitors and district nurses, and they may well feel that they are not prepared to spend money on this activity. Continuing Education is a major aspect of the College of Nursing activity, but if this source of income becomes reduced, it raises questions about the long-term viability of some Colleges of Nursing.

NATIONAL VOCATIONAL QUALIFICATIONS (NVQs)

In the past, the NHS employed nursing auxiliaries to assist the professional nurses in their tasks. These personnel were largely untrained, and learned the job by being shown what to do by the trained staff.

The nursing auxiliary has now been replaced by the health care support worker (HCSW), who undergoes training within the NVQ framework. The National Vocational Qualifications (NVQs) system is a type of credit accumulation and transfer scheme which is concerned with awarding credit for the demonstration of competent performance. The NVQ framework was designed to reform vocational qualifications by offering a coherent model of qualifications that facilitated comparison between vocational awards as well as facilitating transfer and progression within and between occupational areas (NCVQ, 1991).

It is clearly to the advantage of patients and clients to have ancillary staff who have undergone recognized NVQ training. It may be thought, at first glance, that the introduction of NVQ training would be anything but controversial, but there are professional nursing implications that need to be explored. The balance between professionally qualified nurses and health care support workers within an area is termed skill-mix, and it is this concept that is at the centre of the controversy. For example, it has been argued that it is better use of NHS resources to employ two health care support workers rather than one district nurse, and that is it also much less expensive to train the two NVQ level workers than to train the other as a nurse for three years and then a further full-time year to become a district nurse. This model would lead to far fewer professional nurses in employment, and their role would be to supervise and manage the health care support workers who would be responsible for carrying out the majority of the patient/client care. This would entail a major shift in the role of the professional nurse, from a direct provider of care to a supervisor of other workers care, and this is a shift that many nurses find unacceptable. It may also be unacceptable to patients/clients, who have a right to expect their care to be delivered by a professional nurse.

REFERENCES

DFE (1993) *Higher Quality and Choice: The Charter for Higher Education*, Crown Copyright.

HMSO (1989) *Working for Patients, Education and Training, Working Paper 10*, HMSO, London.

NCVQ (1991) *NVQ Briefing Pack Portfolio*, NCVQ, London.

Fundamentals of educational psychology | 2

The profession of teaching, like those of nursing and midwifery, draws upon many other disciplines for its body of knowledge. One of the most important of these contributory disciplines is psychology, especially the branch called 'educational psychology'. This chapter outlines some of the fundamental principles of educational psychology as a basis for subsequent chapters. However, the reader needs to be aware that the majority of research in educational psychology is focused on the teaching and learning of children, so a degree of caution is advisable when attempting to relate such studies to adult students in nursing and midwifery education.

The science of modern psychology has its roots in the discipline of philosophy and this link is very much in evidence when one examines the variety of explanations that psychologists offer in their attempts to make sense of the world. These explanations are influenced by the particular models or metaphors through which psychologists view man and his environment and these have led to a variety of approaches or schools of psychology. One such philosophical metaphor is that of reductionism, which postulates that all things can be reduced to simple, indivisible parts; this atomistic view of the world led to an analytical way of explaining things, i.e. by breaking down wholes into their constituent parts or substages. In biology, these indivisible parts are cells, in physics, they are atoms and in psychology these units of behaviour are called stimuli. Another philosophical concept that has been influential in science is the notion of causal explanation, in which things are explained using only a simple cause–effect relationship. Effects are determined entirely by causes and this approach has been termed deterministic, which implies that everything happens according to physical laws. These philosophical notions of reductionism and cause–effect are inherent in the work of the early psychologists, beginning with the founding of the Leipzig psychology laboratory by Wilhelm Wundt in 1879. Wundt had been impressed by the advances gained in other fields of science by the use of the scientific method, so he attempted to apply this to the field of psychology. His approach was to use a method he termed analytic introspection, in which the subject of the experiment was presented with visual or auditory stimuli and then requested to report the sensations and images he experienced. Wundt carefully controlled the stimuli so that he could generalize the results to other situations, and this belief in the structuring of an individual's mental processes into sensations and images gave rise to the name 'structuralist' for this school of thought.

SCHOOLS OF PSYCHOLOGY

Behaviourism

Behaviourism is a reductionist approach which, whilst denying the value of introspective methods, emphasizes the importance of associations between a stimulus and a response. The concept of mind was rejected as being unnecessary for explaining behaviour. J.B. Watson envisaged the mind as a 'black box', concentrating instead on observable stimulus – response connections. The behaviourist position was further developed by Pavlov (1927), Thorndike (1931) and Skinner (1971) to become the main paradigm in psychology until the 1950s.

Cognitive psychology

During the time Watson was describing behaviourism, a group of German psychologists were propounding an alternative approach called Gestalt psychology, which emphasized the organizational processes in the mind. They rejected reductionist views, arguing that the whole was greater than the sum of its parts. This early approach was cognitive, in that it emphasized internal mental processes rather than observable, measurable behaviour. However, it was largely overshadowed as an approach until the advent of the digital computer in the late 1950s, when interest was revived in the study of mental processes. This new cognitive psychology represents a paradigm shift away from behaviourism towards expansionism and systems thinking (Ackoff, 1973). Expansionism is the opposite of reductionism, in that it sees a whole as made up of interrelated systems that are interdependent upon each other. It uses a synthetic mode of thinking, where components are explained in terms of their contribution to the total system. Table 2.1 draws together some of these key differences between cognitive and behaviourist psychology.

Table 2.1 Philosophical comparison of behaviourist and cognitive psychology

Behaviourist	Cognitive
Reductionism: all things reducible to indivisible parts.	*Expansionism*: focuses on wholes.
Analytic thinking: breaking down into constituent parts.	*Synthetic thinking*: role of parts in relation to whole system.
Causes and effect explanation: effects determined entirely by causes.	*Teleological explanation*: uses purposes and goals to explain things.
Determinism: everything happens according to physical laws.	*Free-will*: man is free to make choices.

Humanistic psychology

This approach involves the study of man as a human being, with his thoughts, feelings and experiences. This is in direct contrast to behaviourism which studies man from the point of view of his overt behaviour, disregarding his inner feelings and experiences. The humanistic approach differs from cognitive theory also, in that the latter is concerned with the thinking aspects of man's behaviour, with little emphasis on the affective components. Exponents of humanistic theory claim that the other two theories omit some of the most significant aspects of human existence, namely feelings, attitudes and values.

INDIVIDUAL PSYCHOLOGICAL DIFFERENCES

Learning theories have attempted to provide explanations about learning that apply to people in general, but in reality, there are no 'people in general' because every individual is unique. At best, the general approaches can provide insight into some of the phenomena that are likely to be associated with learning, but any given individual will differ in the degree to which such phenomena manifest themselves. It is of little practical use to consider theories of learning in isolation from the individual who is the consumer of education and indeed, from the environmental context within which he or she operates. Students are likely to exhibit marked differences in a number of characteristics such as personality, motivation, intelligence, cognitive style and language and these individual differences will affect learning. The social context in which students operate is another important determinant of learning; such factors as socialization, group interaction and social labelling are important variables for the nurse teacher to consider.

Personality

Personality is a particularly difficult concept to define since any definition reflects the individual stance of the person defining it. Krahe (1992) suggests three basic components of the term 'personality' that are generally accepted by researchers regardless of their theoretical orientation:

1. personality is the reflection of individual uniqueness;
2. personality is enduring and stable; and
3. personality and its reflection in behaviour are determined by forces or dispositions assumed to reside within the individual.

This definition shows the difference between idiographic and nomothetic approaches to the study of personality: the former looks at an individual; the latter seeks laws that can be generally applied.

Freudian psychoanalytic theory

Sigmund Freud was born in Austria in 1856, the son of a cloth merchant. His father was almost 30 years older than his mother, who was his third wife and doted on Sigmund, her first-born child. Sigmund studied medicine at the University of Vienna and researched into physiology and cerebral anatomy. He was influenced by Charcot's use of hypnotism and became interested in neurotic disorders, developing his theory of psychoanalysis that was to achieve world-wide fame. Freud considered that there were two observable aspects of mental life or psyche – the brain and consciousness. In 1923, he developed a formal model of the structures that fill the gap between these, identifying them as the id, the ego and the super-ego. The id is the source of psychic energy that resides in the inherited instincts of Eros (life drive) and Thanatos (death drive); the energy of the former is called the libido and the latter comprises self-destructive drives and aggression. The id operates on the 'pleasure principle', which involves the pursuit of pleasure, the avoidance of pain and is irrational, impulsive and demanding. The ego, in contrast, operates according to the 'reality principle' and its function is to express the demands of the id in accordance with the demands of society, blocking or delaying gratification until an appropriate time for its release. The super-ego is somewhat equivalent to conscience and is an internalized sense of right or wrong that judges actions.

Psychoanalytic theory lays great emphasis on the development of the libido, whose energy focuses on the regions of the body called the erogenous zones. The first of these to develop is the mouth, from which the infant derives satisfaction by sucking and feeding – the oral stage. The second stage of development is the anal stage, which occurs at about the age of two to three, with pleasure being derived from the expulsion of faeces. The third stage is termed the phallic stage, in which sensation is focused on the genitals. Male infants sustain erections, which draw their attention to their genitals, leading to the awareness that females do not possess a penis. The child fears that he may lose his penis also, a phenomenon termed 'castration anxiety' by Freud. His father is seen as a rival for his mother's affection and the fantasy that the child will kill his father and possess his mother is termed the 'Oedipus complex'. These conflicts are normally resolved slowly by the identification of the male child with the father. Female children develop somewhat differently during the phallic stage, with the concept of 'penis envy' being paramount. The father becomes the 'love object' and antipathy develops towards the mother, a term called the 'Electra complex'. Again, these conflicts are gradually resolved by identification with the parent of the same sex.

Following these three stages, there is a period of latency until puberty, when the genital stage occurs. Here, sensation remains in the genitals, but assumes its adult nature through intercourse rather than auto-eroticism.

Freud developed the concepts of fixation and regression in relation to these stages of development; the former implies remaining at a particular level when seeking satisfaction at a later stage of development, such as when a person who is fixated at the oral stage continues to seek satisfaction by chewing gum or smoking. Regression implies the return to an earlier stage of development, such as overeating when under stress.

There is a further aspect of Freudian theory called consciousness, which has three levels: the preconscious, the conscious and the unconscious. The first relates to things that we are aware of, the second, to the things we are able to become aware of if we attend to them and the third, to the things that we are not normally aware of. The three aspects of personality, the id, the ego and the super-ego, operate below conscious level, although the ego and super-ego are partially in the conscious level.

In the Freudian system, then, personality is seen as consisting of three components:

1. the id, an inherited instinctual component that comprises sexual and aggressive impulses;
2. the ego, which serves to find ways of gratifying id impulses within the context of external reality; and
3. the super-ego, which acts as an internalized system of values derived from society.

These three components are in a constant state of conflict with each other, with the ego serving to prevent unacceptable id impulses from entering consciousness. It does this by a number of defence mechanisms;

- repression means that the unacceptable desires are prevented from gaining access to the conscious;
- denial occurs when the individual behaves as if nothing has happened, even after serious occurrences such as the death of a loved one;
- reaction formation is the adopting of behaviours diametrically opposite to those of the unconscious impulse, such as disguising hostility by extreme politeness;
- projection involves the attribution to other people of the unacceptable impulses;
- rationalization consists of finding plausible reasons for the unacceptable impulses without being aware of the real unconscious reasons;
- displacement is commonly thought of as 'kicking the cat', where hostility is displaced to a weaker or more acceptable object;
- sublimation is the channelling of unacceptable impulses into other forms of expression such as art.

Hence, these defence mechanisms serve to protect the individual from anxiety, but if they break down, the person is likely to regress to earlier forms of behaviour.

A number of variations grew out of Freud's theory as a result of several of his colleagues developing their own psychoanalytic theories. These included Carl Jung, Alfred Adler and the neo-Freudians Karen Horney and Erich Fromm.

Psychoanalytic theory has always been controversial and has been criticized on a number of grounds. In a most telling critique, Eysenck

(Eysenck, 1985, p. 208) condemns the non-scientific approach adopted by Freud and his followers:

> Psychoanalysis is at best a premature crystallization of spurious orthodoxies; at worst a pseudo-scientific doctrine that has done untold harm to psychology and psychiatry alike, and that has been equally harmful to the hopes and aspirations of countless patients who trusted its siren call. The time has come to treat it as a historical curiosity and to turn to the great task of building up a truly scientific psychology.

Eysenck's criticisms are summarized in his four rules, which he suggests should be followed by anyone wishing to understand psychoanalysis.

1. Do not believe anything written about Freud or psychoanalysis, particularly when it is written by Freud or other psychoanalysts, without looking at the relevant evidence.
2. Do not believe anything said by Freud and his followers about the success of psychoanalytic treatment.
3. Do not accept claims of originality, but look at the work of Freud's predecessors.
4. Be careful about accepting alleged evidence about the correctness of Freudian theories; the evidence often proves exactly the opposite.

Trait or dispositional theories

Traits are relatively permanent aspects of personality that affect people's behaviour and are seen as points lying along a continuum between poles. There are two influential trait theorists – R.B. Cattell and Hans Eysenck. Cattell used a multivariate approach to personality in that he attempted to examine the interrelationships between a number of variables at the same time, a technique termed factor analysis. He first identified all the words in the dictionary that described behaviour and then used a sample of subjects who were rated for these trait elements. Cluster analysis revealed 50 surface traits, which were factor-analysed to reveal 16 source traits – the basis of the 16PF personality test. Cattell used data from observers, questionnaires and objective measures to arrive at his 16PF test and it is possible to construct a profile of personality based upon the individual's performance in the test. The categories for the 16PF test are given in Table 2.2.

Cattell drew a number of conclusions about the application of his work to education:

- outgoing and adaptable students who are warmly related to the teacher learn more quickly;
- students who are more emotionally balanced and less easily upset learn more easily;
- those with greater conscientiousness will make more progress for the same degree of intelligence;
- more dominant students learn more slowly;

- introverts show more vocabulary and grammatical skills than extroverts; and
- docility is associated with passing examinations.

Cattell's work has been criticized because of the inability of other researchers to replicate his findings.

Eysenck's theory of personality, like Cattell's, utilizes factor analysis as a statistical technique to isolate the dimensions of personality. His work has isolated three unrelated and orthogonal dimensions of personality called

introversion/extraversion,
neuroticism/stability, and
psychoticism/stability.

A typical extravert is sociable and outgoing, whereas an introvert is quiet and inward looking. Eysenck views personality as being biologically inherited but arising out of interaction with the environment, pointing out the similarities between the traits identified by factor analysis and the typologies of body humours identified by Galen. The Eysenck Personality Questionnaire is used to measure personality and reveals scores on each of the dimensions, which can be then compared with published norms. The educational implications of Eysenck's theory are not clear cut:

- students withdrawing from college for academic reasons tend to be extraverts, whereas those withdrawing for psychiatric reasons tend to be introverts;
- introverts tend to become bored and fatigued more easily than extraverts;
- excitement tends to interfere with an introvert's performance whilst it enhances that of an extravert;
- stability is related to academic success; and

Table 2.2 Cattell's 16PF personality factors

Reserved	——	Outgoing
Less intelligent	——	More intelligent
Affected by feelings	——	Emotionally stable
Humble	——	Assertive
Sober	——	Happy-go-lucky
Expedient	——	Conscientious
Shy	——	Venturesome
Tough-minded	——	Tender-minded
Trusting	——	Suspicious
Practical	——	Imaginative
Forthright	——	Shrewd
Self-assured	——	Apprehensive
Conservative	——	Experimenting
Group-dependent	——	Self-sufficient
Undisciplined self-conflict	——	Controlled
Relaxed	——	Tense

- there is a correlation between attainment and extraversion in school-children.

Trait theories have been criticized on the grounds that behaviour is much more variable from situation to situation than trait theorists accept and that it is likely that teaching style has greater influence on learning than personality traits.

Rogers' self theory

Carl Rogers, one of six children in a close family, was originally destined to become a religious leader. However, after three years at theological college, he transferred to psychology, spending several years with delinquent children before moving into counselling and psychotherapy. His approach belongs to the humanistic school of psychology and focuses on the subjective nature of the self-concept. This approach emphasizes that people should be seen in terms of how they see themselves and the world around them – their phenomenal field. This is termed the 'internal frame of reference' and this is the best point from which to understand a person's personality; empathy is the relating to another person's internal frame of reference.

Rogers views the person as having a self-actualizing motive, which is a basic tendency to achieve one's full potential and reach fulfilment. The self-concept begins to develop when the infant can distinguish its 'self' from other aspects of the environment and self is often divided into two components – actual self and ideal self. The former is self as it is and the latter, self as one would like it to be and Rogers suggests that the individual strives for consistency between self and experience. Individuals attempt to behave in ways that are consistent with their self-concept, but discrepancies result in states of incongruence, leading to psychological maladjustment.

Rogers distinguishes between internal and external locus of evaluation; internal locus implies that the individual relies on his own values to make choices in life, whereas an external locus implies that he uses other people's values. Increasing maturity and growth leads to a move from an external locus of evaluation to an internal one, with the individual becoming responsible for himself. Self-acceptance is a necessary prerequisite for accepting other people and Rogers uses the term 'fully functioning person' to describe the individual who has become what he truly is.

Rogers' theory has several applications to education – the quality of the relationships between teacher and student is paramount and empathic relationships will foster genuine learning. He has formulated a 'law of interpersonal relationships' for two people willing to be in communication – the greater the communicated congruence of experience, awareness and behaviour of one of them, the greater will it be for the other. This law emphasizes the importance of reciprocal congruence and is the keystone for much of Rogers' psychotherapy. In Rogerian psychotherapy, the therapist must not be the expert, since this implies an external locus of control. Rather, he functions as a facilitator who uses unconditional positive regard for the client, helping him to use his own resources. There is, however, growing disillusionment with this approach, as studies fail to support the claimed relationship between therapist conditions and outcome, i.e. facilitators' skills are not related to outcome.

Kelly's personal construct theory

George Kelly, the son of a Presbyterian minister, graduated in mathematics and physics before studying educational sociology. He became interested in psychotherapy and developed his theory of personal constructs (Kelly, 1955).

Personal construct theory is an unusual personality theory in that it is neither traditional philosophy nor traditional psychology in orientation. Kelly proposes that each individual views the universe in his own unique way and that he actually creates these ways of seeing by the use of constructs. A construct can be likened to a pattern or template with which the individual attempts to match the realities of the universe. Kelly maintains that because the universe is constantly changing, it follows that these constructs must be continually altered over a period of time – no construct can ever be right and therefore man is always trying to make better constructs with which to view the world. He can extend his repertoire of constructs in order to view the world more clearly, or he can modify his existing ones to match reality. Constructs are bipolar, possessing similarity and contrast dimensions. For example, hot and cold, wet and dry, and constructs may be subsumed under superordinate constructs. The process of creating new constructs may be psychologically painful, especially if there is much personal investment in existing ones. It may take prolonged psychotherapy to assist an individual to restructure his constructs, since it is these that determine his ways of relating to other people and his adjustment to the environment.

Personal construct theory has a very clear underlying philosophy called 'constructive alternativism', which states that everything in the universe is open to a number of alternative interpretations, rather than some fixed immutable truth. Man views the universe through his own unique system of constructs and is best studied in the context of his time on earth. Kelly always resisted attempts to classify his theory under one of the schools of psychology, but it deals with essentially cognitive aspects of perception. He emphasized the nature of man as the scientist, who attempts to predict and control events in the same way that scientists do, by his use of constructs. The whole purpose of constructs is to anticipate events and each individual attempts to expand his construct system so that he can better anticipate events. An individual's personality is thus seen as his personal constructs plus his feelings and actions.

Personal construct theory forms the basis of the 'repertory grid technique', which is designed to elicit an individual's constructs and their interrelationships. Subjects are asked to indicate from a list of roles or titles the way in which two people on the list are alike, but different from a third. This gives the similarity and contrast dimensions, and over the course of the test, the subjects' own constructs are elicited without contamination by the views of the experimenter. This aspect of the repertory grid technique is important, since it differs markedly from other forms of test which are generated by the experimenter; subjects are free to reveal their own constructs. Kelly's repertory grid technique has had wide application in education, particularly in eliciting the ways in which teachers view their students.

However, Kelly's theory has been criticized for its lack of emphasis on feelings and for its vagueness on how an individual knows which constructs to use to make the best predictions.

Locus of control theory

This theory emphasizes the importance of the individual's expectancy in the occurrence of behaviour and was formulated by Rotter (1954). His general formula for the probability of occurrence of a given behaviour is

$$NP = f(FM, NV)$$

i.e need potential (NP) is a function (f) of freedom of movement (FM) and need value (NV).

An example from nurse education might be useful here to clarify this formula. Let us assume that a particular nurse teacher has always had good relationships with the principal of the College of Nursing and Midwifery; in other words, this nurse teacher has a high freedom of movement for such relationships, since freedom of movement means the expectation of success based upon previous experience of the situation. The college is then incorporated into the local university, and a new dean of health is appointed. The likelihood of the nurse teacher behaving in a similar way in this new context will depend upon the freedom of movement and also how much the nurse teacher values a relationship with the new dean. A further factor involved in this probability is the notion of perceived control over the outcome of the behaviour; the nurse teacher may attribute the outcome to either internal or external factors. If the behaviour towards the new dean proves successful, the nurse teacher may attribute this to internal factors such as his or her personal charm or social skills, or alternatively it may be attributed to external factors such as being lucky to have such an approachable dean.

This concept of perceived control is the cornerstone of 'locus of control theory' (LOC) and Rotter devised a test that measures whether an individual has an internal or external locus of control. This test is called the internal–external locus of control scale (I–E scale). Individuals with an external locus of control believe that they have little or no control over events in life, whereas those with an internal locus of control believe that they control their own destiny. A number of important claims are made for locus of control theory in a variety of social applications. Lefcourt (1982) suggests that an internal locus of control may well serve as a defence against unquestioning obedience to authority, by enabling an individual to maintain a sense of responsibility. With regard to learning, internals may be more efficient at processing information, more inquisitive and receptive to their surroundings.

Learned helplessness

A phenomenon related to locus of control is that of learned helplessness (Seligman and Maier, 1967). This was discovered in a series of experiments on the effects of inescapable shock on the subsequent escaping behaviour of dogs. In the first experimental procedure, dogs were placed in a harness that limited their movements and were then given aversive electric shocks through the hind feet, the dogs being unable to prevent or escape from the shocks. In the second procedure, dogs were placed in a two-way shuttlebox that had a grid floor through which electric shocks could be administered. In this case, though, the animals could escape the stimulus by crossing to the other side of the box; indeed, they could escape the stimulus altogether if they responded to a prior warning signal by crossing to the other side. Seligman compared the effects of the shuttlebox on dogs that had previously received no shock treatment and also on dogs who had been in the harness and had received inescapable shocks. The results were strikingly different; the previously untreated dogs reacted by barking and running until they escaped the shock, whereas the dogs who had been subjected to inescapable shock previously, made a very passive response to the shock. The conclusion of the experimenters was that these dogs had learned helplessness from their experience of inescapable shock in the previous experiment. These findings have also been observed in human beings who have been subjected to inescapable aversive stimuli such as loud noise.

Type A personality and coronary heart disease

Rosenman, Friedman and Straus (1964) developed a 'susceptibility to coronary heart disease (CHD) profile' based upon a study of patients who had experienced the disease. They found that patients behaviour exhibited common characteristics as follows:

    extremely competitive
    high achieving
    aggressive
    hasty
    impatient
    restless
    explosive speech patterns
    tension of facial muscles
    under time pressure and the challenge of responsibility

The patients who exhibited these behaviours were classified as 'Type A' personality, and subsequent studies have confirmed the link between

CHD and Type A personality. A second type of personality was identified, Type B, a more relaxed type who had low risk of CHD. Health psychologists have developed interventions to change Type A behaviour, with good results.

Motivation

Motivation is a cognitive construct that is used to explain the causes of behaviour. Theories of motivation attempt to explain the reasons why people behave in one way rather than another and are thus more concerned with 'why' rather than 'how'. Motivation to learn is seen as an important variable in educational psychology and a number of approaches are examined in this section.

Instinct theory

The main exponent of this approach was William McDougall, who believed that man was motivated by certain innate tendencies to action, which he called instincts. This highly mechanistic view saw man's behaviour as a product of innate forces acting from within him. For example, a gregarious instinct caused him to seek the company of others, and an acquisitive instinct made him want to acquire things. Most behaviour was thus explainable by reference to a particular instinct, but the theory fell out of favour when it was realized that this approach explained nothing about behaviour as such. However, another school of psychology, ethology, still maintains that some human behaviour is instinctual. Ethology is concerned with the study of animals in their natural settings, rather than in the artificial surroundings of the laboratory and one of the founders of this school was Konrad Lorenz. He demonstrated that animals possess certain fixed-action patterns, which can be triggered off by innate releasing mechanisms and the phenomenon of imprinting is an illustration of this.

Imprinting is a kind of learning that occurs in young animals within two days of birth, or hatching, and consists of the animal following the first moving object it encounters. This is normally the parent and the process has survival value to the species, in that the young animal follows, and remains close to, the parent. Lorenz demonstrated that imprinting will occur on the first moving object, even if this is a human being or an inanimate object, but that it is difficult or impossible after two days, when fear of strange objects has developed. Bowlby (1970) describes the attachment behaviour of the newborn infant towards a preferred figure as a form of imprinting. Lorenz considers imprinting to be an example of a fixed-action pattern, which is triggered off by the sight of the parent moving. Tinbergen has also described such patterns in the male stickleback, in which fixed-action patterns of attack or courtship are released by the red underside of another male, or the swollen abdomen of the female respectively. Eibl-Eibesfeldt has summarized the innate releasing mechanisms in man, citing examples such as the cues in an infant's appearance, which trigger off caring behaviour in adults.

Another theory that utilizes the concept of instinct is that of Freud. His psychoanalytic theory sees man as being motivated by two basic instincts or drives, Eros and Thanatos. The former are life drives and are divided into ego drives, which are concerned with self-preservation, and libido, which is concerned with sexual drive and preservation of the species. Thanatos is composed of self-destructive drives and aggressive drives, and constraints imposed on these by self or society result in their repression below the level of consciousness. Such repressed drives function as unconscious motivators of behaviour.

Drives, needs and incentives theory

Drives are internal states of an organism that arise as a consequence of some form of need, either biological or non-biological. Biological needs are things like food and water, whereas other forms of need are cognitive, emotional or social. Drives act to motivate people to satisfy the particular need in question, but in addition to drives, there are external things called incentives, which also motivate people and thus, motivation can be seen as being a joint product of these two forces. Incentives are used a great deal in industry and commerce in the form of bonus payments or commission, which staff can earn provided they reach certain target levels of performance. Clarke L. Hull (1943) developed a complex system of postulates and theorems to account for motivation and learning in which drive is seen as an aroused state that causes or impels an individual to action. The response of the individual results in drive reduction, which reinforces the response and a secondary drive may develop if the original drive stimulus is paired with a neutral one a sufficient number of times.

Most real-life situations are characterized by multiple motivation where the individual is motivated by a number of different motives. These may be in harmony, thereby increasing the strength of motivation or they may be in conflict, with some producing a positive incentive and others a negative incentive. This has been described as 'approach–avoidance conflict' and there are three types (Bourne and Ekstrand, 1985):

1. approach–approach conflict – conflict between two equally desirable courses of action;
2. avoidance–avoidance conflict – the choice is between two negative motivators, neither of which is desirable; and
3. approach–avoidance conflict – incentives have both positive and negative components, such as eating and weight gain.

One of the major problems with 'needs and drives theory' is that it does not explain why animals or people try to achieve things that are not associated with biological deficits, such as watching television and reading books. This has led to a move in psychology away from 'needs' and towards 'incentives' as a way of explaining motivation.

Maslow's theory of human motivation

Abraham Maslow was one of seven children and he was a rather shy and nervous child. His father was a rather colourful character who liked to drink and fight. Maslow began by studying the law but then changed to study psychology, eventually becoming a trained therapist. He published his 'theory of human motivation', in which there are five classes of need arranged in hierarchical order, from the most basic up to the highest level (Maslow, 1971). Each class of need is stronger than the one above it in the hierarchy, in that it motivates the individual more powerfully when both needs are lacking. Gratification of needs is a key concept in this theory; when a need is gratified at one particular level, the next higher need emerges. The needs are arranged in a hierarchy as follows:

self-actualization
  esteem
    belongingness and love
      safety
        physiological

Physiological needs are the most basic and include hunger, thirst, sleep, maternal needs, etc. An individual dominated by these needs sees everything else to be of secondary importance and this can occur to such an extent that he or she no longer sees anything beyond the gratification of them. The next class is the safety needs, which include security, stability, protection, the need for order and structure, etc. and above this come the belongingness and love needs, including affection, friendship and sexual needs, although the latter can be classified with physiological needs also. Esteem needs are concerned with strength, achievement, mastery and competence and also include reputation, prestige and dignity. Self-actualization is the highest class of needs and is concerned with the fulfilment of one's potential. This will vary greatly from person to person, according to how he or she perceives that potential. There are two further classes of need that Maslow originally included in the hierarchy – the need to know and understand and the aesthetic needs. These are now seen to be interrelated to the basic needs, rather than to separate classes. The order of these remains fixed for most people, but there are exceptions. For example, some people prefer assertive self-esteem more than love. There are examples in life where lack of basic needs seems to be subjugated to the attainment of self-actualization, as with monks who fast for lengthy periods. Maslow examined the lives of well-known public figures and came up with a list of shared characteristics, which are hallmarks of self-actualizing individuals:

- more efficient perception of reality;
- acceptance of 'self' and others;
- spontaneity, simplicity and naturalness;
- problem-centring;
- quality of detachment, a need for privacy;
- autonomy, independence of culture and environment;

- continued freshness of appreciation;
- peak experiences;
- deeper, more profound interpersonal relations;
- democratic character;
- philosophical, non-hostile sense of humour;
- creativeness; and
- transcendence of any culture.

There are not many studies that focus on Maslow's theory, but there is some support for the dominance of basic needs.

Achievement motivation

Achievement motivation was first explored by McClelland and Atkinson in the middle 1950s using the 'thematic apperception test' (TAT) (McClelland *et al.*, 1949). The subject's need for achievement is referred to as 'n ach' and is tested by showing a series of ambiguous pictures about which the subject has to make up a story. The assumption is that the subject's own wishes and thoughts are projected into the picture and are thus a measure of achievement motivation. Achievement motivation appears to be a relatively stable phenomenon over time and there are a number of studies that show that subjects with high 'n ach' do better on tests of problem-solving and mathematics and that, in school and in business, the high 'n ach' individual performs better.

There are at least two factors involved in achievement – the need for success and the fear of failure – and both are present in everyone. The resultant motivation depends upon the relative strength of the two aspects. If the motivation is predominantly the need for success, then the student is likely to keep trying in the event of initial failure. If, on the other hand, he she is motivated predominantly by fear of failure, then they will be put off by initial failure, but encouraged by initial success. The balance between these two aspects will influence the choice of problems that students select. Students with low 'n ach' tend to select either very difficult or very easy problems, whereas those with high 'n ach' select moderately difficult ones.

In teaching students, it is likely that high 'n ach' individuals will benefit from more challenging assignments, stricter marking and feedback; low 'n ach' individuals will respond to less challenging assignments, more flexible marking and avoidance of failure in public.

Attribution theory of motivation

Weiner (1979) formulated 'attribution theory', which puts the emphasis on an individual's search for understanding as the key factor in motivation. In social settings, people are continually trying to understand both their own and other people's behaviour and they do this by making attributions about such behaviour. With regard to his or her own successes and failures in learning, each individual attributes this to a number of

Table 2.3 Weiner's attribution theory of motivation

| | Internal to individual | | External to individual | |
	Stable	Unstable	Stable	Unstable
Controllable	Typical effort	Immediate effort	Teacher bias	Unusual help from others
Uncontrollable	Ability	Mood	Task difficulty	Luck

factors and Weiner identifies eight of these major causes, as outlined in Table 2.3. The stable/unstable dimension is related to future expectations; if the student perceives success or failure as related to stable factors, this will confer a degree of predictability for future outcomes. The internal/external dimension is related to student's feelings; if outcomes are seen to have external causes then likely feelings are gratitude and perhaps surprise if the outcome is successful, whereas unsuccessful outcomes may lead to anger and surprise. Internal causes, on the other hand, may lead to feelings of guilt or incompetence if outcomes are unsuccessful and to pleasure and contentment if successful. The controllable/uncontrollable dimension is closely associated with motivation to perform tasks; students are less likely to undertake tasks when they feel that such a task is uncontrollable by their own efforts. Conversely, they are more likely to attempt tasks that are seen to be under the control of their own actions. The greatest problems of motivation arise when students attribute their lack of success to internal, stable, uncontrollable factors such as their own ability, which is perceived as being beyond their power to change.

Intelligence

Intelligence is a notoriously difficult concept and definitions fall into two categorizes: it is a biological, genetically determined, low-level attribute of the human nervous system; or it is a culturally determined, experientially driven attribute of high-level cognitive function (Anderson, 1989). There is some doubt that the construct exists at all. Howe, (1990), for example, argues that definitions of intelligence are descriptive, not explanatory, and suggests that

> for the important task of helping to discover the underlying causes of differing levels of performance, there is no convincing evidence that the concept of intelligence can play a major role. So far as explanatory theories are concerned, the construct seems to be obsolete.

Intelligence is not something that is achieved or attained, rather, it is a cognitive ability that enables an individual to learn and to adapt to his environment. It is that capacity of people commonly referred to as 'native wit' and needs to be distinguished from the concept called 'education'. A person can be highly intelligent, yet uneducated, since education and knowledge are attainments rather than abilities. Of course, intelligence is important in education and it may transpire that many well-educated people are also highly intelligent, but the two concepts need to be seen as interrelated rather than identical. Another point of difficulty lies in the nature of intelligence – whether it is some sort of overall, global ability or a multidimensional concept. Wechsler (1958) defines intelligence as 'the aggregate or global capacity of the individual to act purposefully, to think rationally, and to deal effectively with his environment' and this definition falls into the global category. Spearman (1927) believed that there were two factors that constitute intelligence – a general factor called 'g' and a number of specific factors termed 's'; the general factor 'g' accounts for the correlation between scores on intelligence tests and the specific factors 's' are specific to a given test.

Cattell (1971) proposed two kinds of intelligence – fluid and crystallized. Fluid intelligence is genetically determined and corresponds to Spearman's 'g', whereas crystallized intelligence is determined by the environment and learning. Fluid intelligence reaches its maximum in individuals by their mid-twenties, but crystallized intelligence continues to increase throughout life. Cattell believes that the quality of an individual's fluid intelligence will influence the development of crystallized abilities such as vocabulary.

Using factor-analytic techniques, Thurstone (1938) identified seven primary mental abilities:

1. verbal comprehension,
2. memory,
3. word fluency,
4. number,
5. perceptual speed,
6. spatial, and
7. reasoning.

These mental abilities show wide variation between individuals and to some extent, contradict the notion of a general factor of intelligence.

Guilford (1967) has developed a model of intelligence that envisages ability as consisting of three components – the 'faces of intellect': mental operations, contents and products. Mental operations are processes used by the individual to deal with information, and the combination of operations, content and products are given 120 cognitive abilities. Table 2.4 shows the categories of these three 'faces'.

A very recent approach to intelligence is that known as 'artificial intelligence' (AI) which has been defined as 'the use of computer programs and programming techniques to cast light on the principles of intelligence in general and human thought in particular' (Boden, 1977). This involves the use of computer simulation to develop theories about human cognitive processes such as language or problem-solving and the approach has been termed 'theory development' by Miller (1978) to contrast with the standard approach in psychology, which is 'theory demonstration'. Theory demonstration involves a written explanation of some specific aspect of cognitive performance and the subsequent experimental testing of it. Theory development or AI, on the other hand, are

Table 2.4 Guilford's model of intellect

1.0	Mental operations	
	1.1 Cognition	Understanding of information
	1.2 Memory	Storage and retrieval of information
	1.3 Divergent production (thinking)	Creativity and variety
	1.4 Convergent production (thinking)	Correctness or conformity
	1.5 Evaluation	Making judgements
2.0	Contents	
	2.1 Figural	Information in form of sensory representations
	2.2 Symbolic	Letters and numbers, music, etc.
	2.3 Semantic	Information in form of meanings
	2.4 Behavioural	Interpersonal perception
3.0	Products	
	3.1 Units	Smallest items of information
	3.2 Classes	Concepts
	3.3 Relations	Principles and rules
	3.4 Systems	Larger combinations of principles and rules
	3.5 Transformations	Changes in existing information
	3.6 Implications	Expectations or predictions

explanations stated in the form of computer programs, which address more general aspects of cognition by attempting to model human cognitive processes prior to experimental testing. One of the advantages of this approach is that great clarity is required in the formulation of the program, otherwise it will not work. The main differences between the two approaches is that theory demonstration emphasizes parsimony as a criterion for a theory, i.e. an explanation that explains the phenomenon more economically is better than one which is more complex. With the AI approach, sufficiency of the theory is the main criterion and there is more tolerance of alternative theories. There are many computer programs in existence that can simulate aspects of human cognition and this artificial intelligence is demonstrated in their ability to translate language, to play chess and to solve complex problems with great speed.

Testing intelligence

Intelligence tests are a source of great controversy among both psychologists and the lay public and this stems largely from the social and racial implications of their use in educational testing. Three main tests have been developed over the years: the Binet–Simon test, the Stanford–Binet test, and the Wechsler tests.

The Binet–Simon test This test was developed in France to identify children who needed special education and consisted of a scale of test items for children aged between three and thirteen years. The underlying assumption is that there is an average mental level for each age and test items were devised to measure this. If a child could answer items from a higher age-bracket than his own, he was said to have a mental age higher than his chronological age. If, on the other hand, he could only answer items from a lower age-bracket than his own, his mental age would be less than his chronological age. This notion was developed by Stern to produce a ratio that is called the 'intelligence quotient' (IQ). It utilizes the concepts of mental age (MA) and chronological age (CA) to calculate an individual's intelligence relative to the average, using the formula

$$IQ = \frac{MA}{CA} \times 100$$

Thus, if a child is aged eight years, but can only answer test items that an average five-year-old could answer, then his IQ is

$$\frac{5}{8} \times 100 = 62.5$$

Since the average IQ is 100 (MA=CA), this child would be considered mentally retarded. Another child may have a mental age of ten and a chronological age of eight, giving an IQ of 125, which indicates superior intelligence.

The Stanford–Binet test This was developed in America by Terman, to give a standardized test for use in that culture and consisted of a series of revisions of the Binet–Simon test, including the first use of the concept of IQ.

Wechsler tests There are three tests used here and each is designed to measure both verbal and non-verbal intelligence.

1. WAIS-R: Wechsler adult intelligence scale (revised version)
2. WISC-R: Wechsler intelligence scale for children (revised version)
3. WPPSI: Wechsler preschool and primary scale of intelligence

Wechsler developed his adult scale because of the problems of measuring the IQ of adults using the Stanford–Binet test. The concept of mental age depends upon the notion that intelligence increases along with chronological age in children, but there is no evidence that this continues beyond adolescence; this would result in an adult's chronological age increasing steadily, whereas his or her mental age may remain the same, leading to a progressively declining IQ. Wechsler overcame this by introducing the deviation IQ, which compares the individual's score with standardized norms for his age group and is expressed in standard deviation units. It is clear that, in considering the usefulness of intelligence tests, we must be sure that the test is measuring ability rather than attainment, since the latter is very much influenced by environmental factors. In practice, however, this is very difficult to ensure and many criticisms are levelled at the cultural bias of tests. In any test, the two main criteria are its validity and reliability, i.e. does the test measure what it is supposed to measure and does it measure this consistently. Intelligence tests do correlate highly with each other, so reliability is high, but this does not prove that validity is equally high. It may well be that these tests are measuring something consistently, but that 'something' is not intelligence. All the tests rely on teachers' opinions about students' ability and this can be unreliable; also, the tests assume a normal distribution of intelligence within the population and this may not be the case. Many of the criticisms centre around the importance of heredity and environment in the determination of intelligence and this will be discussed next.

The nature–nurture controversy

The current controversy is concerned with the relative contribution to intelligence of genetic and environmental factors and has caused such division that social scientists are classified as 'hereditarians' or 'environmentalists'. The hereditarian viewpoint does acknowledge that some contribution is made by environmental factors; what is disputed is the relative contribution made by each. One of the main hereditarians, Arthur Jenson argues that a genetic viewpoint must be considered for two pressing reasons. He claims that, first, environmentalist approaches have failed to provide satisfactory explanations for the results of IQ tests and second, that it is common sense to suppose that mental traits are genetically determined because so many physical characteristics are so determined. The main support for his arguments lies in the concept of heritability (H2) estimates, which attempt to measure the extent to which genetic and environmental factors explain differing performance in IQ tests. The higher the H2 estimate, the more genetic influence. For example, Jensen claims that the H2 estimate for intelligence is 0.80 for white Americans, which implies that 80% of the variance in IQ is attributable to genetic factors, the rest being environmental. This is a population statistic, however, and no conclusions can be drawn about any particular individual within that population. Jensen also claims to be able to falsify every argument put forward by environmentalists to explain the gap between IQ scores of black and white Americans.

Another proponent of the hereditarian view is Eysenck, who uses results from studies with twins to support his points. Twins are classified into monozygotic (identical) or dizygotic (fraternal); the former are produced from the same ovum that has split into two and thus share the same genetic material; the latter are from different ova and are therefore no more alike than ordinary siblings. In twin studies, the amount of resemblance on a given trait between monozygotic over dizygotic twins is taken as evidence of genetic influence. Eysenck and Kamin (1981) quote numerous studies in which a high positive correlation is found between the IQ of monozygotic twins, but not for dizygotic twins, whose scores are much the same as ordinary siblings. Of course, this may be due to environmental influences such as having identical twins dress the same, but further evidence comes from monozygotic twins reared apart. There are high positive correlations between the IQ of monozygotic twins raised apart in some studies and also a high correlation with the IQ of their natural parents.

Another argument put forward by Eysenck is that of the phenomenon of 'regression to the mean'. It applies to any trait that is less than 100% inherited and is described as the tendency for offspring of parents with some extreme characteristic to possess the same characteristic but in a less extreme way. Thus, the children of high-IQ parents tend to have lower IQ than those parents, but still have higher IQ than the population mean. Eysenck uses this phenomenon to counteract the environmentalist argument, since an environmental hypothesis would expect that the children of bright parents should be in an environment conducive to development and should therefore develop IQs higher than their parents. In contrast, children of dull parents show regression to the mean, which means that their IQs are higher than their parents, despite the 'unconducive environment' that might exist in the family.

A final argument put forward by Eysenck concerns the use of biological measures of intelligence. These measures, in Eysenck's words 'provide the most convincing proof to date of the correctness of the genetic model of intelligence' (Eysenck, 1981, p. 67). He quotes the work of Jensen on 'reaction time tests'. Subjects are given various tasks that require a response such as pressing a button. He found that the speed of reaction correlated highly with IQ. Another biological measure is that of evoked potentials on the electroencephalograph (EEG). Evoked potentials are characteristic sets of waves on the EEG, evoked by stimuli such as sudden flashes of light or sounds. Eysenck claims that there is a high correlation between those evoked potential patterns and the IQ of the individual. In fact, he goes as far as to suggest that these results show a 'concrete, measurable, biological basis for IQ' (Eysenck and Kamin, 1981, p. 72).

The environmentalists emphasize the importance of social and physical surroundings and events in determining the intelligence of an individual. First, we examine a theory by Stinchcombe (1969), which proposes that intelligence is not a constant 'dispositional property' but rather layers of cognitive structures, or styles of reasoning. These layers of cognitive structure are well-ordered, in that a five-year-old's IQ score consists of answered questions at the four and five-year-old level rather than a random selection from other ages. Stinchcombe states two factors that would then determine the cognitive functioning, namely, the capacity of the individual to abstract and his or her inclination to abstract. The former is the individual's IQ and the latter is the socialization function of society. Stinchcombe quotes studies in which correlations can be found between the IQ of foster parents and foster children and between teachers' IQ and the achievement of their pupils. He then defines the level of civilization of a group by the average level of cognitive function used to solve its problems. He hypothesizes that rural lifestyles do not provide the experience of analysis at an abstract level, whereas the city dweller is exposed to this sort of experience. Hence, he explains the low IQ scores of rural dwellers and of negro communities, the latter not being allowed to develop their own schools and 'civilizing institutions'.

Another major figure in the environmentalist mould is Leon Kamin. He argues against the hereditarian viewpoint of intelligence, quoting the terrible effects of eugenics movement on such things as immigration quotas and the American sterilization laws (Kamin, 1981). A genetic explanation of intelligence has led to consigning of many students to the 'educational scrap heap' and he maintains that the genetic arguments can all be explained in terms of environmental effects, or of poor or fraudulent data. He does not actually state an environmentalist theory as such, but relies chiefly on criticizing the arguments of the genetic viewpoint.

SOCIAL PSYCHOLOGY

Nurse education takes place in a social context that includes colleagues, teachers and patients. The student may belong to a number of groups in the hospital setting, e.g. a particular set, a certain ward team and a group of friends living on the same floor of the halls of residence. The practice of nursing takes place in the presence of others, so it is worthwhile looking at group performance as an influence on learning.

Audience effects and coaction effects

The mere presence of an audience may facilitate or hinder behaviour. For example, many actors and athletes feel that they need an audience in order to perform to their fullest ability, and this effect is supported by studies. The effect of having someone actually performing a task with another person has also been studied extensively and Allport (1924) concludes that the presence of a co-worker enhances the speed and quality of work on simple tasks. On the other hand, the presence of others can exert an inhibitory effect on behaviour and this has been demonstrated in a number of interesting studies. Latane and Darley (1968) showed the effect of the presence of other people on an individual's reaction to emergency situations. They conclude that people are less likely to intervene in an emergency if other people are present and this can be explained by diffusion of responsibility. If a person is alone when he or she encounters an emergency, then that person is solely responsible for his or her actions. If, however, other people are present, each individual may feel that their own responsibility is reduced and this makes them less likely to become involved.

Two important concepts in groups are roles and norms and these have considerable bearing on the classroom climate. Roles are actions within a given status and examples of roles are those of the teacher as an authority figure and the learner as subordinate. Norms are standards or values of behaviour, which may be formal or informal. Formal norms in a group of students may be imposed by the teacher or the college, whereas informal norms develop from within the group as a result of interaction over a long period. There is evidence that norms may develop over a short period; in a classic study on group norms, Sherif (1936) demonstrated the rapid convergence to a group norm of individuals' opinions regarding the extent of apparent movement of a spot of light in a darkened room. There is a substantial body of knowledge that demonstrates the importance of the social environment in relation to learning outcomes. Fraser and Fisher (1982) in a large-scale study found significant correlations between students' perceptions of the classroom environment and learning outcomes.

Socialization

From early infancy, individuals learn the values, knowledge and patterns of behaviour that make them a member of their particular society; the process by which an individual undergoes induction into these expected behaviours or roles is termed socialization, and is a lifelong process involving transmission of culture. Primary socialization begins in infancy and is mediated through the immediate family; sex roles, social class, morals and manners are all part of this early socialization process. Once the child commences school, the process of secondary socialization begins and this is influenced not only by teachers but by peers; the latter exert a powerful effect as the child moves into adolescence, when peer-group pressure may result in behaviour at variance with the child's family or society.

A particular kind of secondary socialization is that termed occupational socialization, which involves the induction into specific occupational roles after leaving school. The culture called nursing has a powerful influence on new members, socializing them into the role of nurse, with all its attendant values and behaviours. In the past, there was great emphasis on conformity and obedience to superiors and a very rigid code of personal and professional behaviour. This has altered to a certain extent over the last few years, but nursing may still seem rigid and inflexible in comparison with other professions.

Socialization may begin in anticipation of future rules and this anticipatory socialization is important in facilitating the eventual uptake of such roles. Many girls are socialized into nursing from an early age by means of play, especially that associated with hospitals and caring. The mass media is a powerful influence on such socialization and may well be responsible for sex-role stereotyping and racism. Television, newspapers and even children's books often portray nursing as being the exclusive preserve of women; indeed, women are largely portrayed in occupations such as nursing, teaching, domestic work and catering, rather than in engineering or medicine. In television advertisements, the 'boss' is invariably a man and the secretary a woman, which helps to perpetuate the notion that men are the leaders and decision-makers, whilst women are the assistants.

Individuals are not the passive recipients of socialization processes; rather, there is a two-way exchange of behaviour involved. Even very young infants can influence parental behaviour by the type of crying they emit, and by the use of smiling (Schaffer, 1974). Much socialization occurs by imitation of modelling behaviour; a young child copies the behaviour of the adults around him and new nurses copy the professional behaviours of the trained staff in their vicinity. In Chapter 4 (p. 97), the work of Bandura on social learning theory is outlined and this has relevance to the discussion on socialization, because imitation is a central concept in the theory.

Labelling theory and expectancy effect

In sociological terms, labelling is the assigning of an individual to a category as a means of classifying his behaviour or state. Hence, 'ill' is a label used to distinguish people who are not healthy; 'vandal' is a label that distinguishes people who exhibit antisocial behaviour involving damage to property. Labelling, then, involves classifying people who deviate from what is considered to be normal; the term 'deviance', however, is used to indicate a negative social evaluation. Primary deviance is the assigning of a label to particular behaviours or states that society judges to be deviant; these behaviours are socially defined and will vary between different cultures. The behaviours that a society considers deviant may change over the course of time; in the UK, it used to be considered deviant to attempt suicide, or to live as a couple without being married, whereas nowadays these behaviours are seen in quite a different light. Once society has assigned a label to an individual, certain consequences may occur and these are termed secondary deviance. When a person is labelled 'deviant' he or she becomes stigmatized or disgraced in the eyes of society; depending upon the nature of the deviance, the individual may be shunned or worse – this is particularly true for labels such as 'rapist'. Many diseases, however, can stigmatize the sufferer, especially mental illness, epilepsy, AIDS and even such problems as deafness or blindness. Indeed, it can be argued that the diagnosis of such conditions in itself constitutes labelling of primary deviance, setting in train a series of predictable social consequences.

A second major effect of labelling is that of changes in the individual's self-concept; as a result of social reactions to the original label, the affected person begins to respond in a way that is compatible with that label. In other words, he comes to believe that he is what the label says he is and produces stereotyped behaviour that accords with it. This phenomenon has been termed 'the self-fulfilling prophecy' – a prophecy that comes true solely because it has been made. For example, society labels a youth as 'violent' and people begin to react to him according to his label; eventually, the youth begins to accept the label and behaves in a violent way. Obviously, there must have been an initial episode that led to the label, but it may have been a 'one-off' incident entirely untypical of the individual.

The notion of self-fulfilling prophecy has been explored in education, where it is known as 'teacher-expectancy effect'. There is a good deal of evidence about the effect of people's expectations on certain outcomes; experimenters have to be cautious when interpreting results because such results may be due to the 'Hawthorne effect' – a variation in subjects simply due to the fact they are being observed. The presence of an observer in a nursing lecture may have either positive or negative effects on the performance of students that are totally unrelated to the style of teaching given. The notion of self-fulfilling prophecy in education was explored in a study by Rosenthal and Jacobson (1968) called 'Pygmalion in the Classroom'. In this study, carried out in an American school, teachers were given false information about some of the children in their classes; these children were purported to have unusual academic potential and were called 'spurters', but in reality they were randomly selected from the total class. The children were given tests of non-verbal intelligence at the start of the experiment and again at four months and eight months and results showed that the 'spurters' had gained significantly more in terms of IQ than the other children. This was ascribed to the fact that teachers' expectations of the 'spurters' had acted as a self-fulfilling prophecy, which made them achieve more. The study has been criticized on methodological grounds, but there is some support from other studies that teacher-expectancy can influence learning.

Sociometry

Sociometry, as the name implies, is concerned with the measurement of social relationships within groups and its principal tool is the sociogram. Each group member is asked a question about which other group members they would like to work with in a given situation, or which members they would not wish to work with. The members' choices are plotted in the form of a sociogram, as illustrated in Figure 2.1.

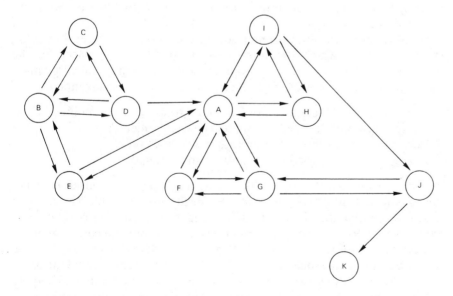

Fig. 2.1   Example of a sociogram.

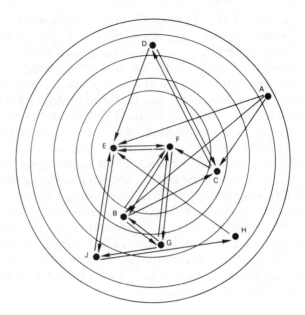

Fig. 2.2   Target sociogram.

Each student is represented a letter (A–K) and the arrows drawn joining the letters indicate the direction of choice for each of the eleven students. There are a number of typical structures revealed by a sociogram (Figure 2.1): the most popular student (A) – who receives six out of the eleven choices – is called the 'star'; other typical structures shown are 'mutual pairs', 'triangles' and 'chains'. It may also be possible to identify an 'isolate', who is not chosen by anyone, or who decides not to make choices.

An alternative way of plotting a sociogram is to use a target sociogram (Figure 2.2), in which the most popular students are placed in the innermost circles and the least popular in the outermost ones, giving a clear indication of choices. Sociometry has a number of advantages:

1. sociograms show relationships from the group members' point of view;
2. choices are uninfluenced by the teacher/experimenter;
3. sociograms can show subgroupings in classes; and
4. sociograms are easy to collect, either in writing or verbally.

There are some disadvantages, however, that need to be borne in mind; many teachers may find the notion ethically unacceptable to use with students, particularly if 'social engineering' is used on the basis of data from sociometry. Intermediate relationships are not indicated, giving a rather 'black-and-white' picture of the relationships in the group. The actual design of the sociogram depends as much on artistic talent as on rational rules, so that two sociograms from the same data may give quite different impressions. Also, for groups of more than about 15, sociograms become impossibly complex.

Another way in which sociometric data can be analysed is by use of sociometric indices, and these can be of use when comparing the same individual in a variety of groups. Sociometric indices reduce the great amount of visual detail in a sociogram into relatively simple numerical values that allow comparison. The following are examples of indices.

- Individual's Choice Status (CSi)

$$CSi = \frac{\text{number of persons choosing } i}{N-1}$$

- Individual's Rejection Status (RSi)

$$RSi = \frac{\text{number of persons rejecting } i}{N-1}$$

- Group Cohesion (CO)

$$CO = \frac{\text{number of mutual pairs}}{\text{possible number of mutual pairs}}$$

The use of indices may give the impression that sociometry is an 'exact science', whereas the reliability of positive choices leaves much to be desired (Harper, 1968). The validity is also questionable, in that choices may reflect the day-to-day changes rather than deep group structure. Perhaps the old maxim about 'analysing data with a microscope that was gathered with a rake' needs to be borne in mind when considering sociometric indices!

Teaching styles

There is no such things as an ideal teaching style, since individual teachers differ widely in personality and approach to teaching. Nevertheless, research has shown that it is possible to categorize teaching styles to some degree, and the common classifications are discussed next.

Getzels and Thelen's teaching styles

Getzels and Thelen (1960) describe three teaching styles: nomothetic, idiographic and transactional. The nomothetic leader is one who places emphasis on the requirements of the institution rather than on the individual. Education is perceived as the handing down of information. The idiographic style is the opposite to this, in that the individual is stressed rather than the institution and education is seen as assisting him to learn what he is motivated to learn. There is an intermediate style called transactional, which implies an appreciation of the limitations of the individual and the institution, and attempts to make a sensible compromise between the two.

Bennett's teaching styles

Neville Bennett (1976) analysed nearly 500 junior school teachers by both observation of classroom activities and interviews about educational issues and teaching methods. He categorized these teachers into three types (formal, mixed and informal) based upon their approach to the following aspects:

1. integration or separation of subjects;
2. pupils given choice of work and/or seating;
3. use of testing and grading;
4. teacher's class control and discipline; and
5. use of class or small-group teaching.

Having classified the teaching styles of teachers, Bennett then classified primary school children into groupings according to personality testing and proceeded to correlate the pupils' progress, pupil type and teacher style. Bennett concluded that the teaching style was more influential than the effects of personality type, but the study has been the subject of extensive criticism on the grounds of methodological and statistical problems.

ORACLE and teaching styles

The 'observation research and classroom evaluation' project (ORACLE) was carried out at the University of Leicester (Galton and Simon, 1975). In total, 58 classrooms were observed, from inner-city, urban, village and housing estate areas. The project used systematic observation plus interviews with teachers, and four teacher styles and four pupil styles were identified. The four teaching styles were as follows.

1. *Individual monitors* (22% of the sample): teachers showed a high level of one-to-one interaction with pupils.
2. *Class enquirers* (15% of the sample): teachers showed a high proportion of class teaching.
3. *Group instructors* (12% of the sample): teachers interacted with groups of pupils rather than individuals.
4. *Style changers* (50% of the sample): teachers were able to change their teaching style in a number of ways.

The ORACLE project found that teaching style was the most important variable in pupil progress and the results showed the characteristics of successful teaching to be:

1. a high level of teacher–pupil interaction;
2. a high level of task statements and questions by the teacher;
3. regular feedback to pupils;
4. encouragement for pupils to work by themselves;
5. use of higher-order and open-ended questions; and
6. avoidance of the overuse of instructions.

REFERENCES

Ackoff, R. (1973) Science in the systems age: beyond IE, OR and MS. *Operational Research*, **21**, 661–71.

Allport, E. (1924) cited in J. Davis (ed.) (1969) *Group Performance*, Addison Wesley, Massachusetts.

Anderson, M. (1989) New ideas in intelligence. *The Psychologist*, **3**, 92–4.

Bennett, N. (1976) *Teaching Styles and Pupil Progress*, Open Books, London.

Boden, M. (1977) *Artificial Intelligence and Natural Man*, Harvester Press, Brighton.

Bourne, L. and Ekstrand, B. (1985) *Psychology: Its Principles and Meanings*, Holt, Rinehart and Winston, New York.

Bowlby, J. (1970) *Attachment*, Penguin, Harmondsworth.

Cattell, R. (1971) *Abilities: Their Structure, Growth and Action*, Houghton Mifflin, Boston.

Eysenck, H. (1985) *Decline and Fall of the Freudian Empire*, Penguin, Harmondsworth.

Eysenck, H. and Kamin, L. (1981) *Intelligence: The Battle for The Mind*, Pan, London.

Fraser, B. and Fisher, D. (1982) Effects of classroom psychological environment on student learning. *British Journal of Educational Psychology*, **52**, 374–7.

Galton, M. and Simon, B. (1975) Observation research and classroom learning evaluation. University of Leicester.

Getzels, J. and Thelen, H. (1960) A conceptual framework for the study of the classroom as a social system, in *The Social Psychology of Teaching*, (eds A. Morrison and D. McIntire), Penguin, Harmondsworth.

Guilford, J. (1967) *The Nature of Human Intelligence*, McGraw Hill, New York.

Harper, D. (1968) The reliability of measures of sociometric acceptance and reflection. *Sociometry*, **31**, 219–27.

Howe, M. (1990) Does intelligence exist? *The Psychologist*, **3**(11), 490–3.

Hull, C. (1943) *Principles of Behaviour*, Appleton Century Crofts, New York.

Kamin, L. (1981) *Intelligence: Battle for the Mind*, Pan, London.

Kelly, G. (1955) *The Psychology of Personal Constructs*, Vol. 1, Norton, New York.

Krahe, B. (1992) *Personality and Social Psychology: Towards a Synthesis*, Sage, London.

Latane, B. and Darley, J. (1968) Group inhibition of bystander intervention in emergencies. *Journal of Personality and Social Psychology*, **10**, 215–21.

Lefcourt, H. (1982) *Locus of Control: Current Trends in Theory and Research*, 2nd edn, Erlbaum, New Jersey.

Maslow, A. (1971) *The Farther Reaches of Human Nature*, Penguin, Harmondsworth.

McClelland, D., Clark, R., Roby, T. and Atkinson, J. (1949) The effect of need for achievement on thematic apperception. *Journal of Experimental Psychology*, **37**, 242–55.

Miller, L. (1978) Has artificial intelligence contributed to an understanding of the human mind? *Cognitive Science*, **2**, 11–128.

Pavlov, I. (1927) *Conditioned Reflexes*, Oxford University Press, Oxford.

Rosenman, R., Friedman, M. and Straus, R. (1964) A predictive study of CHD. *Journal of the American Medical Association*, **189**, 15–22.

Rosenthal, R. and Jacobson, L. (1968) *Pygmalion in The Classroom*, Holt, Rinehart and Winston, New York.

Rotter, J. (1954) *Social Learning and Clinical Psychology*, Prentice-Hall, New Jersey.

Schaffer, H. (1974) Early social behaviour and the study of reciprocity. *Bulletin of the British Psychological Society*, **27**, 209–16.

Seligman, M. and Maier, S. (1967) Failure to escape traumatic shock. *Journal of Experimental Psychology*, **74**, 1–9.

Sherif, M. (1936) *The Psychology of Social Norms*, Harper, New York.

Skinner, B. F. (1971) *Beyond Freedom and Dignity*, Alfred Knopf, New York.

Spearman, C. (1927) *The Abilities of Man: Their Nature and Measurement*, MacMillan, New York.

Stinchcombe, A. (1969) Environment: the cumulation of effects is yet to be understood. *Harvard Educational Review*, **39**, 511–22.

Thorndike, E. (1931) *Human Learning*, Appleton Century Crofts, New York.

Thurstone, L. (1938) Primary mental abilities. *Psychometric Monographs*, No I.

Weiner, B. (1979) A theory of motivation for some classroom experiences. *Journal of Educational Psychology*, **71**, 3–25.

Weschler, D. (1958) *The Measurement and Appraisal of Adult Intelligence*, 4th edn, Williams and Wilkins, Baltimore.

Adult learning: cognitive perspectives | 3

The first part of this chapter takes a general approach to human information-processing and outlines the following key aspects: the human memory system, perception, thinking, problem-solving, and psychomotor skills. The second part adopts a more specific focus by outlining the human psychological development theories of Piaget and Levinson, followed by a range of cognitive theories of learning including Ausubel, Bruner, Gagne, Kolb, and Schon.

THE NATURE OF HUMAN COGNITION

Cognition is the term given to internal mental processes such as thinking, learning, problem-solving, remembering and perceiving. According to Smythe *et al.*, (1987), cognitive psychology is concerned with 'the acquisition and use of knowledge, and with the structures and processes which serve this'. Cognitive psychology is undergoing a major revival owing to the advent of digital computers and the interest in flow charts of computer processes such as feedback control. The computer has provided an analogy for the workings of the human mind, or more accurately, computer programs have provided the analogy. Psychologists are less interested in the 'hardware', i.e. the physiology of the individual than they are in the 'software' or 'programs' that underlie his or her thinking. There is a branch of psychology called artificial intelligence (AI) in which the aim is to devise programs that will make computers simulate intelligent behaviours such as reading or translating. It is from this interest in the way computers process information that the main conceptual model in modern cognitive psychology has developed, namely the information-processing approach.

The information-processing approach

There are a number of different theories that take an information-processing approach, but there are elements common to all. Information-processing approaches postulate a flow of information through the system with this flow taking a finite amount of time. Some parts of the system have a limited capacity for processing information and there are overall control processes that govern the flow; Figure 3.1 shows the basic components.

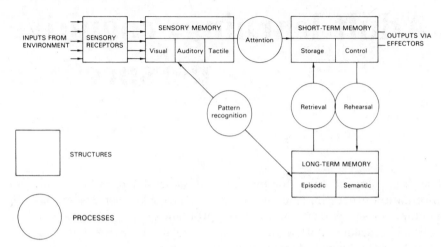

Fig. 3.1 Basic structures and processes of an information-processing system.

The flow of information begins in the sensory receptors, which detect stimulus inputs from the environment and transfer them to the sensory memory. This records all stimuli encountered in a form similar to the actual stimulus: visual stimuli in iconic form, and auditory stimuli in echoic form, i.e. as an auditory echo. The sensory memory registers stimuli for only about one second and so we are not aware of this process. It does, however, allow time for further processing if the particular stimuli are given attention. When stimuli are attended to, the next stage in information flow is to the short-term memory, which has both storage and control functions, but is very limited in capacity. Information can be transferred to long-term memory by further processing, particularly rehearsal. Information required for outputs must first be retrieved from long-term memory and put back into the short-term memory, from whence it can be used to generate outputs via effector organs. There is one other pathway in the flow of information that connects the sensory registers with long-term memory. This is not a direct pathway for storage of stimuli, but it is hypothesized that whenever a stimulus enters the sensory registers, contact is made with long-term memory to see if the stimulus has been encountered and stored before. This process is called pattern recognition.

So far we have examined the flow of information from the external environment through the system, but information can also arise from within an individual, i.e. from his or her own memory. Thus, people often sit and think about things and their thoughts may trigger off a course of action, with a flow of information through the system. This kind of processing is termed 'knowledge-driven' or 'top-down' processing; the processing of stimuli from the environment is termed 'data-driven' or 'bottom-up' processing. The information-processing approach is applied to a variety of aspects of cognition and the next section examines these in relation to nurse education.

THE HUMAN MEMORY SYSTEM

Figure 3.1 shows an information-processing system with three distinct kinds of memory: sensory, short-term and long-term. One of the most influential three-storey models of memory is the Atkinson–Shiffrin (1971) model. These three kinds of memory may indeed be separate systems within the brain, or merely different kinds of storage within the same system. Nonetheless, each of the three memory systems has distinctive characteristics outlined below.

Sensory memory

The sensory memory registers incoming stimuli for a very brief period. It is a high-capacity system that registers all sensory inputs in their original form – visual stimuli as images or icons, and auditory stimuli as echoes of the sounds. Visual stimuli last for about one second and auditory stimuli for about four seconds, and we are unaware of these stimuli. However, when a stimulus is registered in sensory memory, contact is made with long-term memory to check whether there is an existing pattern for that stimulus. The role of sensory memory is to prolong stimuli just long enough to allow for selective attention to important ones.

Short-term memory

This is also termed working memory, primary memory and short-term store and is characterized by a limited capacity for storage, of about seven chunks of information. The term 'chunks' is deliberately vague and applies to any unit that is familiar to an individual (Miller, 1956). Hence a chunk may be a single word or a single letter and it is possible to increase the amount of data in short-term memory at any one time by incorporating more information into each chunk. In addition to this storage function of short-term memory there are control processes such as rehearsal, which can be divided into maintenance rehearsal and elaborative rehearsal (Craik and Lockhart, 1972). Maintenance rehearsal consists of going over and over the material in short-term memory in order to keep it there; it does not affect the long-term recall of the material. Elaborative rehearsal, on the other hand, processes the material much deeper by relating it to existing material in long-term memory. Short-term memory is also involved in the processes of both thinking and language by providing the working area for these, hence the alternative name, working memory. It is likely that information is coded in the form of both acoustic and articulatory codes in working memory; the former involves the sound of a word and the latter involves the way it is pronounced. Baddeley and Hitch (1974) and Baddeley and Leiberman (1980) describe working memory has having a 'central executive' and two slave systems, the 'phonological (or articulatory) loop' and the 'visuo–spatial sketch pad'. The central executive has an overall co-ordinating and control function; the phonological loop is concerned with speech-based information, and the visuo–spatial sketch pad with spatial information.

Long-term memory

There appears to be no limit to the capacity of long-term memory and information stored here has been subjected to considerable processing. Craik and Lockhart (1972) have suggested a levels-of-processing approach, which states that there is a variety of levels at which information is processed, from the physical characteristics of the stimulus through to the identification of meaning of the stimulus. Deeper-level processing results in better remembering of information, because it allows more elaboration of the stimulus, i.e. more links are made with relevant information already existing in long-term memory. This means that the information has been subjected to considerable top-down processing and is therefore more susceptible to distortion and bias. It seems likely that there are two kinds of information stored in long-term memory – episodic knowledge and semantic knowledge. Episodic knowledge is associated with particular events in time and space, such as the memory of an encounter with a particular student, whereas semantic knowledge consists of general concepts unrelated to specific events or episodes (Tulving, 1972). Autobiographical memory differs from other knowledge structures in the degree of self-reference and the sensory/perceptual nature of the knowledge stored (Conway, 1991).

Representation of knowledge in long-term memory

It is useful to distinguish between declarative knowledge and procedural knowledge; the former is about 'knowing that' and the latter is about 'knowing how'. Declarative knowledge consists of knowledge of factual information and can be transmitted verbally to others. Procedural knowledge, on the other hand, is concerned with knowing how to do something, such as administering an injection, and is often more difficult to explain. Indeed, the most effective way of explaining procedural knowledge to someone is by demonstrating the procedure to them and this is the basic way of teaching a psychomotor skill.

Current research suggests two main theories about the way in which knowledge is represented in long-term memory, the 'propositional code theory' and the 'dual-code theory'. Propositional code theory (Anderson and Bower, 1973; Pylyshyn, 1973) states that information is coded in the form of propositions, i.e. the smallest unit that can be judged true or false. Propositions contain a central relationship called the predicate and a number of arguments, and are thus units of knowledge that can stand as separate assertions. All sentences are composed of propositions, and computers can store information in this form also. According to this theory, information in long-term memory is stored in terms of the meanings of propositions rather than their exact words, hence the term

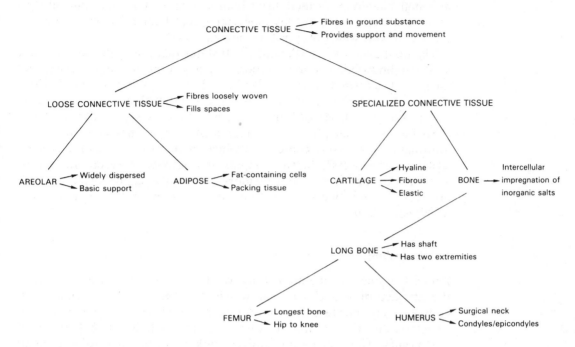

Fig. 3.2 Simple two-dimensional network hierarchy in semantic memory.

'semantic' memory. Information is thus organized into a network of propositions that is hierarchically arranged via nodes and connections.

Figure 3.2 shows how a simple two dimensional network hierarchy for 'tissues' in semantic memory might appear. The spatial orientation of the nodes is irrelevant, in that it is the connections that matter not the location. (Propositions can also be represented in three dimensions.) It is claimed that these networks can represent both perceptual and linguistic information in long-term memory and that this single-code explanation is more parsimonious than the dual-code theory.

Network systems have been utilized in several computer models, the earliest being that of Collins and Quillian (1969). This computer model is called Teachable Language Comprehender (TLC) and it assumes that knowledge is represented in the form of propositional networks. The TLC theory was tested by giving subjects sentences (such as the following) to verify and then measuring their reaction times.

1. A canary is a canary.
2. A canary is a bird.
3. A canary is an animal.

Subjects, according to the theory, should take longer to verify the third sentence because more nodes have to be traversed than in the first or second sentences, and this indeed was the finding. However, later work has shown that this is not always the case; for some concepts, the search is faster for sentences with more nodes to traverse. The sentence 'A dog is a mammal' should be verified faster than 'A dog is an animal', but subjects found the latter more quickly, suggesting that familiarity plays a part in the speed with which propositions are searched.

The dual-code theory (Paivio, 1969) states that there are two different kinds of knowledge representations in long-term memory, verbal and imagery. If information is encoded in both modes, there is a much better chance of remembering it; some words are easier than others to encode with imagery, such as words that describe concrete concepts like 'forceps'.

So far in this chapter the discussion of memory has been within an information-processing context, in which memory is seen as intervening structure or processes between inputs and outputs. A recent alternative approach to theorizing about memory is discourse analysis (DA), which involves the study of discourse in talk or written text (Edwards, Potter and Middleston, 1992).

Remembering

An early pioneer of memory study was Ebbinghaus who used himself as the subject of experiments in which he used nonsense syllables to eliminate any interference from previous knowledge of the words to be remembered. One group of very effective techniques is that called mnemonics. These make the subject think about the item to be remembered by using some kind of scheme. The following offers a selection of these techniques.

Method of loci

In this method, the student first imagines a familiar place such as home or work and chooses a sequence of rooms to remember. He then pictures an item to be remembered in each room until his whole list of items has been used. When he wishes to recall the list, he simply does a mental walkabout through his house to find the items in their locations.

Natural language mediation

This mnemonic is useful for learning unfamiliar words, such as many of those encountered in nursing, and consists of turning the strange word into one that the student already knows and which relates to the new word. For example, if a student is trying to learn the name of the drug streptomycin, he might think of 'strapped the mice in', which implies containment of the spread of the pest.

Key word method

This can be helpful when learning the vocabulary of a foreign language; the student first chooses a French word such as pain (bread) and then makes a visual image of a loaf of French bread 'crying out in pain'.

Acronyms

These are lists of letters arranged vertically to form a word, with each letter itself forming the first letter of a horizontal word. For example, the curriculum components might be remembered thus:

A (aims)
C (content)
M (methods)
E (evaluation)

Forgetting

There are three stages of memory: encoding, storage and retrieval. Encoding involves putting representations into the memory system, storage is maintaining these in memory, and retrieval is the recovery of memories from the memory system. There are a number of explanations for forgetting, but all of them involve either the original memory trace not being available, or being available but not accessible. The latter is termed 'tip of the tongue' (TOT) phenomenon and is a familiar experience for most people.

Interference theory

This states that forgetting is due to interference from other memories. Retroactive interference occurs when new learning material interferes with that previously learned. Student nurses may attend two or three lectures during an afternoon and the first one may be forgotten due to retroactive interference from the ones that followed it. Proactive interference means the opposite; the second lecture of the afternoon is largely forgotten due to interference from the first.

Encoding specificity theory

The key point of this approach is that all forgetting occurs because the cues that were present when the memory was encoded are not present when it is retrieved. It is claimed that the best cues for remembering something are the cues that were present when the memory was encoded. It is well-established that when someone visits a place where they lived as a child, the context cues the recall of memories long thought to have been forgotten.

Consolidation theory

In this theory, the idea is that every experience sets up a trace in the brain and this trace needs to be consolidated if the information is to be remembered. Hence, the trace can be destroyed before it has had time to be consolidated, as in electroconvulsive therapy and retrograde amnesia following head injury.

PERCEPTION

In order to discuss the processes involved in perception, we need to refer back to the diagram of the information-processing system in Figure 3.1. It can be seen that sensory inputs from the environment are first registered in the sensory receptors such as the cells of the retina in the eye. These receptor cells transform the physical stimulus into electrical impulses and transfer it to the brain. Sensation is the term given to the initial processes of reception of the stimulus by the sense organ, whereas perception is used for the processes that occur centrally in the information-processing model. Perception can be defined as an organized process in which the individual selects cues from the environment and draws inferences from these in order to make sense of his experience. Each of the components of this definition will now be outlined, beginning with the notion of organization.

When a particular stimulus such as the letter 'T' impinges on the cells of the retina, the information is transmitted to the cells of the visual cortex and it is here that the process of perception begins. These cortical neurones are designed to respond to particular types of stimuli or patterns, with some responding to vertical lines, some to horizontal, others to acute angles and so on.

Selfridge (1959) constructed a model of perception that he called 'Pandemonium', in which the various detector neurones are envisaged as little demons who do specific jobs inside our heads. These 'demons' are organized hierarchically at different levels, with the most important ones at the top and those doing the least work at the bottom. These bottom-level demons merely record the stimulus and then the next level of demon takes over and looks for evidence of special features such as acute angles, curves and the like. These feature demons then hand over to the cognitive demons that represent each letter of the alphabet and the appropriate ones are activated by the particular stimulus in question. The final demon is called a decision demon and his job is to decide which of the cognitive demons is correct, thus making the final perceptual recognition of a letter 'T'. This is called 'bottom-up' processing, but there is also some 'top-down' processing in the form of prior expectations or set. This predisposes the system to perceive things in a certain way.

The next component of the definition is selectivity and this is concerned with attention. Of the many thousands of stimuli that are registered by the receptors each day, only a certain selection go through to the level of awareness. Take watch straps as an example; normally we are not aware of the presence of the watch, even though the pressure will be registered by the skin receptors. Hence some selecting mechanism must be working that keeps the sensation from being perceived. The criteria for selection will normally include the following:

- new or unusual stimuli;
- changing stimuli;
- very high-intensity stimuli such as bright lights or loud noise;
- motives- or needs-related stimuli, such as the sight of a restaurant sign when you are hungry and searching for somewhere to eat.

The definition also refers to cues from the environment and these cues are used in perception of movement, depth, objects and people. Cues for objects are such things as shape, size, colour, texture, smell and taste. If I saw a large, square, red object coming towards me I would use those cues to make the inference it was a bus, especially as my past experience has led to my being correct on previous occasions when I encountered the stimulus.

Movement cues include the covering and uncovering of background and a change in the shape or sound of the object. Cues for depth perception are both monocular and binocular; the former include nearer objects occluding far ones and convergence of lines. Binocular cues are due to stereoscopic vision, in that each eye sees things from a different angle and when superimposed gives depth cues.

Perception tries to keep things constant, so that when we perceive a bus going along the road, we are not aware of any change, even though its shape and size will alter as it recedes into the distance. This perceptual constancy can lead to illusions if the stimuli are ambiguous.

Gestalt laws of perception

It was mentioned earlier that 'top-down' processing occurs in perception and one of the early descriptions of this was by the group known as the Gestalt psychologists. The three main exponents of this school were Max Wertheimer (1880–1943), Kurt Koffka (1886–1941) and Wolfgang Kohler (1887–1967). Their work was originally concerned with the study of perception, but this became closely involved with a theory of learning. Gestalt psychology developed in the opposite direction to stimulus–response theory, its exponents decrying the piecemeal analysis of behaviour as an explanation of learning. The Gestalt view was that people see things as unified wholes, not as separate components, the German word 'Gestalt' meaning 'pattern' or 'configuration'. These patterns, or 'Gestalten', tend to stand out distinctly from the background against which they are seen, giving rise to the concept of figure and ground in perception. The Gestalt psychologists formulated laws of perception, which govern whether or not a particular stimulus will be perceived as figure rather than ground. The laws are as follows.

Law of similarity

Stimuli which are similar to one another tend to be grouped together in one's perception. In Figure 3.3, the observer tends to see alternate rows or columns of dots and crosses rather than 25 items in a square.

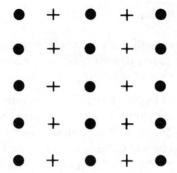

Fig. 3.3 Law of similarity.

Law of proximity

Stimuli that are closer together tend to be grouped into patterns. The example in Figure 3.4 is seen as four pairs of vertical lines rather than eight separate ones.

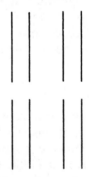

Fig. 3.4 Law of proximity.

Law of closure

Areas that enclose space tend to form 'Gestalten', and thus stand out against the background. In Figure 3.5(a), the four pairs of lines can be made to form a unified whole by adding two incomplete lines to the inner four lines. Closure also occurs with six lines, as in Figure 3.5(b).

Koffka considered that these laws of perception could also be seen as laws of learning, with application to the teaching situation. This is further elaborated in the section on problem-solving later in this chapter.

Perception and nurse education

There are a great many implications for nurse education in both teaching and practice-based learning. In practice settings, students need to be taught about the factors that affect their perception of things, particularly the influence of 'top-down' processing, which might make them miss cues

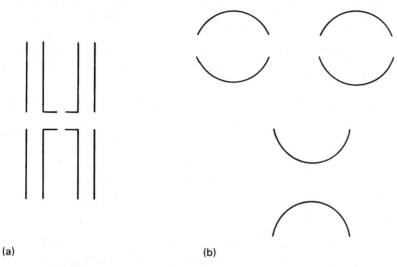

(a)   (b)

Fig. 3.5 Law of closure.

that patients might emit. Nurses need to recognize that a patient's perception may be altered by illness and must make the necessary allowance for this by giving more frequent explanations and reassurance, in case the patient may not have perceived the message. Selective attention will operate in clinical areas where patients may be kept awake by jangling drug keys or the sound of a trolley. Some patients may become disoriented and so experience perceptual distortion; the nurse's role in this case is to reduce stimulation by maintaining a quiet, dark environment. In teaching, it is important to use methods that hold the attention of the students with, for example, bright visual aids and changes of activity at frequent intervals. The teacher should maintain a central position as 'figure' separate from the 'ground' of background noise and distractions. The teaching should be for 'insight' rather than always giving factual information, so that students experience 'penny-dropping' when learning concepts.

THINKING AND CONCEPT FORMATION

Concepts can be defined as 'objects, events, situations or properties that possess common criterial attributes and are designated by some sign or symbol' (Ausubel, Novak and Hanesian, 1978). A concept is thus a category or class of objects, rather than an individual example, each member of that class sharing one or more common characteristics.

- The word 'cell' represents a concept, in that it stands for a class of things that possess a number of common qualities or attributes, such as a cell membrane, cytoplasm, nucleus and so on.
- The words 'Florence Nightingale' do not represent a concept, since there is only one example of this individual.

The common characteristics that members of a concept share can be either structural or functional attributes or both.

- The concept 'bandage' contains a wide variety of shapes and sizes, but the functions are largely identified as support, pressure and securing of dressings.

In order to qualify as a member of a particular concept group, an individual example must possess certain key characteristics called critical attributes. Without these, the individual example cannot be classified as one of the concept in question.

- The concept 'myocardial infarction' is a class of events that includes chest pain, vomiting, pain in the arms, breathlessness and myocardial necrosis.

Individual examples (i.e. patients), exhibit much variation in these features making it difficult to decide the critical attributes of this concept; it is possible to suffer from a myocardial infarction without experiencing pain, vomiting or breathlessness, so it seems that the only critical attribute of the concept is myocardial necrosis. The concept 'angina pectoris' may share the attributes of chest pain and breathlessness, but lacks the critical attribute of myocardial necrosis and hence does not belong to the class of concepts called 'myocardial infarction'.

Concrete and abstract concepts

Concepts that can be observed are termed 'concrete' whereas those that are not observable are termed 'defined' or 'abstract'. 'Liver' is an example of a concrete observable concept, whereas 'intelligence' is an abstract one. Abstract concepts tend to be more difficult to learn than concrete concepts. Concepts form hierarchies, with the most inclusive ones at the top and the more specific ones below and they also cluster together with other related concepts.

Schemata

The work discussed so far has referred largely to simple concepts, whereas in real life, most information-processing involves connected sequences of events such as reading of connected discourse. Schema theory attempts to explain the inferences we make when processing events and was first introduced by Bartlett (1932). Definitions of 'schema' are:

- an implicit mental theory about the world which we need in order to see or understand (Oatley, 1978);
- large, complex units of knowledge that organize much of what we know about general categories of objects, classes of events and types of people (Anderson, 1980); and
- a relatively abstract representation of objects, episodes, actions or situations which contains slots or variables into which specific instances can be fitted in a particular context (Doyle, 1983).

From this range of definitions, it can be seen that schemata are larger units of knowledge than propositions. A number of different theorists have adopted schema theory (Minsky, 1975; Rummelhart and Ortony, 1977; Schank and Abelson, 1977). People have schemata for a large range of familiar events and they use these to fill in gaps and make inferences in conversations or stories. Schemata do not represent specific objects, but rather they represent general categories; propositions represent specific things or people.

The work of Elinor Rosch has shed much light on the nature of schemata for natural categories of events in the real world. She has postulated that instances of a category share certain family resemblances and it is these which define whether the instance is a member of the category. Some category members are seen as more typical of the category than others. For example, apples are more typical fruits than rhubarb, since more fruits grow on trees than in the ground. There is often wide disparity in subjects' agreement of category members. Schema theory states that people are aware of which features in the environment tend to go together, and that these features are noticed and remembered. Schemata tend to be incomplete, in that they leave some features unspecified, namely, those features that are considered irrelevant.

Rummelhart and Ortony (1977) suggest that there are four essential characteristics of schemata. First, schemata have variables and may have different variables on different occasions, depending on the context of the schema. (For example, the schema for 'take' might have three variables – a recipient, an object and a donor – in one context and only one variable in another, such as in 'taking one's time'.) Second, schemata can embed into each other, i.e. schemata are represented in terms of other schemata, these others being termed sub-schemata. Only the names of these are represented though, since this avoids the problem of having every piece of knowledge included with every schema. Third, schemata vary in their levels of abstraction; this is the characteristic that most differentiates schemata from propositions. Schemata can be seen as parcels of information at many different levels of abstraction, from simple concepts to very inclusive aspects of comprehension. Last, schemata represent knowledge; schemata are not merely dictionary entries, but abstract representations of knowledge. Schemata, then, constitute the 'basic building-blocks of the human information-processing system' and play a key part in the process of comprehension. Understanding of something involves the selection of schemata that will satisfactorily account for the information being processed.

CRITICAL THINKING SKILLS

Pathway aims within HE are of two kinds: the specific aims of the pathway in relation to its subject area; and the more general educational aims that apply to all pathways. The latter are more general and include development of skills in communication, problem-solving, evaluation, and critical thinking. At honours degree level, the emphasis is very much on higher-order cognitive skills: 'Programmes must stimulate an enquiring, analytical approach, encouraging independent judgement and critical self-awareness' (CNAA, 1992). Whilst these general aims apply to all courses in HE, specific aims for individual pathways within healthcare also tend to emphasize the acquisition of higher-order cognitive skills. For example, validation documents for Project 2000 courses tend to contain reference to the development of students' skills of critical enquiry, analysis, critical awareness, critical thinking, and evaluative skills.

At post-registration level, typical outcomes are the ability of students to reflect upon and critically evaluate their own professional practice. These aims, although couched in a variety of terms, can be classified as generic critical thinking skills. Burnard (1989) states: 'The need to develop critical ability in all nurses, both during basic training and beyond it, seems to be a fundamental requirement in the development of modern nursing.'

The word 'critical' is a very common term in education, but it has a very different connotation from the lay use of the word. In society, the term is equated with 'criticism', which carries negative overtones from childhood and schooldays. In this context, it usually meant hostile or unkind comments about aspects of an individual's behaviour, and this notion may carry through to adult life. Critical thinking is very different from criticism, in that it is basically a positive activity. To question established assumptions may be interpreted as undermining them, but in reality such critical appraisal of situations is a positive and necessary process for growth and development to occur within a society or an organization. Critical thinking is not confined solely to learning in higher education, but permeates all the activities of adult life including interpersonal relationships and work.

Components of critical thinking

It is useful to define critical thinking as a core concept consisting of a number of abilities – the ability to:

1. define a problem;
2. select relevant information for problem-solving;
3. draw inferences from observed or supposed facts;
4. recognize assumptions;
5. formulate relevant hypotheses;
6. make deductions, i.e. draw conclusions from premises;
7. make interpretations from data; and
8. evaluate arguments.

There is some variation in the literature with regard to these components; Brookfield (1987) for example, identifies the four components discussed below.

Identifying and challenging assumptions

Critical thinkers ask awkward questions in order to identify and challenge the assumptions which underlie issues and problems.

Challenging the importance of context

Critical thinkers are aware that beliefs, actions, and established practice reflect the context in which they are set, both cultural and professional. For example, opinions about the standard of appearance for nurses and midwives may be based upon the norms of a generation or more ago, such as a particular view of what constitutes an acceptable hairstyle. Modern hairstyles that are entirely appropriate in a social context may be perceived as being 'unprofessional' in a nursing or midwifery context. The same may be said about so-called 'designer-stubble' in male nursing or medical staff.

Imagining and exploring alternatives

Critical thinkers have the ability to imagine and explore alternatives to established ways of thinking or behaving, because they are aware of the assumptions and the context of issues or problems.

Reflective scepticism

Reflective thinkers take a sceptical view of established dogma and practices, carefully scrutinizing them and questioning their current validity. For example, this approach is encouraged in Project 2000 courses, but may be perceived as threatening by qualified nurses whose own professional education did not foster such an approach. Hence, their reflective scepticism needs to be handled with some sensitivity by students if they are to avoid conflict with qualified colleagues.

Tests of critical thinking

There are a number of tests of critical thinking in common use and although these tests contain different sorts of items, there is considerable overlap within them. One example is the Watson–Glaser critical thinking appraisal (Watson and Glaser, 1961). This tests the subject's ability on five aspects of critical thinking: inference; assumptions; deduction; interpretation; and evaluation of arguments.

Inference

This is a conclusion based upon facts or observations. For example, by looking at a post-operative patient's facial expression and body posture, a nurse may infer that he or she is in pain. However, there may be other, equally plausible, explanations, such as anxiety about whether their job will still be there when they are well enough to leave hospital.

Assumptions

These are something assumed or taken for granted. For example, a nurse may assume that a post-operative patient will wish to be given analgesia as soon as pain is experienced. However, the patient may have a negative attitude to taking any form of drug, and so reject the offer of analgesia.

Deduction

This consists of drawing conclusions from stated premises. Either the conclusion follows from the statements, or it does not. For example, from the two statements

> Some nurses look untidy.
> Being untidy is unprofessional.

It is possible to deduce the conclusion that 'some nurses are unprofessional'. However, the conclusion that 'unprofessional nurses look untidy' does not follow from the two statements given, since unprofessional nurses may well look tidy, and yet have other shortcomings that contribute to their unprofessionalism.

Interpretation

This involves judging whether or not a conclusion follows, beyond a reasonable doubt, from the facts given. Let us take a purely hypothetical example; suppose a survey of professional misconduct within the Barsetshire Region found that female nurses were involved in 34 cases of complaints from patients, but male nurses were involved in only 22 cases of complaint. The following conclusions might be drawn.

A: There were more complaints by patients against female nurses than male nurses in Barsetshire.
B: Patients are generally more satisfied with male nurses than female nurses.

Conclusion A follows beyond a reasonable doubt, since it a factual statement supported by the evidence of the numbers involved. However, conclusion B does not follow beyond a reasonable doubt, as it makes unwarranted generalizations from the given data e.g. its takes no account of the number of male/female nurses – 34 may represent 1% while 22 represents 5%.

Evaluation of arguments

When attempting to make important decisions about an issue or problem, it is necessary to be able to distinguish between strong and weak arguments. Watson and Glaser use two criteria for a strong argument: it must be important, and it must be directly related to the issue or problem. If one of these is absent, then the argument is considered to be weak.

Critical thinking and nurse education

From the foregoing discussion, it is apparent that nursing and midwifery curricula espouse the importance of critical thinking. How then can the nurse teacher facilitate its development in students? Brookfield (1987) offers a useful ten-point checklist for this.

1. *Affirm critical thinkers' self-worth*: it is important when teaching critical thinking to maintain an atmosphere of psychological safety, whereby students thinking can be challenged, but they are not made to feel threatened or insulted.
2. *Listen attentively to critical thinkers*: during training the teacher must attend carefully to students' verbal and non-verbal signals, so that interventions are both appropriate and sensitive to the situation.
3. *Show that you support critical thinkers' efforts*: students do not become critical thinkers overnight; their initial efforts need support and encouragement if they are to progress, and there is a delicate balance between this and the necessary degree of challenge and 'upset' that is important for critical thinking skills development.
4. *Reflect and mirror critical thinkers' ideas and actions*: trainers can foster the development of critical thinking by using reflection techniques that let the student see how their behaviours and attitudes are perceived by others.
5. *Motivate people to think critically*: there is a delicate balance between motivating students to think critically, and helping them to estimate the risks involved in criticizing and destabilizing established practices. It would be naïve to think that by simply criticizing the status quo, change will automatically follow. In reality, established organizational practices and systems tend to be relatively entrenched, and critical thinking may result not in change, but only in the loss of the critical thinker's job.
6. *Regularly evaluate progress*: one of the important roles of the trainer is to encourage students to engage regularly in reflective evaluation of their critical thinking skills, so that behaviour patterns are identified and insights gained.
7. *Help critical thinkers to create networks*: networking is a common educational strategy, and is akin to self-help groups. Students should be encouraged to network with other students who are developing critical thinking skills, so that experiences and insights can be shared and analysed.
8. *Be a critical teacher*: teachers themselves can adopt a critical thinking approach to their teaching by questioning assumptions, promoting inquiry, and experimenting with new ideas during their teaching.
9. *Make people aware of how they learn critical thinking*: this focuses on helping students to understand their own learning styles in relation to critical thinking, such as how they sustain their motivation, how they integrate new ideas and experience, and how they approach new areas of knowledge.
10. *Model critical thinking*: observing a good role model can help students

to become critical thinkers, so teachers should model these skills during their everyday teaching.

PROBLEM-SOLVING SKILLS

Problem-solving is a good example of the interrelationship of all the components of an information-processing system of cognition. This section addresses two approaches to problem-solving: the Gestalt approach, and an information-processing approach.

The Gestalt approach and insightful learning

The kind of learning described by Gestalt psychology is called learning by insight (or insightful learning), in which the student's perception of a situation or problem undergoes a restructuring, and he or she sees the aspects of the situation in a new relationship to one another. This new relationship forms a unified whole, or Gestalt, which is meaningful to the student, who is then said to have insight into the problem or situation. Kohler demonstrated insight learning in the chimpanzee during a series of classic experiments in Tenerife during World War I. In one experiment, the chimpanzee was placed in a cage which had a banana suspended out of reach and several boxes scattered around. It was impossible to reach the banana by standing on only one of the boxes and the animal would manifest trial and error behaviour, including great restlessness. Suddenly it would pile the boxes one on top of the other, and climb up to the banana. Kohler noticed that this sudden activity often followed a period when the animal had been sitting quietly, not attempting to reach the fruit. He interpreted the behaviour of the chimpanzee as that of gaining insight into the problem, by seeing the banana and the boxes in a new relationship that was meaningful and thus perceiving the solution to the problem.

The laws of proximity and closure can be said to be at work in the insightful learning of the chimpanzee, the former being shown by the fact that all the aspects of the problem, namely the banana and the boxes, must be in the animal's visual field at the same time for insight to occur. Closure is suggested by the sudden awareness of the relationship between the boxes as a means of climbing to the banana, bringing the previously unrelated boxes into a complete, closed Gestalt.

This sudden insight into the problem or situation applies to human learning also and has been termed the 'aha' phenomenon. Most people have had, at some time, the experience of suddenly grasping or understanding a problem that has previously perplexed them and have uttered the expression, 'Aha, now I understand.' The cognitive restructuring that occurs in insightful learning is said by the Gestalt psychologists to occur also in rats who are running in a maze. They achieve insight into the correct path to the food by a series of partial insights, gained by discovering that certain patterns of movement are non-productive, whilst others lead to food.

Problem-solving as information-processing

The other main approach to problem-solving research is information-processing, which seeks to explain the sequence of operations that subjects use in solving problems. The problem situation is termed the 'problem space', and is composed of an 'initial state' in which the individual is currently in, a 'goal state' which is the desired end state, and one or more 'operators' which are a set of operations that transform the initial state into the goal state (Smythe *et al.*, 1987).

Stages of problem-solving

Howard (1983) gives the following stages:

1. encode the problem in the working memory;
2. search the long-term memory for a plan or production system;
3. execute the production system; and
4. evaluate the results.

This sequence may or may not be successful, depending upon the problem.

When individuals carry out problem-solving tasks, they tend to exhibit similar types of phenomena, such as rigidity, incubation and insight, and 'satisficing'. Rigidity implies that subjects tend to become entrenched in one particular way of seeing a problem, which prevents them from finding a solution. They are also influenced by perceptual set, which makes them respond to the problem as they have done in the past, even if this is not appropriate to the current problem. Incubation and insight refer to the lapse in time between tackling the problem initially and going back to it later, if unsuccessful. There is an increased chance of arriving at a solution after incubation; indeed, it very often results in a 'penny-dropping' insight into the problem. 'Satisficing' is a word meaning that people tend to settle for good choices rather than seeking better ones.

Conditions of learning for problem-solving

Gagne (1985) suggests there are both intrinsic and extrinsic conditions for problem-solving. The conditions within the student that must be met are:

- recall of relevant rules that have been learned previously;
- possession of verbal information organized in appropriate ways, i.e. schemata; and
- cognitive strategies previously learned.

The extrinsic conditions in the learning situation are:

- verbal instructions by the teacher to stimulate recall of rules.

Problem-solving and nurse education

Gagne (1985) suggests that the most effective problems for student learning are those that are novel to the students and within their capabilities. Barrows and Tamblyn (1980) recommend problem-based learning as a strategy in teaching health studies and define it as learning that results from the process of working towards the understanding or resolution of a problem. Problem-based learning is different from other problem-solving teaching strategies, because the problem is given to the student prior to any form of input; usually, traditional methods involve the giving of information followed by the application of that information by use of clinical problems. Problem-based learning starts with the problem, and students have to find out what they need to know in order to solve it. This approach is very much a discovery-type approach and can be very motivating (Allen and Murrell, 1978).

Problem-based learning lends itself well to computer-assisted learning, with the use of simulation and case method. Students are given basic data about a patient and are then asked to produce a suitable care plan. Having selected a series of interventions, the nurse can check to see whether in the real case, the ones chosen were actually selected for the patient.

Problem-solving is closely related to the nursing process, which is often termed a problem-solving cycle but is better described as a problem-identification cycle.

PSYCHOMOTOR SKILLS

In Chapter 2, the difference between declarative knowledge and procedural knowledge was identified, the latter being knowledge about how to do things. This procedural knowledge is an essential part of motor skills, forming the mental part of the term psychomotor skills. Motor skills are an extremely important aspect of the practice of nursing, since nursing science is largely a practical endeavour, but the notion of skill pervades the whole of society; indeed, the concept of social class is very much influenced by the degree of skill of the occupations in each category of the Registrar General's classification. Motor skills are concerned with movements and a skilled person exhibits certain characteristics over a novice as outlined in Table 3.1.

Human motor skills can be divided into three broad categories (Oxendine, 1984):

Table 3.1 Characteristics of a skilled performance

Accuracy	Skill executed with precision
Speed	Movements siwft and confident
Efficiency	Movements economical, leaving spare capacity available
Timing	Accurate timing and correct sequential order
Consistency	Results are consistent
Anticipation	Can anticipate events very quickly and respond accordingly
Adaptability	Can adapt the skill to current circumstances
Perception	Can obtain maximum information from a minimum of cues

1. *maturation-dependent skills*, such as crawling, walking and speaking;
2. *educational-related skills*, such as writing, reading and observation; and
3. *intrinsic-value skills*, such as recreational and vocational skills.

It might be useful, at this point, to look at some definitions of motor skill:

1. a persistent change in movement-behaviour potentiality as a result of practice or experience (Oxendine, 1984);
2. a learned ability to bring about a predetermined result with maximum certainty and minimum time and effort (Fitts and Posner, 1967).

Table 3.2 gives some of the terms commonly used in relation to motor skills.

Obviously, not all motor performances need to be learned from scratch, as many of the component skills will already have been mastered. Take the example of a nurse learning how to do a drug round; although she will not have done the motor performances before, such as taking a medicine pot to the patient, she will have acquired the skill of picking up and carrying a small container of fluid without spilling since childhood. Hence, the nurse teacher needs to consider the entry behaviours that students bring to the motor-skill learning situation. Three dimensions of motor skills are commonly identified in the literature: fine/gross, continuous/discrete, closed/open looped.

Fine versus gross   Gross performance involves the whole body, or large muscles, such as in lifting a patient. Fine performance involves fingers and wrists, as in removing sutures.

Continuous versus discrete   The former involves continuous adjustment and corrections to stimuli, such as the continuous movements of external cardiac massage, while the latter is a movement made in response to an external stimulus, such as switching off a patient's nurse-call button.

Closed-looped versus open-looped   Closed-looped performance relies entirely on proprioceptive feedback, so could be performed with eyes closed, whereas open-looped is affected by external stimuli. For example, the painless removal of sutures requires some reaction from the patient, which indicates comfort or otherwise.

Table 3.2 Terminology of motor skills

Procedure	An intellectual skill consisting of rules for sequencing actions
Motor skill	Ability required for the execution of a procedure
Motor performance	Execution of an overt action
Total skill	Total motor performance with characteristics of a procedure
Part skill	Sub-component of a total skill
Ability	Capacity to execute something

Learning motor skills

Motor skills, unlike other forms of learning, require practice in order to be learned and practice consists of repetition of a procedure under specific conditions. These conditions are that the students must intend to learn the skill and they must obtain feedback about their performance. The reason why motor skills require practice is because of the importance of kinaesthetic feedback from the students' own body and this takes time to produce skilled, efficient movements. It is useful to distinguish between physical and mental practice; the former means the actual physical repetition of the procedure, whereas the latter involves thinking about the skill in between practice sessions. Mental practice or imagery is not a substitute for physical practice, but evidence suggests that it is a very useful way of encouraging skills learning when used in conjunction with it. Reminiscence is the term used to describe improvements in performance occurring without physical practice and may be due to mental practice.

The acquisition of a motor skill normally follows a smooth curve when plotted against the time and the number of trials. The occurrence of plateaux, in which the student seems to stay at the same level of performance, are fairly rare. There are also no obvious stages, but Fitts and Posner (1967) suggest that there are three processes that occur, in the following order:

1. the cognitive phase, which is really concerned with the learning of the procedure, and the more complex the skill, the longer this period will take;
2. the associative phase, in which the part-skills are taking on the characteristics of skilled performance and interfering responses are eliminated; and
3. the autonomous phase, during which the skill becomes automatic and can occur without the student thinking about it.

The frequency and distribution of practice can affect learning of motor skills; distribution can be divided into massed practice and distributed practice, the former having little or no rest from beginning to end of practice and the latter having practice sessions separated by rest periods or by longer intervals of time. Distributed practice is generally more effective for learning motor skills, possibly because of the avoidance of boredom, fatigue or loss of attention. Simple tasks, however, are better learned in one session, and short practice periods are preferable to long ones. Of course, student motivational level will influence the amount of practice they can accommodate.

One of the key features of practice pointed out earlier was that it must occur with feedback to the students about their performance in order to help them improve. (Thorndike (1931), in a classic experiment asked subjects to draw four-inch lines whilst blindfolded and they were not told how close to four inches their efforts were. There was much variability in line length drawn, but no trend towards improvement over the trials.) Feedback can be classified as intrinsic or extrinsic. Intrinsic feedback is feedback arising within the performer and is further subdivided into reactive and operational feedback: reactive feedback consists of the kinaesthetic feedback from the performer's body muscles and joints; and operational feedback is the observation of the effect of the action by the performer, also termed knowledge of results (KOR). Extrinsic feedback is external to the performer and is also termed augmented feedback; it can be done by teachers, peers or coaches and may be done concurrently during the performance, or terminally when it is finished.

When student nurses learn a new skill, it is likely that there will be some element of transfer from previously learned skills; transfer means that a previously learned skill has a positive or negative influence on the new one, and this is termed pro-active transfer. It is also possible for the new skill to influence the old one, a phenomenon called retroactive transfer. Transfer of skill may be specific or non-specific; specific aspects that are transferred in nursing are such things as lifting patients without injuring oneself, whereas general transfer occurs with less obvious things such as problem-solving ability.

Positive transfer of skills is enhanced by similarity between them, and also if well-learned responses can be used in the new skill. On the other hand, well-learned habits may interfere with new responses, as in driving a car with different controls. There is evidence to suggest that an understanding of the underlying principles will enhance transfer to a different activity.

Teaching a motor sklll

Teaching motor skills involves the same principles as any other form of teaching, namely, an atmosphere conducive to learning that is free from threat or stress. There must be opportunity for feedback and analysis of the performance and the use of videotaped microteaching can be invaluable in this respect. Teachers must appreciate that learning a skill requires time and that individual students will differ in the amount of time they require. Nurse teachers need to utilize intensive skills-learning laboratories to ensure that students become proficient before transferring the skills to the real setting under supervision. Another point to be borne in mind is that nursing procedures involve more than motor skills; Gagne (1985) classifies procedures as intellectual skills or rules for determining the sequence of actions and thus students need to learn the procedural rules as well as the motor skills aspects.

When planning to teach motor skills, the teacher will have to consider the level at which the student must learn the skill. When we consider the characteristics of a skilled performance as outlined in Table 3.1, it becomes obvious that students cannot achieve this level for every skill they learn; indeed, experienced nurses will vary in their relative degree of skill amongst the nursing procedures they practise. There will be some motor skills that students must learn to the highest level and others where an intermediate level is acceptable. A useful point of reference for levels of skills is the notion of taxonomies of motor skills; in Chapter 12 (p. 279), the taxonomy of Simpson (1972), is outlined in relation to curriculum objectives and this can provide guidance for the teacher. The taxonomy has seven levels as follows:

1. perception – concerned with perception of sensory cues;
2. set – concerned with readiness to act;
3. guided response – skills performed under guidance of instructor;
4. mechanism – performance becomes habitual;
5. complex overt response – typical skilled performance;
6. adaptation – skills can be adapted to suit circumstances; and
7. origination – creation of original movement patterns.

It would seem that many nursing skills learned by students will be geared at level 3 or 4 and that the higher levels may only be reached when the student has practised as a qualified nurse for some time. Skills at level 3 are commonly taught in specialist areas, where the student is allowed to perform under guidance having first been shown how to do a procedure. For example, the skills of dialysis may be taught at this level during a student's allocation to a renal clinical area, but there is no expectation that the student nurse will achieve a highly-skilled performance during the brief allocation period. The same can be said for other clinical specialisms such as intensive-care units, neonatal units and the like.

The teaching of motor skills involves the provision of information and the opportunity for practice under supervision. The following checklist for teaching a motor skill, includes the key points which will then be explained in further detail:

1. provide an atmosphere conductive learning;
2. carry out a skills analysis to determine part-skills and elements;
3. determine the sequence of the procedure;
4. assess entry behaviours of students – these need not be taught again;
5. model the skill by demonstration or film, at normal speed;
6. teach the sequence of the procedure;
7. teach the motor skill by either whole-learning or part-learning method;
8. allocate sufficient time for practice;
9. provide augmented feedback on performance;
10. prompt student to use intrinsic feedback; and
11. encourage transfer of existing similar skills by pointing out similarity.

The provision of an atmosphere conducive to learning has already been discussed and its importance noted. Skills analysis is a useful way of identifying the part-skills that comprise the total motor skill. Table 3.3 shows a task analysis for the motor aspects of the procedure of performing a surgical dressing. These motor skills are further subdivided into part-skills and elements, and it can be seen that the elements consist of many previously learned entry behaviours such as moving the bed table and pulling curtains. Determining the sequence of the procedure is important and it may be forgotten that students must remember this as well

Table 3.3 The procedure of performing a surgical dressing

Total motor skill	Part-skills (tasks)	Elements*
1.0 Preparation of work area	1.1 Clearing space	1.11 Pushing locker away 1.12 Moving bed table
	1.2 Screening	1.21 Holding curtain and pulling it round
	1.3 Closing windows	1.31 Pulling window cord
	1.4 Stopping smoking	1.41 Requesting all patients in vicinity to stop
	1.5 Positioning patient	1.51 Asking if possible to lie recumbent 1.52 Removing pillows 1.53 Folding bedclothes 1.54 Loosening clothing 1.55 Covering with blanket
2.0 Preparation of equipment and trolley	2.1 Hand-washing 2.2 Cleaning trolley 2.3 Collecting equipment 2.4 Setting trolley 2.5 Taking to bedside	
3.0 Performance of dressing	3.1 Opening bags 3.2 Loosening dressing 3.3 Hand-washing 3.4 Opening packs 3.5 Removing dressing 3.6 Cleaning wound 3.7 Applying dressing	
4.0 Organization of trolley	4.1 Closing pack 4.2 Closing bags 4.3 Securing bags	
5.0 Ensuring patient's comfort	5.1 Attending to position	
6.0 Clearing of trolley and equipment	6.1 Removing from bedside 6.2 Disposal of soiled dressings 6.3 Disposal of instruments 6.4 Hand-washing 6.5 Clearing equipment 6.6 Cleaning trolley 6.7 Hand-washing	
7.0 Returning to patient	7.1 Assist with clothing 7.2 Assisting with position 7.3 Offering drink, newspaper, etc. 7.4 Removing screens 7.5 Returning tables, locker, etc.	
8.0 Recording and reporting	8.1 Writing report 8.2 Reporting verbally to nurse in charge 8.3 Comparing report with previous one	

* Elements are stated only for section 1.0 of the total motor skills.

as the motor skills. Entry behaviours need to be identified, since they are already learned and hence do not need to be taught again.

Modelling of the skill can be done by an actual demonstration or by film or videotape and it gives the students an overall impression of the skill they are aiming at.

There is some controversy as to whether skills should be taught in their entirety (whole-learning), or divided into part-skills, with each part being taught separately first and then combined into a whole – part-learning. The disadvantage of whole-learning in that it may be difficult to comprehend large units of procedures if taught together. However, part-learning may waste time because the student has to learn the part-skills first and then learn to combine them together. It may also be boring for the student if the part-skills are simple. The advantages of whole-learning are that it may be:

- more meaningful, as perceived as whole;
- more efficient, as students can identify the aspects which need further practice within the whole;
- more effective for students who already have a background in the skill;
- better for highly-motivated students; and
- better for older students.

The advantages of part-learning are that it may:

- help to motivate students, as each part-skill provides immediate achievement;
- by its small-step nature act as a reinforcement for learning;
- be better for younger students;
- be better for students lacking a background in the skill; and
- help to improve specific responses for part-skills.

Another area of controversy is that of massed practice versus spaced practice; massed practice involves continuous practice until the skill is learned, whereas spaced practice may spread the practice over a period of time, with rest in between. There is no evidence that one is better than the other, but there are obvious pitfalls associated with massed practice, such as boredom and fatigue. As we have seen earlier, feedback is a crucial aspect of motor-skills learning, without which no improvement can occur. The teacher needs to encourage students to become aware of the intrinsic feedback from their own muscles and joints, which informs them about the position of limbs and the action of movements. Information gained from their own observation of their actions will also help the students to learn a skill and here again the teacher may use questioning to ascertain whether each student is able to self-evaluate outcomes. The main role of the teacher is in providing augmented feedback in the form of verbal guidance both during and on completion of the motor performance. The nurse teacher can teach for transfer of learning by using a variety of techniques to make the student understand the principles underlying the skill. Existing skills must have been well-learned if they are to transfer positively to the new skill, and the similarities need to be pointed out to the students.

THEORIES OF HUMAN PSYCHOLOGICAL DEVELOPMENT

There is a wide variation in the age of students in nursing and midwifery education, which can range from teenage through to pre-retirement depending upon the nature of specific programmes. It is certainly common to find students, both pre-registration and post-registration, in their thirties and forties and this may itself present certain difficulties in relation to learning. Older students may lack confidence in their academic and study ability, especially if they have not been engaged in formal study for some considerable time. If older students are in the minority within a group, they may feel marginalized or isolated from the younger students. It is not always easy to bridge the 'generation gap' and mix freely with a younger group, so teachers may need to offer additional support to older students if they become isolated. On the other hand, the younger students may benefit enormously from the experience and stability of the older students. It is important for the nurse teacher to have a basic understanding of psychological development across the lifespan, as it may provide insights which help to explain the behaviour of both young and older students within nurse education. This section outlines approaches to psychological development from two theorists, Piaget and Levinson.

Piaget: stages of cognitive development

Piaget's work focuses on the intellectual development of the individual and his or her adaptation to the environment (Piaget and Inhelder, 1969). For adaptation to occur there must be some form of organization within the individual, and these two processes work interdependently and in parallel.

Schemas

The internal organization of an individual consists of schemas, which are ways of giving meaning to, and dealing with, aspects of the environment that are encountered. They can be likened to mini-theories that develop as a result of the infant's interactions with the environment. In early infancy, schemas equate to reflexes but as development progresses these schemas become more complex, and this occurs through two processes: assimilation and accommodation. When children encounter a new situation they try to assimilate it into their existing familiar schemas but if the latter are inadequate then their schemas have to be modified to accommodate the new situation. For example, a child's schema for 'dog' may include all smallish, four-legged animals such as cats and foxes, but as accommodation progresses these become schemas in their own right. Hence, the child's knowledge of the world is modified and extended by the processes of assimilation and accommodation, and these processes are in balance with one another; Piaget calls this balancing process equilibration – a dynamic process that prepares the child for new learning. In Piagetian theory, motivation is intrinsic and arises from the application of schemas to the environment.

Stages of cognitive development

Cognitive development is seen by Piaget as consisting of four stages.

1. Sensorimotor (birth – 2 years)
2. Pre-operational (2–7 years)
3. Concrete operational (7–11 years)
4. Formal operational (12 years and up)

Sensorimotor stage (birth – 2 years)   At birth, the infant is equipped only with basic reflexes and these serve as the first schemas, hence thinking equates with doing. Gradually 'self' becomes differentiated from objects, and intentional behaviour begins at eight months or so. The infant begins to understand that objects exist even when they cannot be seen; this object permanence is an important characteristic at this stage since it demonstrates that a mental representation of the object must be present. It also indicates the beginnings of a move away from the egocentric focus of early infancy.

Pre-operational stage (2–7 years)   This stage is called pre-operational because the child is unable to use mental rules or operations for transforming information. He or she is still egocentric – focusing on general aspects instead of on the individual aspects of a situation. This is strikingly demonstrated in the child's lack of conservation; for example, if presented with two balls of clay of equal size, the child will indicate that they are the same size. If one ball is then rolled into a cylindrical shape, the child will say it has more clay. Lack of conservation also applies to numbers: if two rows of coins are evenly spaced-out, and then in one row the coins are spaced closely together, the child will indicate that the original row contains more coins. Thus, the child lacks reversibility, i.e. the ability to understand that if an operation is reversed it reverts back to its original state.

Concrete operational stage (7–11 years)   In this stage, the child develops conservation, and the ability to undertake mental operations. However, these operations are limited to the here-and-now; in other words, the child cannot reason hypothetically.

Formal operational stage (12 years and up)   This final stage is characterized by the ability of the child to reason hypothetically, i.e. he or she can focus on the form of a problem without being limited to the concrete aspects as in the previous stage.

Levinson: adult development model

Levinson's (1986) model of adult development identifies four major periods or eras.

1. Pre-adulthood (0–22 years)
2. Early adulthood (17–45 years)
   (a) early adult transition (17–22 years)
   (b) entry life structure for early adulthood (22–28 years)
   (c) age 30 transition (26–33 years)
   (d) culminating life structure for early adulthood (33–40 years)
3. Middle adulthood (40–65 years)
   (a) mid-life transition (40–45 years)
   (b) entry life structure for middle adulthood (45–50 years)
   (c) age 50 transition (50–55 years)
   (d) culminating life structure for middle adulthood (55–60 years)
4. Late adulthood (60 + years)
   (a) late adult transition (60–65 years)

The eras are relatively stable periods, but the periods of transition between stages are characterized by turmoil. The era of early adulthood, which marks the adolescent's entry to the adult world, is a time for exploring possibilities and for the beginnings of stability in life. The age 30 transition is a period of settling down, of taking a more serious approach to life and work. The transition stage into middle adulthood or mid-life has become synonymous with the term 'mid-life crisis'. For some 80% of Levinson's sample this transition period was extremely stressful and characterized by self-doubt and a realization that their career progression had probably reached its limit. In the mid-life era, there are added pressures such as elderly parents to worry about, the beginnings of physical decline such as the need to wear spectacles, and children becoming independent young adults. There may be a positive side to mid-life, though, such as being financially more secure, and enjoying life as a couple again after children have left home.

SPECIFIC COGNITIVE THEORIES AND PERSPECTIVES ON LEARNING

A number of influential learning theorists have taken a cognitive approach in an attempt to explain how people learn, and those with application to adult learning are included here.

Ausubel: assimilation theory of meaningful learning

The psychologist David P. Ausubel is somewhat unusual among educational psychologists in that he focuses very much on presentational methods of teaching and also on the acquisition of subject matter in the

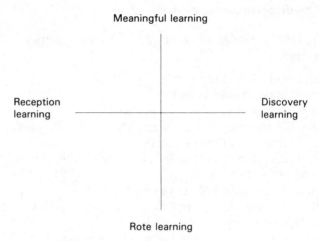

Fig. 3.6 Ausubel's dimensions of learning.

curriculum. He draws a distinction between psychology and educational psychology, the former being concerned with problems of learning whilst the latter is an applied science, the function of which is to study those aspects of learning that can be related to ways of effectively bringing about assimilation of organized bodies of knowledge.

Ausubel (1978) distinguishes between types of learning by using a model consisting of two orthogonal dimensions of learning; one on the continuum from rote to meaningful learning; and the other on the continuum from reception to discovery learning (Figure 3.6). These dimensions are unrelated and it can be seen that the diagram consists of four quadrants:

- meaningful reception learning,
- rote reception learning,
- meaningful discovery learning, and
- rote discovery learning.

Ausubel maintains that most classroom learning is of the reception type, in which information is presented in its final form to the student. Discovery learning, on the other hand, consists of allowing students to discover for themselves the principles of content. Discovery learning may fall at any point on the continuum and it is more usual to find a form of guided discovery learning in use in the classroom. Whilst acknowledging the place of discovery learning, Ausubel claims that it is simply not feasible for transmitting large quantities of knowledge, since discovery learning requires greater time and resources. The second, unrelated, dimension is rote/meaningful; rote learning is defined as any learning that does not meet the criteria for meaningfulness.

Types of meaningful learning

There are three types of meaningful learning.

1. *Representational or vocabulary learning* All other types of learning depend upon this basic form, which consists of the learning of single words or what is represented by them.
2. *Concept learning* Ausubel defines concepts as 'objects, events, situations or properties that possess common criterial attributes and are designated by some sign or symbol'. He identifies two kinds of concept acquisition, the first occurring in young children, called concept formation, and the second occurring in school children and adults, called concept assimilation.
3. *Propositional learning* In this form of learning, it is not simply the meaning of single words that is learned, but the meaning of sentences that contain composite ideas. Syntax and grammatical rules must also be understood.

Ausubel takes pains to point out that there is a difference between meaningful learning and the learning of meaningful material. In order for material to be learned meaningfully, it is necessary to meet three criteria.

1. The student must adopt an appropriate learning 'set', which is a disposition to approach a learning task in a particular way. In the case of meaningful learning, the student must adopt a set to learn the task in a meaningful, as opposed to a rote, fashion.
2. The learning task itself must have logical meaning, in that it can be related to the student's own cognitive structure in a sensible way. This cognitive structure is said to provide anchorage for the new information, with both components being modified in the process of assimilation.
3. The student's own cognitive structures must contain specifically relevant ideas with which the new material can interact.

Rote learning, on the other hand, can be considered as any learning in which these conditions are not present. For example, the student may adopt a set to learn the material in a word-for-word fashion, in which case the new material would be linked to the existing structure in a simple, arbitrary way without any real interaction. Such linkage prohibits the direct use of existing knowledge and in addition, the word-for-word nature of learning will place limits on the amount of material that can be learned and retained. Ausubel considers that pure rote learning plays little part in everyday classroom learning beyond elementary school level.

These conditions form an integral part of Ausubel's assimilation theory, which states that most meaningful cognitive learning occurs as a result of interaction between new information that the individual acquires and the specifically relevant cognitive structures that he or she already possesses. This interaction results in the assimilation or incorporation of both the new and the existing information to form a more detailed cognitive structure. Figure 3.7 shows this process; the new information is not simply added to the old in a cumulative way – rather, it acts upon the existing information and both are transformed into a new and more detailed cognitive structure. The pivotal nature of this idea to Ausubel's theory can be seen in his statement (1978, p. 163):

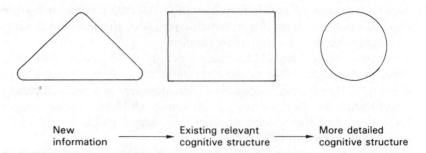

New information → Existing relevant cognitive structure → More detailed cognitive structure

Fig. 3.7 The process of assimilation of information.

If I had to reduce all educational psychology to just one principle it would be this: 'The most important single factor influencing learning is what the student already knows. Ascertain this and teach him accordingly.'

Assimilation theory forms the basis of Ausubel's ideas on the organization of instruction and the main variables affecting learning are outlined below.

1. Cognitive variables
   (a) The student's previous knowledge of related ideas – seen to be important to the learning of new material, and forms the basis of the notion 'transfer of learning'
   (b) Developmental readiness, which is the stage of cognitive development the student has reached
   (c) Intellectual ability of the student
   (d) Practice
   (e) Arrangement of instructional materials in order to facilitate learning
2. Affective/social variables
   (f) Motivation and attitudes
   (g) Personality
   (h) Group and social factors
   (i) Teacher characteristics

One of the key strategies for learning advocated by Ausubel is the concept of 'advance organizer', a strategy introduced in advance of any new material in order to provide an anchoring structure for it. This strategy is based on the assimilation theory, which, as we have seen, states that new information is subsumed or incorporated into an anchoring structure already present in the student. Typically, an advance organizer consists of ideas that are similar to the material that is to be learned, but are stated at a higher level of generality and inclusiveness, so that the new material may then assume a subordinate relationship to the advance organizer. The concept is similar to an overview (or summary), except that the latter is presented at the same level of generality or inclusiveness. Advance organizers form the link between the student's previous knowledge and what is needed to be known, before any meaningfully learning can take place. A further advantage is that it provides a highly specific anchoring structure because the content is virtually identical to the material that follows, although to be effective, it must obviously be potentially meaningful and capable of being understood.

The process of forgetting meaningfully learned material is also explained by Ausubel in terms of assimilation theory. Learning, as we have seen, consists of the interaction between new information and knowledge already present in the cognitive structure of an individual. During the process of assimilation, this new information gradually loses its discrete identity as it becomes part of the modified anchoring structure; this process is termed obliterative subsumption. This gradual loss of separate identity ends with the meaning being forgotten when the idea falls below the threshold of availability. This threshold forms a level below which an idea cannot be retrieved, but the level is subject to variation, e.g. due to anxiety.

Ausubel's theory and nurse education

How effective are advance organizers in practice? Barnes and Clawson (1975) reviewed 32 students involving the use of advance organizers and found that 12 reported significant effects and 20 were non-significant. They analysed the studies according to selected variables, finding that length of treatment was not critical and that the ability levels of students had no differential effects on learning. Similarly, no clear pattern emerged in relation to the grade level of the students or to the types of organizer. They concluded that the efficacy of advance organizers had not been established. Ausubel, however, states that Barnes and Clawson failed to take into account the fact that most studies did not analyse the students' relevant subsumers nor the conceptual material to be learned. Meena (1980) reports a study in which advance organizers were used prior to information presented in an instructional film; results showed that learning and retention were significantly superior for the organizer groups. Nicholl (1978) studied the effects of advance organizers on a cognitive social-learning group, but the results were not significant.

The most obvious application of assimilation theory is that of advance organizers for lectures. As was pointed out earlier, an advance organizer is a form of introductory material, introduced and taught to the students in advance of the main body of the lecture, and its purpose is to provide the necessary specific anchoring structures for the information presented in the main body of the lecture. In order to do this, the advance organizer must fulfil certain criteria.

1. It must form a bridge between what the student already knows and the new information to be encountered in the lecture.
2. The advance organizer must be more general and inclusive than the material that follows it in the main body of the lecture; it must abstract out from that knowledge the key essence of the lecture.

3. It must be taught and learned just like any other information, either immediately prior to the lecture, or some time in advance of it.

One of the difficulties of grasping the concept of an advance organizer is that Ausubel only ever gave one example, because the organizer must relate intimately to the teacher's subject matter and thus cannot be written by anyone else. In order to see how the organizer is structured, it is always necessary to have the subject matter of the lecture available as well. Figure 3.8 shows an example of an advance organizer for a lesson on the circulatory system, including the lesson plan for the main lecture.

The advance organizer is taught at the beginning of the lecture, and is then followed by the main body of informations the advance organizer contains all the elements of the lecture that follows it, but at a much more abstract level. For example, it talks about 'certain cells' rather than giving specific names; the names are introduced later in the lecture. The advance organizer also contains information that the student already knows, i.e. the transport systems of society and so forms a bridge between this prior knowledge and the new information about the circulation. Another example of an advance organizer is given in Chapter 17 (p. 406), where it is used in a lecture on shock and haemorrhage.

The principle of meaningful learning can be applied at all levels of nurse education and it is particularly important to ascertain students' prior knowledge when working in the clinical setting. A few minutes spent clarifying what the student understands about the nursing care of a patient will be rewarded by providing a framework upon which further explanation can be hung.

Nurse teachers should try to discourage students from learning material in a rote fashion and instead, encourage them to learn it meaningfully, by ask them to try to explain the material to a fellow student.

Bruner: discovery learning

The work of Jerome Bruner (1960) has had a profound influence on educational thinking and he is particularly associated with 'discovery learning'. Bruner sees the learning of a subject as involving three processes.

1. *The acquisition of new information*: this usually builds on something that is already known, albeit tentative or vague.
2. *Transformation of information*: new information is analysed and processed so that it can be used in new situations.
3. *Evaluation*: all aspects of the processing of information are evaluated to check whether they are correct.

Subject matter is usually broken down into a series of units or learning episodes and each episode involves the three processes above.

Structure of a subject

According to Bruner, the purpose of learning is that it should be useful to us in the future and this occurs by the process of transfer. Transfer of

Introduction
Good morning and welcome to this lecture on the circulatory system. Before we begin I would like to include some introductory material to help you understand the lecture.

Advance organizer
You are all very familiar with the notion of transport systems in society; for example, road, rail, air and sea transport. Any transport system has a number of basic components as follows:

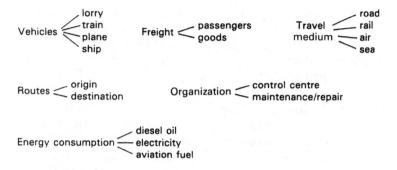

The circulatory system in the body is another example of a transport system with the same basic components. We can usefully examine the system using these components as follows:

Vehicles: In the bloodstream, certain cells act as vehicles for transporting substances, as does the liquid part of the blood, called *plasma*.

Freight: Many 'goods' are transported in the blood, including foodstuffs, oxygen, chemical messengers and waste products.

Travel medium: The liquid part of the blood is the transport medium.

Routes: There are many routes involved in the circulation. For example, oxygen originates at the lungs (the supplier) and its destination is the tissue cells (the consumer).

Organization: There is a complex organization of circulation, both from central control in the brain to local control in the tissues.

Energy Consumption: Like all other body systems, the circulation burns up glucose to make energy.

Main body of lecture

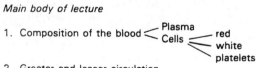
1. Composition of the blood

2. Greater and lesser circulation
3. Functions of blood
4. Control of circulation

Fig. 3.8 Example of a lesson plan with advance organizer for 'the circulatory system'.

learning can occur in two main ways – transfer of specific skills or transfer of general principles. This latter type of transfer is fundamental to the educational process and is dependent upon a thorough understanding of the structure of subject matter. This concept of structure is explained by Bruner (1960, p.7) as follows:

> Grasping the structure of a subject is understanding it in a way which permits many other things to be related to it meaningfully. To learn structure, in short, is to learn how things are related.

Structure, then, involves the basic patterns and ideas of the subject, but not the details or specific facts. If students understand the structure, they should be able to work out for themselves much of the fine detail. The structure is made up of concepts or categories and Bruner sees learning as a process of categorization of objects. Classes of objects are seen to be characterized by common properties, and it is these properties that are used as a basis for identifying new objects that are encountered. The new object is compared with the properties of a category, to see if it belongs there. If the object fits a particular category, then we infer that it possesses the characteristics of that category. A category has certain distinguishing properties that differentiate it from other categories and it also has a certain order in which the characteristics are combined. For example, the category 'bed' has the following components: frame, legs, headboard, footboard, mattress, pillows, blankets and counterpane. These characteristics are assembled in a certain order, such as the legs underneath, the mattress on the frame, the pillows and blankets on top, etc. There are also limits of acceptance for objects to fall within a category. For instance, a bed would still be a bed if there were no headboard, but it would not constitute a bed if there were no frame.

When categorizing an object, an individual tends to follow a sequence of four stages. The first involves isolating the object from its background, a process called primitive categorization. A search for cues then follows, which may be conscious or unconscious, and the individual attempts to categorize the object using cues available. He or she may employ a conscious cue search by saying, 'I wonder what this can be.' Having made a cue search, the individual makes a tentative categorization and this then narrows down the search to those cues that will confirm the tentative categorization. This is termed confirmation check. The fourth stage involves ceasing the search for cues and additional cues are more or less ignored. This stage is called confirmation completion and the object is identified and categorized.

Coding systems for information

The learning of more complex information is explained by Bruner in terms of coding systems. A coding system is a set of general categories that an individual uses to classify and to group information about the world. These systems are hierarchically arranged, with the more specific information in the lowest categories. As one rises in the hierarchy, each category is more general and less specific than the one below, and to recall a specific item, it is necessary to recall the coding system of which it is a

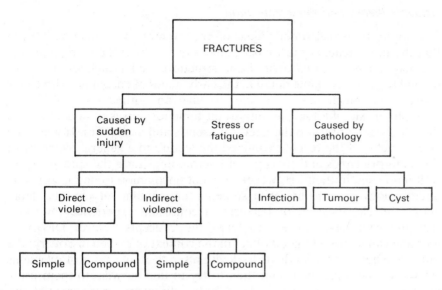

Fig. 3.9 Coding system for fractures.

member. Thus, the general principles of a subject are contained in the upper parts of the hierarchy of a category and in transfer of learning, these previously learned coding systems are applied to new events or objects. Figure 3.9 shows a coding system for fractures, with the most general concept at the top, namely fractures and progressively finer subdivisions or subordinate concepts.

Acquisition of coding systems is influenced by a number of factors, including the learning 'set' of an individual towards a learning task, and motivation of the student. In addition, there must be mastery of the specific aspects of a situation before the principles can be combined into a more general or generic coding system, and this acquisition of generic coding systems is enhanced by a variety of learning situations, especially discovery-learning situations.

Discovery learning

Discovery learning involves students in discovering the structure of a subject through active involvement and can be divided into pure discovery and guided discovery. The former is virtually impossible to organize, since it involves no direction whatsoever, so the latter is preferable. The role of the teacher is to pose questions or problems that stimulate students to seek answers in an active discovery way. One of the great obstacles to this kind of learning in nurse education is the pressure on students always to produce the correct answers to questions, and this runs counter to the notion of intuitive thinking. Intuition involves making an educated guess about phenomena before one has the complete data, and can be very motivating for students because they then have to check whether their hypothesis was correct or not.

Bruner's theory and nurse education

The implications of Bruner's ideas on the structure of subject matter are that the nurse teacher must ensure that any new material being taught is first explained in terms of its basic structures and principles. It is not helpful to give lots of fine detail in the early stages of encounter with a new subject and much more sensible, to give an outline only. Take the example of microbiology, an important topic for nurses to understand so that they can appreciate the need for asepsis and antibiotics. It would be good practice if the teacher confined the lecture to a general overview of the main principles and concepts of microbiology until the students were well-immersed in them. However, it is not uncommon to find lectures on microbiology given to first-year students that contain very specific detail about the classification of bacteria, a confusing experience for those students who have not encountered the concepts before. Discovery learning can be used to good effect in the context of guided discovery; the nurse teacher can ask students to devise a series of questions or problems related to the topic areas and then to try to find answers to them using whatever resources are available. Another discovery approach is to use practical laboratory sessions to generate activities and then to ask students to try to explain why things happened.

Gagne: the conditions of learning and theory of instruction

Robert Gagne does not propose a theory of learning *per se*, but focuses on the conditions of learning. Using an information-processing model, he analyses these conditions and develops a theory of instruction based upon them. Learning is defined as 'a change in human disposition or capability that persists over a period of time and is not simply ascribable to processes of growth' (Gagne, 1985). Thus growth is seen very much as being genetically determined, whereas learning is seen as being mainly under the control of environmental influences that interact with the individual. Any learning situation can be seen as having a number of elements, namely the student, the stimulus, the contents of the student's memory and the response or performance outcome. Such a learning situation or occurrence is described by Gagne (1985, p. 4) as follows:

> A learning occurrence, then, takes place when the stimulus situation together with the contents of memory affect the student in such a way that his or her performance changes from a time before being in that situation to a time after being in it. The change in performance is what leads to the conclusion that learning has occurred.

Learning capabilities

Gagne believes that it is possible to make sense of all the different learning outcomes that people make during a lifetime by organizing them into five performance categories, each representing a different kind of learning capability.

1. Intellectual skills
    (a) Discrimination
    (b) Concrete concepts
    (c) Defined concepts
    (d) Rules
    (e) Higher-order rules
2. Cognitive strategies
3. Verbal information
4. Motor skills
5. Attitudes

Prototypes of learning

The five varieties of learning capability include some elements that Gagne terms 'prototypes of learning'; these are commonly identified phenomena of learning that constitute basic forms of learning by association. They include

classical conditioning,
operant conditioning,
verbal-association learning, and
'chaining'

and are seen as basic forms because they comprise only parts of specific capabilities and are insufficient to explain all aspects of complex learning. Hence, association is seen as an important aspect, since its various forms constitute some of the components of the five learning capabilities. These prototypes are discussed in Chapter 4.

Having emphasized the importance of association learning as a basic component of all types of learning, we now examine the five varieties of learning capability in more detail.

Intellectual skills

It is useful to think of intellectual skills as forming a hierarchy in which any particular skill requires the prior learning of those skills below it in the hierarchy, as illustrated in Figure 3.10.

The dependence of intellectual skills on the basic prototypes is shown and each level consists of progressively more complex skills. These intellectual skills are what is referred to as 'procedural knowledge' (i.e. knowledge about how to perform such things as mathematical calculations) and are typified by rule-governed behaviour. Rules state relationships between things and are composed of simpler components called concepts, which in turn depend on the ability to discriminate between various characteristics of things.

Discrimination   Young children learn to respond to collections of things by learning the differences between them, a process called discrimination.

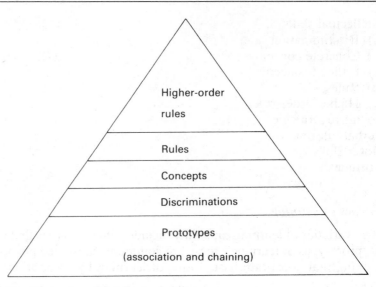

Fig. 3.10 Hierarchy of intellectual skills.

Discrimination learning involves perceiving differences in size, shape, colour, texture, etc. and multiple discriminations have to be made when there is more than one stimulus present. Student nurses and midwives may have to learn to discriminate between the various kinds of tissue when using a microscope. This is usually taught by presenting examples and non-examples of a particular tissue, a process called 'contrast practice'. When the student is making multiple discriminations, there is a danger of confusion between stimuli and interference in the learning of discriminations.

Concrete concepts Discrimination learning is confined to specific stimuli, whereas concept formation allows the student to respond to collections of things by classifying them into categories sharing common abstract properties. Unlike prototypes and discriminations, concepts are capable of being generalized to other situations and hence they free the student from control by specific stimuli. Once a student nurse has acquired the concept of a 'pressure sore', this can be applied to any example on all areas of the body, provided that the concept adequately represents the range of pressure sores possible. It may be that students have inadequate concepts for some classes of phenomena, so these need to be developed and extended by appropriate instruction.

Gagne describes three stages in the learning of a concrete or observable concept: discrimination, generalization and variation in irrelevant dimensions. The first stage involves the student in discriminating between one object and another, e.g. a capsule and a tablet. The next stage involves generalization of the discrimination, in which the student discriminates between the capsule and a variety of tablets of various shapes, sizes and colours. The final stage involves variation in the size, shape and colour of the capsules, as well as the variations in the tablets and if the student can identify all the capsules, then he or she has acquired the concept of a 'capsule'. This attainment can be tested by showing the student nurse a capsule and a tablet, neither of which have been seen before; if the student nurse can identify the capsule, he or she has attained the concept by identifying a novel instance.

The learning of a concept can be made much easier by the use of language, i.e. verbal cues or instructions; indeed, many of the concepts used in nursing are learned verbally by attending lectures or by reading. Concepts learned in this linguistic manner need to have concrete references to the real world if students really are to understand them. Such concrete reference can be made by the use of practical work in laboratories or clinical settings.

Defined concepts In the previous section, concrete concepts were referred to by Gragne as concepts-by-observation; certain concepts, however, can only be learned as definitions, since they do not actually exist as concrete entities, for example, health or empathy. A definition is a statement that expresses rules for classifying objects or events and consists of 'thing-concepts' and 'relational concepts'. The definition of an object consists of four parts:

1. a thing-concept that is superordinate;
2. a set of characteristics of the above,
3. a relational concept indicating the use of the object; and
4. a thing-concept that is the object of the verb above.

Figure 3.11 illustrates the components of the definition of the concept of a 'syringe'.

Many concepts are themselves relations and the components of these definitions are slightly different:

1. a relational concept that is already known by the student;
2. a thing-concept that is the object of the above, and
3. modifier words that are the characteristics of the relation.

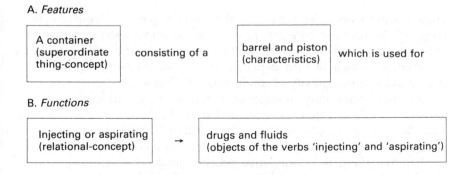

A. *Features*

| A container (superordinate thing-concept) | consisting of a | barrel and piston (characteristics) | which is used for |

B. *Functions*

| Injecting or aspirating (relational-concept) | → | drugs and fluids (objects of the verbs 'injecting' and 'aspirating') |

Fig. 3.11 Components of the definition of 'syringe'.

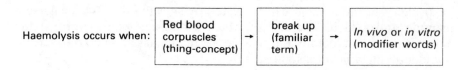

Fig. 3.12 Components of the definition of 'haemolysis'.

Figure 3.12 illustrates the components of the definition of 'haemolysis'.

There is one point of possible confusion between concrete concepts and defined concepts; it is quite common to find that concrete concepts are given definitions, as in the example of syringe, but this does not make them defined concepts. A defined concept cannot be concrete, however, since it is concerned with relations not objects. Defined concepts are taught by pointing out the thing-concepts and the relational concepts to the student and these are then understood, provided the student has already acquired the relevant component concepts of the definition. For example, the term 'diffusion' can be defined as 'the continual intermingling of molecules in liquids or gases', but for the student to understand this concept, he or she must first understand the component concepts of 'intermingling' and 'molecules'.

Rules A rule is defined by Gagne (1985, p. 118) as 'an inferred capability that enables the individual to respond to any instance of a class of stimulus situations with an appropriate instance of a class of performances'. Rules require as prerequisites, the component concepts and these are then put in the correct sequence, as in the rules of grammar or mathematics. Rules are often thought of as statements in lay terms, e.g. the rule book, but it is important to remember that the rule itself is an inferred capability, which is one of the aspects of intellectual skills. However, verbal statements are very useful for learning rules, as in the 'diffusion' example mentioned earlier. Rules are also termed procedures and may consist of long sequences or steps in a particular sequence. Nursing procedure manuals are published that contains a series of rules about the carrying out of various nursing procedures.

Higher-order rules We have seen that rules require prerequisite knowledge of the relevant concepts in order to be understood and that such concept attainment is reliant upon the necessary discriminations made by the student, which in turn depends upon associations between stimuli. The increasing complexity of intellectual skill does not stop at rules, but higher-order rules may develop as a result of the student's problem-solving, resulting in the combination of several rules into a more complex rule. Much learning can be seen in the form of learning hierarchies, with the simpler rules forming prerequisites for more complex ones and this implies that there is a cumulative process involved in learning. Hence, simpler rules are transferred to more complex rules and these higher-order rules tend to be more generalizable in their application.

Cognitive strategies

These strategies exert control over the internal mental processes of learning such as thinking, memory and problem-solving and are independent of content. They are involved in the learning of intellectual skills and other learning capabilities and are often referred to as metacognitive processes or 'learning to learn'. Students use cognitive strategies for attending to stimuli, for encoding and retrieving information in the memory and for thinking and problem-solving, e.g. the use of mnemonics and imagery. Cognitive strategies are easily acquired by students and become better with practice, and there is some evidence to suggest that these skills will transfer to other situations.

Verbal information learning

Verbal learning entails 'declarative knowledge', the kind of knowledge involved in telling or verbalizing, and it utilizes sentences or propositions. There are three forms of verbal learning: names (or labels), facts (or single propositions) and organized verbal knowledge.

Names or labels   These are normally learned at the same time as the concept is acquired, hence only one or two labels or names are learnt at any one time. On occasions, however, it is necessary to learn several names at one time, such as when a nurse teacher meets a new student group and has to remember each name, which can be very difficult.

Facts or single propositions   It seems likely that facts are stored in memory as meaningful propositions rather than as verbatim words in some form of semantic network.

Organized verbal knowledge   This refers to collections of propositions that are organized into connected discourse called prose. It is suggested that a student's previous knowledge is a major influence on the learning of new information from prose texts, due to the previous formation of global schemata for particular situations or events.

Motor skills

Much human learning is to do with movements and a practice discipline like nursing centres around the learning of motor skills and procedures. There are three dimensions of motor skills: fine/gross performance, continuous/discrete movements, and closed/open looped tasks.

Fine versus gross performance   It is possible to distinguish motor skills in terms of the involvement of muscles, gross skills requiring the use of large muscles as in the lifting of patients and fine skills, the use of fingers and wrists, as in the removing of sutures.

Continuous versus discrete   These terms are self-explanatory, the former consisting of continuous movements such as those of external cardiac massage and the latter consisting of single-direction movements, such as the switching off of the nurse call-button.

Closed-looped versus open-looped tasks   The former relies entirely on proprioceptive feedback and can be performed with the eyes closed; the latter involves some kind of external stimulus that influences the movement, such as inflating the cuff on a sphygmomanometer according to the level of the column of mercury.

Motor skills often occur as components of procedures, such as giving a blanket bath or changing a dressing; a procedure consists of a series of rules in sequential order, but also requires certain motor skills in order to be executed. It is therefore incorrect to think of procedures as being motor skills alone, rather they involve both intellectual and motor skills. Practice is a basic requirement for the acquisition of motor skills in order to allow the student to learn from the proprioceptive feedback from his or her own body movements; in addition the student receives feedback both from observing the effects of his or her movements and by augmented feedback from someone else: a teacher or a coach. When attempting to learn a procedure, a student combines a series of part-skills into the total procedure in a particular order and these are known as behavioural chains.

Attitudes

According to Gagne (1985, p. 63), an attitude is 'an internal state that influences (moderates) the choices of personal action made by the individual'. Attitudes are learnt as individuals develop during childhood and adult life. Their relationship to behaviour is not clearly identified, but they serve to predispose the individual to act towards things in a particular way. There are three components of an attitude:

1. the cognitive component consists of the beliefs which an individual holds about the attitudinal object;
2. the affective component is concerned with feelings that the individual has about the beliefs that he or she holds about the attitudinal object; and
3. the behavioural aspect – a predisposition to act in some way – although studies have shown poor correlation between attitudes and behaviour.

A nurse may have a positive attitude towards the elderly, believing that they have a right to be treated with respect and dignity and this belief may be very strongly felt. The nurse may endeavour in his or her behaviour towards the elderly to ensure always that they are treated as individuals and made to feel respected.

The conditions of learning

The learning capabilities outlined above form the cornerstone of Gagne's approach to instruction, since this involves identifying the conditions of learning for each of these capabilities, as well as for the prototypes called association. Gagne suggests that in order to infer that learning has taken place, it is necessary to know not only the changes in performance following instruction, but the capabilities that students already possess prior to instruction. These previously learned capabilities are what Gagne refers to as 'internal conditions of learning', in contrast to 'external conditions of learning', which consist of the stimulus situations outside the student. Both are necessary if learning is to take place and Gagne has described the internal and external conditions necessary for learning in each of the learned capabilities and prototypes. These are outlined in Table 3.4.

Gagne's theory of instruction

Gagne points out that there is a difference between theories of learning and theories of instruction in that the latter utilizes a range of theories of learning in order to establish principles of instruction. The events of instruction are different for each of the learning capabilities. Gagne suggests a sequence of instructional events related to internal processes of learning in an information-processing framework.

1. *Gaining attention* A variety of strategies, including loudness of the voice, gesturing, asking questions, or a practical demonstration of something can be used. Attention-getting devices are applicable to all the learning capabilities.
2. *Informing students of the objective* If students know the objectives of instruction, they will be motivated to learn, so it is important that such objectives are transmitted to them for whichever type of capability that might be being taught. These may be stated in the form of behavioural objectives.
3. *Stimulating recall of prior learning* This is important for all learning capabilities and is commonly done by asking questions of the students.
4. *Presenting the stimulus* This depends upon what is to be learned and can involve printed materials, the presentation of a problem, a description of a strategy or the demonstration of a motor skill.
5. *Providing learning guidance* This consists of conveying the meaningfulness of the stimulus by such devices as relating new information to existing knowledge and giving concrete examples of abstract concepts.
6. *Eliciting performance* Here, the student is asked to demonstrate the application of learning to a novel problem, to ensure that learning has occurred.
7. *Providing feedback* Feedback as to the correctness or otherwise of a student's performance is important for his or her further learning and this can be achieved by a teacher giving verbal feedback or written

Table 3.4 The conditions of learning for prototypes and learning capabilities

Capability	Internal conditions (within the learner)	External conditions (the learning situation)
Prototypes		
Classical conditioning	Presence of a natural reflex in the learner, i.e. unconditioned stimulus results in unconditioned response	(i) Contiguity, i.e. conditioned and unconditioned stimuli must be presented close together (ii) A repetition of the paired stimuli must occur
Operant conditioning	Reinforcement of behaviour is essential	(i) A reinforcement contingency must occur (ii) Contiguity and repetition are also necessary
Chaining	Each stimulus–response association must be previously learned	(i) Learner must state the links of the chain in their correct order (ii) Contiguity, repetition and reinforcement are necessary.
Verbal association	(i) Every link must be previously learned as a stimulus–response association (ii) Mediating connections, i.e. verbal codes, visual and auditory images, must be previously learned	(i) Verbal units must be presented in correct sequence (ii) External cues should be provided, e.g. mnemonics (iii) Student's memory determines the length of the chain he or she is capable of learning at one time (iv) Correct responses must be confirmed to the learner
Learning capabilities 1. Intellectual skills		
(a) Discrimination	Recall of stimulus–response chains to demonstrate discrimination	Selective reinforcement of correct, as opposed to incorrect, responses is required
(b) Concrete concepts	(i) Discriminations must be previously learned (ii) Verbal labels must have been previously learned if verbal instructions are used (iii) Generalization of basic discrimination	Verbal cues should be given, i.e. (i) One example and one non-example of concept (ii) Same example plus various non-examples (iii) Variations in both examples and non-examples (iv) Reinforcement of correct responses and contiguity
(c) Defined concepts	(i) Component concepts must be available in memory (ii) Rules of syntax must be previously learned	(i) Definition should be presented verbally or in writing to act as cue for retrieval of concepts (ii) Examples and non-examples of defined concepts should be given
(d) Rules	Knowledge of the concepts involved in the rule	Verbal instructions as follows: (i) Expected performance outcome should be stated (ii) Teacher should evoke recall of the component concepts (iii) Verbal cues should be given for whole rule (iv) Reinforcement and repetition are required

Table 3.4 *continued*

2.	Cognitive strategies	(i) Understanding of the meaning of self-instruction strategies (ii) Task-related concepts must be previously learned	Discovery by the learner of strategies for encoding, etc.
3.	Verbal learning	(i) Previously learned and organized knowledge in student's memory (ii) Strategies for encoding verbal information	(i) Provision of a meaningful learning context (ii) Making cues for recall as distinctive as possible to avoid interference (iii) Practise retrieving information by review and repetition
4.	Motor skills	(i) Part-skills must be recalled (ii) The procedure (executive routine) must be recalled	(i) Verbal instructions should be given (ii) Pictures in the form of diagrams or video to show movements involved (iii) Demonstration of movements by skilled practitioner (iv) Practice must be allowed (v) Feedback about the performance is important for motor-skills learning, i.e. augmented feedback given by instructor
5.	Attitudes	(i) Concept to which attitude is related must be previously learned (ii) Certain information is necessary to the establishment of an attitude	(i) Human models for attitudes: model should be credible and appealing; recall of relevant information is encouraged; the desired action is indicated to the learner; the model is seen to receive reinforcement (ii) Alternative forms of modelling can be used, e.g. role-play, reading fiction, television and drama, etc. (iii) Reinforcement is given for choice of desired action

comments. Alternative forms can be given by the use of computers or other technology.

8. *Assessing performance* This is typically done by means of a test in which the student is given new examples to work on.

9. *Enhancing retention and transfer* This can be done by giving practice in the relevant capability and by increasing the variety of performance.

Learning is also affected by such variables as the time spent on learning a task and the individual differences in students in terms of motivation, previous knowledge and comprehension.

Kolb: The theory of experiential learning

David Kolb (1984) sees learning as a core process of human development, and makes a distinction between development and simple readjustment

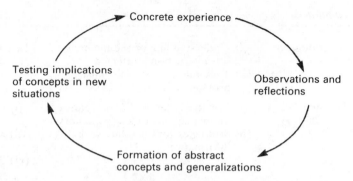

Fig. 3.13 Experiential learning model (Kolb, 1984).

to change. Development results from learning that is gained through experience, and this is the basis of the 'experiential learning model' (or experiential learning cycle').

The cycle, as shown in Figure 3.13, begins with some kind of concrete experience, professional or personal, that the student considers interesting or problematic. Observations and information are gathered about the experience and then the student reflects upon it, replaying it over again and analysing it until certain insights begin to emerge in the shape of a 'theory' about the experience. The implications arising from this conceptualization can then be utilized to modify existing nursing or midwifery practice or to generate new approaches to it.

Generic adaptive abilities

There are four generic adaptive abilities required for effective learning:

1. *Concrete experience (CE)* The students must immerse themselves fully and openly in new experiences.
2. *Reflective observation (RO)* The students must observe and reflect on concrete experiences from a variety of perspectives.
3. *Abstract conceptualization (AC)* The students must create concepts that integrate their observations into logical theories.
4. *Active experimentation* The students must apply these theories in decision-making and problem-solving.

Primary dimensions of learning process

These four generic adaptive abilities consist of two pairs of opposites, forming two primary dimensions of learning:

1. concrete experience – abstract conceptualization; and
2. active experimentation – reflective observation

During a learning situation, the student moves from action to observation to a varying extent according to the nature of the situation, both dimensions being important aspects of the learning process. This approach is compatible with other theories of cognitive development such as those of Piaget and Bruner referred to earlier in this chapter.

The experiential learning cycle and nurse education

Kolb and Fry (1975) identify four learning styles based upon the theory of experiential learning, and these are outlined in Chapter 16 (p. 374). The experiential learning cycle has been influential in curricula for nursing and midwifery, and forms a very useful theoretical basis for the Accreditation of Prior Experiential Learning (APEL), discussed in Chapter 13 (p. 323). However, the model does not have a great deal of empirical support, and it is unlikely that every single learning situation will demand an integrated approach using the four general adaptive abilities.

Schon: the reflective practitioner

Although the concept of reflection was already well-established in education, e.g. Dewey (1933), it was the publication of *The Reflective Practitioner: How Professionals Think in Action* (Schon, 1983) that caught the imagination of nurses and midwives, who saw in Schon's ideas the rationale for practice that they had been seeking. Schon's focus is the relationship between academic knowledge as defined in universities, and the competence involved in professional practice. He argues that professional practice is based upon a 'technical rationality' model which makes erroneous assumptions about the nature of practice, and in so doing reduces its importance in relation to theory. Technical rationality views professional practice as the application of general, standardized, theoretical principles to the solving of practice problems. This top-down view puts general theoretical principles at the top of the hierarchy of professional knowledge and practical problem-solving at the bottom, leading to the current situation in education, i.e. the pre-eminence of theory and the denigration of practice. Schon cites the position of research in relation to practice, with the former conducted in different institutions to those where the profession is practised. He also notes that research is seen to be more prestigious than practice, and we can draw a parallel between this point and the fact that professional educators are seen as more prestigious by the practitioners themselves.

Technical rationality, therefore, views professional practice as a process of instrumental problem-solving, with the assumption that problems are self-evident. Schon, however, argues that in reality practitioners are not presented with problems *per se*, but with problem situations. These must be converted into actual problems by a process of problem-setting, i.e. selecting the elements of the situation, deciding the ends and means, and framing the context.

Technical rationality also fails to take account of the fact that problems encountered in professional practice are rarely standard or predictable. Schon maintains that professional practice involves the use of tacit, intuitive knowledge; the professional practitioner has the ability to reflect upon this knowledge whilst engaged in the activities of practice, and this enables the practitioner to deal with unique, unpredictable or conflicting situations. Schon maintains that practice is the expression of an important form of knowledge and that this knowledge is embedded in action; when something unusual is encountered the practitioner steps back and reflects on what he or she is doing, and thereby restructures understanding. This notion of the reflective practitioner, according to Schon, contrasts markedly with the prevailing model of professional practice, the technical rationality model.

According to Schon, the reflective practitioner is characterized by a range of personal qualities and abilities, such as the ability to:

- engage in self-assessment;
- criticize the existing state of affairs;
- promote change and adapt to change; and
- practise as an autonomous professional.

Schon also distinguishes between the effective and the ineffective practitioner; the former is able to recognize and explore confusing or unique events that occur during practice, whereas the latter is confined to repetitive and routine practice, neglecting opportunities to think about what he or she is doing.

REFERENCES

Allen, H. and Murrell, J. (1978) *Nurse Training: an enterprise in curriculum development*, Macdonald and Evans, Plymouth.

Anderson, J. (1980) *Cognitive Psychology and its implications*, W.H. Freeman, San Francisco.

Anderson, J. and Bower, G. (1973) *Human Associative Memory*, Winston, Washington.

Atkinson, R. and Shiffrin, R. (1971) The control of short term memory. *Scientific American*, **225**, 82–90.

Ausubel, D., Novak, J. and Hanesian, H. (1978) *Educational Psychology; a cognitive view*, Holt, Rinehart and Winston, New York.

Baddeley, A. and Hitch, G. (1974) Working memory, in *The Psychology of Learning and Motivation*, (ed. G. Bower) Vol 2, Academic Press, New York.

Baddeley, A. and Lieberman, K. (1980) Spatial working memory, in *Attention and Performance VIII*, (ed. R. Nickerson), Erlbaum, New Jersey.

Barnes, B. and Clawson, E. (1975) Do advance organizers facilitate learning? *Review of Educational Research*, **45**, 637–59.

Barrows, H. and Tamblyn, R. (1980) *Problem-based Learning: an Approach to Medical Education*, Springer, California.

Bartlett, F. (1932) *Remembering*, Cambridge University Press, Cambridge.

Brookfield, S. (1987) *Developing Critical Thinkers*, Open University Press, Milton Keynes.

Bruner, J. (1960) *The Process of Education*, Harvard University Press, Cambridge Mass.

Burnard, P. (1989) Developing critical ability in nurse education. *Nurse Education Today*, **9**, 271–5.

CNAA (Council for National Academic Awards) (1992) CNAA Handbook, CNAA, London.

Collins, A. and Quillian, M. (1969) Retrieval time from semantic memory. *Journal of Verbal Learning and Verbal Behaviour*, **8**, 240–7.

Conway, M. (1991) Cognitive psychology in search of meaning: the study of autobiographical memory. *The Psychologist*, **4**, 301–305.

Craik, F. and Lockhart, R. (1972) Levels of processing: a framework for memory research. *Journal of Experimental Psychology, General*, **104**, 268–94.

Dewey, J. (1933) *How We Think*, Regnery, Chicago.

Doyle, W. (1983) Academic work. *Review of Educational Research*, **53**(2), 159–99.

Edwards, D., Potter, J. and Middleton, D. (1992) Towards a discursive psychology of remembering. *The Psychologist*, **5**(10), 441–6.

Fitts, P. and Posner, M. (1967) *Human Performance*, Prentice-Hall, Englewood Cliffs, New Jersey.

Gagne, R. (1985) *The Conditions of Learning and Theory of Instruction*, 4th edn, Holt, Rinehart and Winston, New York.

Howard, D. (1983) *Cognitive Psychology*, Macmillan, London.

Kolb, D. (1984) *Experiential Learning*, Prentice-Hall, London.

Kolb, D. and Fry, R. (1975) Towards an Applied Theory of Experiential Learning, in *Theories of Group Processes*, (ed. C. Cooper), Wiley, London, pp. 33–57.

Levinson, D. (1986) A conception of adult development, *American Psychologist*, **41**, 3–13.

Meena, V. (1980) The effect of written and graphic comparative advance organizers upon learning and retention from an audio-visual presentation, dissertation. *Abstracts International*, **40**, 3713–14.

Miller, G. (1956) The magical number seven plus or minus two: some limits on our capacity for processing information. *Psychological Review*, **63**, 81–97.

Minsky, M. (1975) Artificial intelligence. *Scientific American*, summer 1975.

Nicholl, G. (1978) The effect of advance organizers on a cognitive social learning group. *Dissertion Abstracts International*, **38**, 44–75.

Oatley, K. (1978) *Computational Metaphors for Perception, D303*. Open University Press, Milton Keynes.

Oxendine, J. (1984) *Psychology of motor learning*, 2nd edn, Prentice-Hall, New Jersey.

Paivio, A. (1969) Mental imagery in associative learning and memory. *Psychological Review*, **76**, 241–63.

Piaget, J. and Inhelder, B. (1969) *The Psychology of the Child*, Basic Books, New York.

Pylyshyn, Z. (1973) What the mind's eye tells the mind's brain. *Psychological Bulletin*, **80**, 1–24.

Rummelhart, D. and Ortony, A. (1977) The representation of knowledge in memory, in *Schooling and the Acquisition of Knowledge*, (eds R. Anderson, R. Spiro and W. Montague) Erlbaum, New Jersey.

Schank, R. and Ableson, R. (1977) *Scripts, Plans, Goals and Understanding*, Erlbaum, New Jersey.

Schon, D. (1983) *The Reflective Practitioner: How Professionals Think in Action*, Basic Books, New York.

Selfridge, O. (1959) Pandemonium: a paradigm for learning, in *Mechanization of Thought Processes*, HMSO, London.

Simpson, E. (1972) The classification of educational objectives in the psychomotor domain. *The Psychomotor Domain*, **3**, Gryphon House, Washington DC.

Smythe, M., Morris P., Levy, P. and Ellis, A. (1987) *Cognition in Action*, Lawrence Erlbaum Associates, London.

Thorndike, E. (1931) *Human Learning*, Appleton Century Crofts, New York.

Tulving, E. (1972) Episodic and semantic memory, in *Organization of Memory*, (eds E. Tulving and W. Donaldson), Academic Press, New York.

Watson, G. and Glaser, E. (1961) *Watson–Glaser Critical Thinking Appraisal*, Harcourt, Brace and World Inc., New York.

Adult learning: behaviourist and other perspectives

4

Chapter 3 focused on cognitive perspectives on the learning and teaching process. This chapter explores a range of perspectives from a number of schools of psychology, including the influential behaviourist and humanistic approaches.

Behaviourist or stimulus–response (S–R) theories

The term behaviourist derives from the fact that this school considers that only observable behaviour can be used to explain learning. An alternative term is associationist which derives from the belief that learning is a result of an association between a stimulus and a response, hence the term S–R theory.

S–R theory proposes two forms of learning; classical conditioning and operant conditioning. John B. Watson is credited with founding the term behaviourism, and his work on classical conditioning complements that of Ivan Pavlov. The principles of operant conditioning were formulated by B. F. Skinner, although Edward Thorndike had independently developed the concept of reinforcement in learning.

Classical conditioning: the work of Ivan P. Pavlov

Ivan P. Pavlov (1849–1936) was a Russian physiologist who, in the course of his work on digestive secretions, observed phenomena that are fundamental to stimulus–response theory (Pavlov, 1927). His main interest was the control of salivary and gastric secretions and by careful experimentation he established that salivation relies upon two kinds of stimulation. With the first kind, salivation was an unlearned, physiological reflex that occurred after food was introduced into the mouth of the animal. With the second type, salivation occurred when the animal merely caught sight of the food, that is, before the food had actually entered its mouth.

This latter type intrigued Pavlov because he had observed over the course of his work that the dogs had begun to salivate immediately he entered his laboratory. Wondering whether this would occur to other stimuli, he paired a tone on a tuning fork with the immediate delivery of food to the dogs. This pairing was done on a number of occasions and at first the dogs only salivated when food was actually in the mouth, but eventually they salivated after the tone was sounded, but before food had entered the mouth. Pavlov considered that this salivation was a learned response as opposed to an innate reflex and termed the process 'conditioning'. Pavlovian conditioning has since been termed 'classical conditioning' to distinguish it from the other form of conditioning described by Skinner.

The vocabulary of conditioning requires some explanation, as it is fundamental to the behaviourist approach. In the experiments performed by Pavlov the first type of salivation was due to an inherent physiological reflex to the presence of food in the mouth of the dog. This is a natural or unconditioned situation, in which the food is said to be the unconditioned stimulus (US) and salivation the unconditioned response (UR). In the second phase of the experiment, the giving of food to the dog was paired with a tuning fork. After a number of such pairings, the tuning fork, which had previously been a neutral stimulus, now actually functioned as a stimulus for the flow of saliva. This is now a different situation and is called a conditioned situation, as the tuning fork is said to be the conditioned stimulus (CS) and salivation the conditioned response (CR). Although salivation is the response in both unconditioned and conditioned situations, it is considered that the latter response is a new one: hence the term 'conditioned response'. This response is so-called because it is conditional upon the presence of food. If the tuning fork had not been sounded at the same time that food was given to the dog, then the conditioned response of salivation would not occur. In other words, the conditioned stimulus (in this case a tuning fork) serves as a signal to the dog that the unconditioned stimulus (in this case food) is about to occur. Table 4.1 illustrates the sequence of events involved in classical conditioning.

Four further terms are used in connection with conditioning: extinction, generalization, discrimination and spontaneous recovery.

Table 4.1 The process of classical conditioning

Before conditioning	US: presence of food	UR: salivation
During conditioning	US: presence of food in mouth, and CS: tuning fork	UR: salivation
After conditioning	CS: tuning fork (alone)	CR: salivation

US = unconditioned stimulus
UR = unconditioned response
CS = conditoned stimulus
CR = conditioned response

Extinction   If the conditioned stimulus is presented a number of times without being followed by the unconditioned stimulus, then the conditioned response will gradually weaken and eventually become extinct.

Generalization   If a musical tone of a different pitch is used instead of the usual one, the conditioned response will generalize to include the new stimulus, provided that it differs only slightly from the original.

Discrimination   If the experimenter presents stimuli in the form of musical notes of varying pitch, but only presents one of these notes with the unconditioned stimulus, then the animal will learn to discriminate between the notes. Different shapes have also been used to demonstrate discrimination, the animals demonstrating this to a complex degree.

Spontaneous recovery   A conditioned response that has become extinct may often exhibit spontaneous recovery without further training. It is also much easier to recondition an animal to the original response than it was to condition it in the first instance.

Classical conditioning: the work of John B. Watson

John B. Watson (1878–1958) graduated from the psychology school at the University of Chicago, where he had been trained in the skills of animal experimentation. Such experimentation was used to determine the mental qualities of the animals, but seldom led to much agreement among psychologists. Watson noted that observations on the animals' behaviour yielded far more objective data than did the deliberations concerning the animal's mental state. Watson's position can be summarized in three main statements.

1. Introspective methods have no place in the study of psychology.
2. Observations should be made only on the behaviour of an animal, since this was the object of study in the other scientific disciplines. The emphasis was to be on objective experimentation and replication of results, leaving no place for subjective inquiry.
3. Most behaviour is learned by making an association between a stimulus and a response, hence the term stimulus–response (S–R) theory. Experiments in animals can be extrapolated to human beings, as the former differ only in their degree of complexity from man. Watson was convinced that even complex behaviour could be accounted for by this association of stimuli and response, and the publication of Pavlov's work on classical conditioning provided the confirmation he sought.

Watson became famous for his work with Rosalie Rayner on conditioned fear in humans (Watson and Rayner, 1920). By modern day standards their experiments seem ethically dubious although they believed no permanent harm would be done to the child. Their subject was a nine-month old called Albert B. (little Albert!) who showed no fear when

Table 4.2 Classical conditioning of fear in 'little Albert'

Before conditioning	US: loud noise from hammer striking metal bar	UR: fear response i.e. crying and withdrawal
During conditioning	US: loud noise, plus CS: white rat	UR: fear response
After conditioning	CS: white rat (alone)	CR: fear response

presented with a range of stimuli, including a white rat. He did, however, show a fear reaction to a stimulus consisting of a loud noise which Watson made by striking a metal bar with a hammer behind the child. The conditioning process involved presenting the rat to the child, and when he reached towards it the metal bar was struck loudly behind him, causing him to startle and cry. After repeated pairings of the rat and the noise, presentation of the rat alone caused him to cry immediately and to crawl away rapidly. His fear of the rat showed generalization to other furry objects such as a rabbit and a dog. This demonstrated that the child had learned to be afraid of the rat through the process of classical conditioning; the sequence of events is shown in Table 4.2.

Classical conditioning, then, is a basic form of learning that pervades many aspects of daily life, and examples of conditioned reflexes are fear and anxiety.

Operant conditioning: the work of Edward L. Thorndike

The work of Edward L. Thorndike (1874–1949) was concerned with animal learning and in 1898 he formulated his law of effect. This was based on his work with cats in a 'puzzle box'. He confined a hungry cat in a puzzle box and placed food outside the box so that it was clearly visible to the animal. It was possible for the cat to escape from the box by clawing at a cord which released the door. Thorndike observed its behaviour and in particular, the length of time taken to escape. Initially, the cat made various movements in an apparently random fashion, such as scratching at the door, until it succeeded by chance in escaping. It was allowed to eat the food and was then put back in the puzzle box and Thorndike observed that over a period of trials, the animal's movements became less and less random. It managed to open the door in a successively shorter time in each trial, until it eventually opened the door immediately it was placed inside.

The law of effect states that behaviour that results in success or reward is more likely to be repeated than behaviour that does not. Thorndike explained the importance of what he termed the satisfier in reinforcing behaviour. In the puzzle box, the cat was rewarded for the responses that led to escape (because those responses enabled it to obtain the food), whereas responses which did not lead to escape were gradually phased out.

Thorndike also formulated another law, called the law of exercise, which states that knowledge of results must occur before the behaviour can be reinforced.

Thorndike's contribution to learning theory stems from this concept of reinforcement, in which he sees the reward acting as a positive reinforcer for the association between stimulus and response. This is now seen as a form of conditioning called operant conditioning, which was also developed independently by B.F. Skinner.

Operant conditioning: the work of B.F. Skinner

B.F. Skinner has made an important contribution to the study of learning by his work on another form of conditioning called operant or instrumental conditioning. He distinguishes between respondent behaviour and operant behaviour, the former being elicited by specific stimuli and the latter being emitted spontaneously by the organism, such as the random pecking behaviour of pigeons. Classical conditioning involves respondent behaviour, and has only limited relevance for the kinds of academic learning with which education is concerned. This is because the conditioned response can have no effect on the environment; in other words, the animal cannot control the events that occur. For example, the dog in Pavlov's experiments made a conditioned response of salivation, but this response in no way affected the speed of delivery of the food. Operant conditioning, on the other hand, operates on the environment and the learned behaviour is instrumental in controlling events.

The apparatus used for experiments in operant conditioning was the 'Skinner box', a kind of puzzle box containing something that the animal has to manipulate in order to obtain a reward. A great deal of Skinner's work was carried out using pigeons and in a typical experiment the hungry pigeon would be placed in a box containing an illuminated window. In a similar fashion to Thorndike's cat, the hungry bird strutted around in a random manner, pecking here and there until, by chance, it happened to peck at the illuminated window. Immediately, a pellet of food was delivered into a tray beneath the window and this was consumed by the bird. Random behaviour was then resumed until the pigeon happened to peck at the illuminated window again and was reinforced with another food pellet. After a number of trials, the random behaviour would cease, and the pigeon would peck at the window immediately it was put into the box. Skinner described the role of the food pellet as a reinforcer of behaviour, in that the window-pecking behaviour was followed by a food pellet that caused the behaviour to be repeated (to the exclusion of non-reinforced behaviour).

This operant conditioning is clearly different from classical conditioning, in that the pigeon's behaviour actually affects the environment by bringing about delivery of the food pellet. Skinner's view of operant conditioning is that it is not a sequence of stimulus–response connections, but rather that behaviour is spontaneously emitted by the organism. He tends to disregard the role of stimuli. There are four principles in operant conditioning: positive and negative reinforcement, punishment and omission of reinforcement.

Positive reinforcement   This consists of the presentation of some kind of reward following a particular response. The rat is given a food pellet because it presses the lever. This increases the probability of occurrence of the response that precedes it.

Negative reinforcement   In this case, the rat is subjected to an unpleasant stimulus, such as an electric shock, from which it can escape by making a particular response. Pressing the lever of the Skinner box will switch off the current, so the rat will press the lever to escape the unpleasant stimulus. Negative reinforcement increases the probability of occurrence of the response that precedes it.

Punishment   Punishment differs from negative reinforcement in that the unpleasant stimulus occurs after the animal's response, whereas in the latter it occurs before. If the lever in the Skinner box is wired to deliver an electric shock when pressed, then the rate of the lever-pressing response by the rat will decrease. Punishment decreases the probability of occurrence of the response that precedes it.

Omission of reinforcement   If the rat presses the lever but receives no reinforcement, the rate of response will diminish. This is similar to the case of classical conditioning, where absence of reinforcement will lead to the extinction of the response.

  Thus, the central tenet of Skinner's theory is the concept of reinforcement, which he considers to be the main factor in learning. He has done considerable research into patterns of reinforcement and their effects upon the response of the animal and this has led to the concept of 'schedules of reinforcement'. Skinner has classified these schedules into two main types, continuous and intermittent. In the former type, every response by the animal is reinforced, whereas in the latter only some of the responses are. Intermittent reinforcement can be subdivided into:

- ratio schedules, which are determined by the rate of the animal's response; and
- interval schedules, which are determined by the time factor.

In addition, each of these subdivisions may be fixed or variable, giving four possible categories of intermittent reinforcement:

1. *fixed interval* schedule, where the responses are reinforced at a regular interval of time – e.g. every two minutes;
2. *variable interval* schedule, where reinforcement is given at varying intervals of time, some short, others long;
3. *fixed ratio*, where reinforcement is given after a set number of responses, such as every tenth response; and
4. *variable ratio*, where reinforcement is given after varying numbers of responses – e.g. ten, and then four, and then one.

The importance of these schedules lies in the different rates of response that they produce, ratio schedules giving higher rates than interval ones. This can be explained in terms of the animal's influence over the reinforcement, in that the ratio schedule gives the animal the chance to speed up its response so that reinforcement occurs more often. On an interval schedule, the rate of response has no effect on the delivery because reinforcement is dependent on the passage of time. Variable ratio schedules bring about the consistently highest response rates, and the ones most resistant to extinction.

'Shaping' is another concept that Skinner has developed in relation to animal behaviour. Shaping implies the incorporation of novel behaviours, which are not part of the animal's natural responses, into its behavioural repertoire. He trained pigeons to play table tennis by selective reinforcement of the desired behaviours and this involved, in the first instance, reinforcing the bird when it approached the ball. Reinforcement is then given to successive approximations to the desired table-tennis-playing behaviour, such as pecking at the ball, knocking it over the net and finally, getting it into the opponent's trough.

Animals can be trained to perform complex skills by the use of shaping techniques, but Skinner believes that human behaviour is largely reinforced not by primary reinforcers like food or drink, but by secondary reinforcers such as money and prestige. The effectiveness of secondary reinforcement is well illustrated by behaviour modification techniques that use a token economy in learning disability nursing. Patients can be helped to become independent by the selective reinforcement of desired behaviours such as washing and dressing, or can be conditioned to modify problem behaviour. Reinforcement in the form of tokens is given for appropriate behaviours, and these can be exchanged for food, cigarettes or other material goods.

Nurse education and the stimulus–response approach

Stimulus–response theories of learning have come in for a great deal of criticism over the years. For example, Skinner's laboratory experiments seem to have little ecological validity when generalized to human beings, i.e. they ignore the importance of human relationships and the social context in which behaviours occur. It is also difficult to see how stimulus–response connections can account for the infinitely complex skills of language. Another difficulty arises when attempting to use S–R theory to explain how individuals learn by imitating the behaviour of other people. Humanistic psychologists find S–R theory distasteful, as it makes man merely a puppet, the passive recipient of external forces. In addition, the application of reinforcement theory may lead to a situation where the learner will only consider doing something if there is a reward associated with it, i.e. a 'what's in it for me?' attitude. Another objection concerns the ethical issues surrounding the manipulation of human behaviour, in particular the problem of who has the right to control and manipulate another individual's behaviour. However, despite all these criticisms the

S–R approach has had considerable impact on education, and some examples of this are outlined below for nursing education.

Classical conditioning is confined to lower-order learning such as a conditioned fear response. However, this may still influence adult learning, as in the case of a student nurse who fears written examinations because in the past he or she has been humiliated by school teachers when his or her performance has been poor, thus setting up a conditioned fear of examinations. Even though such an experience may have been long ago, it can still be a very powerful emotion. However, the good news is that conditioned reflexes occur for positive feelings as well as negative, and the learned associations between pleasurable events and feelings can serve to make students enjoy the experience of learning.

One application of classical conditioning that has been used in education is systematic desensitization, a commonly used technique for treating phobias such as fear of spiders or heights. A nurse teacher may encounter a student who has learned a conditioned fear response to participating in small-group discussion or seminar, perhaps due to humiliation in the past. The student could be taught relaxation to counter the effects of anxiety and then the particular stimulus that is causing the fear can be presented in a hierarchy of contact. Having first been taught relaxation, the student would then go through the problem situation in a series of small steps, beginning with discussions with one or two other students only, gradually building up to a full group size. However, such intervention may be considered to be beyond the competence of a nurse teacher, and systematic desensitization may be more appropriately carried out by a behavioural therapist.

Another way in which students may be helped by classical conditioning is by the prevention of negative conditioning situations in the first place. Hence, when student nurses are first introduced to the clinical setting, a concerted effort should be made to make them associate the visit with such positive events as a warm welcome, a sense of *esprit de corps* and a general air of interest and helpfulness.

Operant conditioning offers a greater range of educational applications than classical conditioning. In operant conditioning, reinforcement is a fundamental principle and can be used as feedback on learner performance. Knowledge of success is said to act as a reinforcer of behaviour, so it is important to give immediate feedback on performance, in both clinical and classroom settings. The use of praise may be reinforcing, since it acts as a reward, but it is important to vary the type of reinforcement given, so that the behaviour is maintained. This is more difficult than it sounds, for the teacher may appear insincere if he or she thinks too much about the way to respond, e.g. smiling, nodding, praising and the like.

A variable-ratio type of reinforcement produces the highest response rate, so when learning a new response the student should be given reinforcement at frequent intervals and as performance improves, less frequently, until eventually only really good performances are reinforced.

A fixed-interval schedule of reinforcement may be effective when given following periodic tests, or by feedback during daily ward reports. As indicated earlier, behaviour modification is a well-tried technique in clinical psychology, where selective reinforcement is used to shape acceptable behaviours in patients/clients. It has been suggested that teachers may use it in class to encourage acceptable behaviours and to discourage negative ones. If the nurse teacher wishes to shape student nurses to answer questions in class, he or she may praise the students each time they answer a question, regardless of whether or not their answer is correct. Gradually the teacher will begin to praise the students only when the answer is correct. Extinction can be applied to unwanted behaviour such as dominating a lesson or discussion, or coming into class late. If the teacher ignores these behaviours, they may undergo extinction, rather than being reinforced by having attention drawn to them.

Chapter 13 (p. 338) outlines Skinner's concept of programmed learning, an attempt to apply the theories of shaping of behaviour to the process of education. Skinner devised the linear type of programme, in which material is presented in an orderly, logical succession of small steps. Each step requires the student to make a response and if this is correct, the student is said to receive reinforcement from providing such a response. Linear programmes can be obtained in book form, or in a roll that can be inserted into a teaching machine. In the latter type, the student presses a button to indicate his or her response and the programme moves on automatically.

Another educational application of S–R theory is the behavioural objectives approach. This is concerned with the prescription of the outcomes of learning and enshrines the principles of behaviourism. Behavioural objectives are discussed in some detail in Chapter 12 (p. 272).

Social learning (observational learning) theory

Albert Bandura, the main proponent of social learning theory, was a behaviourist psychologist who found the S–R explanation of observational learning unsatisfactory. Social learning (or observational learning) occurs when an individual learns something by observing another person doing it, in other words it is learning by modelling. According to social learning theory, behaviour is seen as a two-way interaction between an individual and his or her environment, that is, both 'people and their environments are reciprocal determinants of each other' (Bandura, 1977). Exponents of this theory view the behaviouristic approach to learning as one that limits the idea of the potential of individuals and their influence over their own behaviour. According to social learning theory, an individual possesses no inherent behaviour patterns at birth other than reflexes, so must learn everything else. Such learning occurs as a result of observing the behaviour of other people, which allows complex patterns to be acquired in a more efficient way than trial and error. Indeed, some behaviours such as language can only be learned, according to Bandura, by observation of human models, as it is highly unlikely that mere reinforcement of random vocalization would lead to the complex use of speech that forms the everyday language of an individual. Learning, then, is envisaged as behaviour acquired by observation of modelling stimuli, providing the learner with a symbolic image of such behaviour, which may serve as a guide. Bandura identifies four processes involved in the observational learning situation: attention, retention, motor reproduction and motivational processes.

Attentional processes These processes are concerned with the characteristics of the model and of the observer. In the former, some of the factors which influence learning are variables such as:

- interpersonal attraction between the model and the observer;
- the usefulness of the observed behaviour; and
- the distinctiveness, complexity and frequency of contact with the modelled stimuli.

Observer characteristics comprise the level of arousal, capacity to process information, the perceptual set and the amount of previous reinforcement.

Retention processes It is obviously important to remember the modelled behaviour if one is to learn from it, so the role of such strategies as rehearsal is crucial. The highest level of learning is achieved when the modelled behaviour is first organized and symbolically rehearsed before actually performing the behaviour.

Motor reproduction processes The learner must be capable of actually carrying out the observed behaviour and of evaluating it in terms of accuracy.

Motivational processes Modelled stimuli are more likely to be learned if the observer sees some value in them, but the role of reinforcement in social learning theory is one of facilitation rather than necessity. It may take the form of external reward (such as money) or self-reinforcement, where the learners reward themselves with something when a predetermined behaviour has been achieved. For example, a person may set a number of personal objectives to achieve for a course and, having attained them, may choose to go out to dinner as a reward. The likelihood of the modelled behaviour being learned is increased when the observer sees the model being reinforced for performing that behaviour. This is termed vicarious reinforcement.

Information can be transmitted by the model in a variety of ways, such as an actual physical demonstration, by pictures, words and the mass media. Abstract modelling is the term used for the process whereby the observer elicits the principles of behaviour from a variety of modelled stimuli and applies them to a situation similar to the ones which were observed. Thus, observation of various models performing a nursing procedure would allow the observer to learn the rules of the procedure and these could then be applied to similar situations.

How does social learning theory explain the development of novel or creative responses? Bandura sees the novel response as a utilization of the qualities of many models, to produce a new creative behaviour. There are a number of characteristics of both the model and the observer that make learning more likely. Experiments indicate that persons who possess status, prestige and power are more effective models for those kind of behaviours. Individuals who are lacking in self-esteem and confidence and those who are dependent tend to be more easily influenced by the behaviours of models who are obviously successful. However, one needs to interpret such results with caution, as many confident people readily adopt behaviour of those whose actions are seen to be of value.

Nurse education and social learning theory

Observational learning is potentially a powerful tool for the nurse teacher in a wide range of applications. One of the important early aspects of nursing which a new student must acquire is that of the professional role and this can be fostered by allowing the student to observe a prestigious trained nurse going about her daily work. The student will be able to observe not only clinical skills, but interactions with patients and other members of the health care team, thus learning about professional attitudes as well as techniques. This strategy has been used in nursing with some success; Kramer (1972) took students into the clinical areas and had them work in the vicinity, but not actually attached to her. The students thus had the opportunity to see her interacting with patients and giving care, and she acted as a model for their observational learning. In a British study in an elderly care setting, Raichura and Riley (1985) used modelling as a strategy for teaching trained staff about care of the elderly. The nurse teacher must also act as a professional model when with students, showing enthusiasm about nursing and the ability to do the job skilfully. A good role model must also be a good practitioner if students are to learn the correct roles. It is a useful idea when working with student groups to pair the students so that the weaker ones are working with the more able students and learning by observation. The teacher should ensure that the more able students are given responsibility, since these high-status students are more likely to serve as models for the others.

HUMANISTIC THEORIES

There is no single theory that represents the humanistic approach, but all theories share a common view that this approach involves the study of man as a human being, with his thoughts, feelings and experiences. This is in direct contrast to the stimulus–response theorists, who study man from the point of view of his overt behaviour, disregarding his inner feelings and experiences. Humanistic differs from cognitive theory also, in that the latter is concerned with the thinking aspects of man's behaviour, with little emphasis on the affective components. Exponents of humanistic theory claim that the other two theories omit some of the most significant aspects of human existence, namely feelings, attitudes and values. Humanistic theory is closely related to the philosophical approach called phenomenology, which asserts that reality lies in a person's perception of an event and not in the event itself. The humanistic viewpoint is summarized by Hamachek (1978):

> It is a psychological stance that focuses not so much on a person's biological drives, but on their goals; not so much on stimuli impinging on them, but on their desires to be or to do something; not so much on their past experiences, but on their current circumstances; not so much on life conditions *per se*, but on the subjective qualities of human experience, the personal meaning of an experience to persons, rather than on their objective, observable responses.

Humanistic theory, then, is concerned with human growth, individual fulfilment and self-actualization and it is claimed that this approach is 'intuitively right', as it agrees with the ideas most people have about what is uniquely human. However, the behaviourist approach is not considered to be wrong; rather, humanistic theory prefers to emphasize the affective aspects of man as being of equal importance to the cognitive and psychomotor elements. There are two main principles that apply to the humanistic approach to learning and teaching, namely teacher–student relationships and the classroom climate. The former stresses the importance of the interpersonal relationship between learner and teacher as a major variable affecting learning and this in turn affects the climate of the classroom. The presence or absence of conflict and tension will depend largely on the quality of relationships within the classroom setting.

Humanistic psychology: the work of Abraham H. Maslow

Abraham H. Maslow (1908–1970) was a major exponent of the humanistic approach to psychology, and has also made a significant contribution to motivation theory with his theory of a hierarchy of needs (see Chapter 2, p. 20). He coined the term 'third force' psychology because he considered the first force to be Freudian psychotherapy and the second to be the stimulus–response school. The latter school, he felt, had little relevance to the human personality: 'these extensive books on the psychology of learning are of no consequence, at least to the human centre, to the human soul, to the human essence' (Maslow, 1971). One of the key concepts he defined was that of 'self-actualization' and he studied the behaviour of people whom he classified as self-actualizers. Maslow stated eight ways in which an individual self-actualizes, and these include 'experiencing fully, vividly, selflessly, with full concentration and total absorption' (p. 44). He mentions the 'peak experience', which is an ecstatic moment that can be brought on by such experiences as classical music and religious experiences. For the humanist, the goal of education is to assist the individual to achieve self-actualization, or, as Maslow puts it, 'to help the person to become the best that he is able to become' (p. 163). This intrinsic approach is in contrast to the extrinsic educational ethic, in which the transmission of factual knowledge is seen to be more important than the development of an individual. The ideal college, according to Maslow, would be one in which the main objectives would be the discovery of one's identity and the destiny or vocation for each person.

Humanistic psychology: the work of Carl R. Rogers

Carl R. Rogers made his reputation as a psychotherapist, developing a new approach that he called client-centred therapy (Rogers, 1951). This involves the therapist in a non-directive role in which the client is encouraged to develop a deeper understanding of his or her 'self'. The role of the therapist is to provide a non-critical atmosphere, in which there is no attempt to interpret for the client, but simply a reflecting back of the statements made in order to assist him or her in developing self-awareness. This concept of client-centred therapy led Rogers to formulate his student-centred approach to learning, which is contained in his most important work on the subject (Rogers, 1969). In this work, he states ten principles of learning.

1. Human beings have a natural potentiality for learning.
2. Significant learning takes place when the subject-matter is perceived by the student as having relevance for his own purposes.
3. Learning which involves a change in self-organization is threatening and tends to be resisted.
4. Those elements of learning which are threatening to the self are more easily perceived and assimilated when external threats are at a minimum.
5. When threat to the self is low, experience can be perceived in differentiated fashion, and learning can proceed.
6. Much significant learning is acquired through doing.
7. Learning is facilitated when the student participates responsibly in the learning process.
8. Self-initiated learning, which involves the whole person of the learner, feelings as well as intellect, is the most lasting and pervasive.
9. Independence, creativity and self-reliance are all facilitated when self-criticism and self-evaluation are basic and evaluation by others is of secondary importance.
10. The most socially useful learning in the modern world is the learning of the process of learning, a continuing openness to experience and incorporation into oneself of the process of change

These principles illustrate Rogers' approach to learning and his emphasis on relevance, student participation and involvement, self-evaluation and the absence of threat in the classroom.

Rogers sees the teacher as a facilitator of learning, a provider of resources for learning, and someone who shares feelings as well as knowledge with their students. Rogers has further articulated his approach to education in his book *Freedom to Learn for the 80s* (Rogers, 1983). He sees learning as being a continuum, with much meaningless material at one end and significant or experiential learning at the other. The former could describe many curricula, which are seen as virtually meaningless by the student for whom they are intended. Experiential learning, on the other hand, has a number of qualities such as personal involvement, self-initiation, pervasiveness, self-evaluation and meaningfulness. Rogers contrasts the kind of learning that is concerned solely with cognitive functioning with that involving the whole person.

Teaching, according to Rogers, is a highly overrated activity, in contrast to the notion of facilitation. Teaching by giving knowledge does not meet the requirements of today's changing world; what is required is the facilitation of learning and change and this calls for a different set of qualities in the facilitator. The most important factor is the relationship that exists between facilitator and learner and Rogers suggests a number of qualities that are required for this: genuineness, trust and acceptance, and empathetic understanding.

Genuineness The facilitator should come across as a real person rather than as some kind of ideal model. Hence it is important that facilitators show 'normal' reactions to their students.

Trust and acceptance The facilitator should demonstrate acceptance of the student as a person in his or her own right as a person worthy of their respect and care.

Empathic understanding Facilitators need to put themselves in the students' shoes in order to see and understand things from their students' perspective.

Rogers suggests that it is possible for the teacher to build into a programme the freedom to learn, which students require. This can be done by using students' own experiences and problems so that relevance is obvious and by providing resources for the students in the form of both material and human resources. The goal of education is that of the student becoming a fully functioning person.

Nurse education and humanistic theories

The humanistic approach to education centres on the relationships between teachers and students, each learner being considered as an individual. The use of forenames between teacher and learner can increase the feeling of identity for the learner and help to reduce barriers to communication. Involvement in decision-making is a further step in helping students to develop a sense of personal value and worth. While it is impossible to involve each learner in major planning decisions, it is useful to have student representatives on course and pathway committees to contribute ideas and suggestions from their peer group or cohort.

Most teachers are aware of the individual differences between students prior to commencing training, but they also need to be sensitive to the fact that they will still have differences at the end of the course. It is important to remain aware that the students are individuals, even though they have been exposed to a common training programme and to encourage them to maintain their unique attitudes and values, rather than aiming for a conformist, homogeneous end product.

The role of the teacher is seen by the humanistic approach as being that of helper and facilitator, rather than a conveyor of information. In other words, the teacher becomes another learning resource for the learner. In order to perform their role satisfactorily, teachers must fully understand themselves, and be flexible in their approach to teaching. The classroom and clinical climate is seen to be of major importance and should be an environment where psychological safety exists and where the students feel at ease. Some of the barriers between teacher and learner may be lessened by the rearrangement of the seating and the use of small-group techniques. These also facilitate the discussion of feelings and values, an aspect that is considered crucial in the humanistic approach.

A specific application of humanistic psychology is in the use of learning contracts, which give the students the opportunity to take responsibility for their own learning. Learning contracts are discussed in the next section, on andragogical theory of learning.

One of the most serious criticisms of the humanistic approach is that it is lacking in empirical evidence to support its claims, relying upon observations and assumptions of human behaviour. In addition, there is concern that this approach may lead to the teacher becoming an amateur psychotherapist with all the attendant dangers. It could also be argued that the emphasis on personal growth and self-exploration in humanistic theories makes them less useful for specific professional education and training in nursing. Nevertheless, it is fair to say that humanistic theories have had a major impact on nursing curricula, perhaps because they embrace a holistic concept of the person that is compatible with the concept of holistic nursing.

ANDRAGOGICAL LEARNING THEORY

Malcolm S. Knowles has developed an approach to the teaching and training of adults termed andragogy (Knowles, 1990). The term is used in the literature as a contrast to pedagogy, literally a leader of children, and Knowles' approach is based upon the differences he perceives between the teaching of adults and children. He maintains that educational systems, including those for adult students, are based on a pedagogical model. Indeed, the dictionary definition of pedagogy reinforces this view: 'the art, science, and profession of teaching'. He notes that all the great teachers in history, such as Socrates and Confucius, were teachers of adults and uses the term andragogy, i.e. a leader of man (adults) to describe his approach. He points out that the term 'adult' has a number of meanings:

Table 4.3 The different assumptions of pedagogy and andragogy

Assumptions	Pedagogy	Andragogy
Learner's need to know	Students must learn what they are taught in order to pass their tests.	Adults need to know why they must learn something.
Learner's self-concept	Dependency: decisions about learning are controlled by teacher.	Self-direction: adults take responsibility for their own learning.
Role of learner's experience	It is the teacher's experience that is seen as important. The learner's experience is seen as of little use as a learning resource.	Adults have greater, and more varied experience which serves as a rich resource for learning.
Learner's readiness to learn	Learner's readiness is dependent upon what the teacher wants them to learn.	Adult's readiness relates to the things he or she needs to know and do in real life.
Student's orientation to learning	Learning equates with the subject-matter content of the curriculum.	Adults have a life-centred orientation to learning involving problem-solving and task-centred approaches.
Student's motivation	Student's motivation is from external sources such as teacher approval, grades and parental pressures.	Adult's motivation is largely internal such as self-esteem, quality of life and job satisfaction.

- biological adulthood is the ability to reproduce;
- legal adulthood is defined by the law;
- social adulthood is the stage at which adult roles are performed; and
- psychological adulthood is when self-direction is assumed.

The two models are based on different assumptions about the learner on six dimensions:

1. the learner's need to know;
2. the learner's self-concept;
3. the role of the learner's experience;
4. the learner's readiness to learn;
5. the learner's orientation to learning; and
6. the learner's motivation.

The different assumption for pedagogy and andragogy are outlined in Table 4.3.

Knowles argues that traditional education conditions the learner to react to teacher stimuli, and this reactive learning does not equip the learner with the skills for lifelong learning. Andragogy encourages a pro-active approach to learning in which enquiry and autonomy feature predominantly. However, pedagogy and andragogy should be seen as parallel, rather than as opposing, models and Knowles acknowledges that both may be appropriate for children and adults depending upon the given circumstances. For example, it might be that a pedagogical or dependent approach involving didactic teaching would be more appropriate when the learner first encounters new or unusual learning situations, provided that an andragogical approach is used overall. Similarly, Knowles believes that andragogy can be appropriate for children, with its emphasis on a classroom climate conducive to learning, and the concept of increasing self-direction and autonomy.

Nurse education and andragogical theory

Two aspects of Knowles' work have had a particularly strong influence on nurse education curricula, his process model for human resources development, and the use of learning contracts.

Process model for human resources development

Knowles uses the term 'human resources development' to cover the whole range of continuing education and training in a wide variety of contexts, and the implementation of the andragogical model involves a 'process model' as opposed to the pedagogical one of a 'content model'. There are seven elements to the process model.

1. Establishing a climate conducive to learning This involves both the physical, and the human and interpersonal environment; the former takes account of the seating arrangements, decor, ventilation and lighting, and the latter such things as the organizational climate, mutual respect, collaboration, mutual trust and supportiveness, openness and authenticity and a climate of pleasure and humaneness.

2. Creating a mechanism for mutual planning It is one of the cardinal principles of andragogy; all those concerned with the educational enterprise should be involved in its planning.

3. Diagnosing the needs for learning According to Knowles, a learning need is a gap between the specified learning outcomes of a programme and the existing state of the learner in relation to these. Andragogy emphasizes the importance of the learner's own perception of this gap, but there may be tension between the needs of participants and the needs of the organization, and this conflict must be negotiated with care.

4. Formulating programme objectives Knowles acknowledges the widely differing viewpoints on the nature of objectives, and cautiously suggests that behavioural objectives might be more appropriate for training, and more process-orientated outcomes for education.

5. Designing a pattern of learning experiences Self-directed learning is central to andragogical design models and involves a choice of learning methods that are appropriate to the learner's objectives.

6. Operating the programme This involves the administration of the learning programme, and the quality of learning resources is a crucial factor.

7. Evaluating the programme Knowles favours a five-step approach to evaluation:

(a) reaction evaluation is on-going evaluation during the programme;
(b) learning evaluation is the gathering of data about the learning outcomes achieved;
(c) behaviour evaluation takes a wider view of the changes in behaviour, culled from supervisors' reports, etc.;
(d) results evaluation is organizational data such as costs, efficiency, absence, etc.; and
(e) rediagnosis of learning needs is really a repeat of step 3 above, and involves helping students to re-evaluate where they are in relation to programme objectives.

Learning contracts

As Knowles points out, individuals have a need to be self-directing in their learning, yet traditional curricula were largely controlled by the educational institution. Learning contracts are a means of reconciling the learning needs of the student and those of other interested parties such as educators and employers. The focus of nurse education is the promotion and maintenance of professional competence; what constitutes such competence is decided not only by the individual nurse but also employers and professional bodies. The needs of each of these key players may well conflict on occasions, and learning contracts provide a useful way of negotiating an acceptable compromise. Knowles offers the following stages for developing a learning contract:

Step 1: Diagnosis of learning needs This involves the students in assessing the difference between their present state of knowledge or skill in relation to an area of learning and the state they aim to achieve in that area. In nursing, this often requires the help of tutors and clinical colleagues.

Step 2: Specifying learning objectives The learning needs, identified in Step 1, are then written as learning objectives such as acquisition of certain knowledge or skills.

Step 3: Specifying learning resources and strategies In this step, the students take each learning objective and identify how they are planning to achieve it, e.g. reviewing the relevant literature.

Step 4: Specifying evidence of accomplishment For each learning objective, the students describe the evidence which they will produce to indicate their achievement, e.g. an essay can provide evidence about knowledge of a topic.

Step 5: Specifying how the evidence can be validated Here the students state the criteria by which the evidence can be judged, and who will do the judging, e.g. an essay might be judged according to level of analysis and synthesis of arguments by a member of the teaching staff of the institution.

Step 6: Reviewing the contract with consultants Once the first draft of the contract is complete, each student should seek the opinions of colleagues such as fellow students, supervisors or teachers about the clarity and relevance of the contract.

Step 7: Carrying out the contract This step involves implementing the contract, and adapting it as necessary as learning proceeds.

Step 8: Evaluating learning In this final step the evidence presented by the student is judged by the person named in Step 5.

Although extensively used as a model in nurse education curricula, Knowles' theory is not without its critics. The different assumptions of pedagogy and andragogy are debatable. For example, the self-directing characteristic of adults is a cornerstone of Knowles' theory, yet experiences with open learning programmes indicate that many adult students find it difficult to unlearn their dependence on tutors and take considerable time to develop self-direction in their learning. Also, Knowles' process model can be seen as prescriptive, and there is a certain naïvety in his assumption that students' needs will be given equal consideration in learning contracts where there is conflict between these and the needs of the organization.

SYNERGOGY

It can be seen from earlier in this chapter that the traditional model of pedagogy has a number of serious weaknesses when applied to adult students in nursing. It fosters dependence in the learner by its reinforcement of the passive role in learning and it may reduce motivation by causing resentment or hostility among adult students. Andragogy, on the other hand, does rely very much on the students' previous knowledge as well as on the key role of the facilitator. Synergogy attempts to capitalize on the best features of both pedagogy and andragogy by making use of expert knowledge, whilst at the same time, encouraging active involvement of the student. Synergogy is 'a systematic approach to learning in which the members of small teams learn from one another through structured interactions' (Mouton and Blake, 1984). It has four fundamental differences from other approaches:

1. it uses learning materials managed by a learning administrator rather than having a teacher who might be seen as an authority figure;
2. students have responsibility for their own learning through active involvement with other students;
3. it rests on the premise that learning that arises from teamwork is greater than that done by the individual alone, i.e. the principle of synergy; and
4. the planned interaction with colleagues acts as a motivator for learning.

Educational success is promoted by three principles that underpin synergogy. The first involves the use of learning materials that serve to give the students direction without inhibiting their self-development. The second principle is that of teamwork. Synergogy relies on teamwork and the authors emphasize the difference between teamwork and group work, the former involving a learning team with clear goals, learning tasks and outcomes as well as procedures for enhancing team effectiveness. The third principle is that of synergy, in which the whole is greater than the sum of its parts. In contrast to ordinary group discussion, synergogy ensures the systematic sharing of knowledge, with its consequent implications for each student's growth and development.

Synergogy can be applied to the learning of knowledge, skills and attitudes and there are four designs for learning:

- team-effectiveness design (TED),
- team-member teaching design (TMTD),
- performance judging design (PJD), and
- clarifying-attitudes design (CAD).

Each is now considered, in turn.

Team-effectiveness design (TED)

This design is concerned with the domain of knowledge and utilizes teamwork to facilitate learning from each other within a team of students. The team-effectiveness design might be chosen as a revision aid, with the following sequence of segments.

Individual preparation by students The total group of students is first divided into teams of five or six students. All students are then given the same material to be studied on an individual basis and this may consist of a learning package extract or other material. Each student then completes the test, which is at the end of the study material and is usually a multiple-choice type test.

Teamwork In this segment, each team must discuss the questions and decide which answers are the best in terms of what the text material contained. A time limit is imposed on this discussion, after which the answer-key is distributed and each team member marks his or her own test. The teams' negotiated answers are also compared with the key and if the teamwork was effective, one would expect that the team score would be better than that of any one individual.

Interpretation of scores The efficiency of any team's score is decided by checking it against the average individual score, a higher team score is positive and a lower team score is negative.

Critique of teamwork In this segment, the teams evaluate how well they functioned as a team in relation to the test.

Evaluation of individual progress Students may take the test or an alternative form of the test at a later date to see how well they have retained the information.

   Thus, the team-effectiveness design offers a system in which students can check their understanding of written materials by comparing it and discussing it with their team members.

Team-member teaching design (TMTD)

This design is also concerned with acquisition of knowledge and consists of each member of a team learning a portion of study material and teaching it to the other members. During the teaching presentation, each successive portion is taught by the particular student responsible for it and other students can then see how their portion fits in with the whole. The sequence is as follows.

Individual preparation by students The selection of material to be learned by each member must be of approximately the same length and capable of being understood on its own, without reference to the other portions.

Team-member teaching Each team member then teaches their portion of the material, following a logical sequence in the order of presentations. Other team members can take notes or ask questions in order to clarify their understanding of the material. After summarizing the material, each team member takes a test on the whole of the material and the individual scores are calculated using the answer key.

Interpretation of scores Each team member's score gives an indication of their understanding of each of the portions of the material. The team's average individual score shows how the group as a whole has understood the material and students can see by their own scores for their particular teaching portion how well they prepared for the task.

Critique of teamwork This involves not only assessing each member's teaching ability, but also the team's use of questions and discussion.

Performance judging design (PJD)

This particular design focuses on the acquisition of psychomotor skills and is therefore of great potential use to nurse teachers. The design gives each team member responsibility for other members' skill development and also for developing criteria by which their own and other students' performances can be evaluated.

Individual performance by students Students are given a task to work on individually, which will demonstrate their current level of the skill in question. This might take the form of a videotape of each student nurse taking someone's temperature by the oral method, so that there will be approximately five recordings of nurses taking temperatures for each team to consider.

Teamwork There are two main aspects to this segment of the design. Firstly, the team meets to decide which criteria should be used to judge effectiveness in taking a temperature orally. They are then given external criteria devised by experts to discuss and to compare with their own criteria, and eventually they have to decide upon a series of criteria that will serve as a basis for evaluating the effectiveness of their team members' performances.

Judging performance Each team member takes one of the examples of performance, i.e. one videotape of another team member and presents it to the rest of the team for comparison with the established criteria. This critique of each member's performance is written down and given to the member in question, so as to have a record of the feedback comments.

Evaluation of progress and upgrading of skills In this segment, each team member is given something comparable to perform individually and each is required to use the previously agreed criteria when performing the task. It may be that the students are asked to take a temperature by the *axillary* method whilst being videotaped and the same process of team evaluation is repeated. Hence, there is a constant cycle of additional performances that can be used to increase the level of skill amongst the team members in all aspects of nursing.

Critique of teamwork Here, team members discuss the effectiveness of the teamwork as in previous designs.

Clarifying-attitudes design (CAD)

This final design, as the name implies, is concerned with attitudes, particularly with those in the public domain. In nursing, attitudes are a legitimate area for educational exploration, particularly in such controversial fields as abortion and acquired immune deficiency syndrome (AIDS). This design is used to help individuals to develop awareness of their own attitudes and also to become sensitive to the alternative attitudes that may exist.

Individual preparation by students In this segment, the individual student first composes a statement of his or her own attitude towards the topic in question and then completes an attitude questionnaire which involves ranking a number of alternative attitude statements. The attitude statement that corresponds most closely to the written statement made by the student at the beginning is noted.

Teamwork The team then attempts to rank the same items on the basis of which is most sound, or most valid, and to come to a consensus of opinion about the order of ranking. This encourages discussion and questioning of individual reasoning and may well expose the basis for holding such an attitude. The difference between the agreed attitudes and the ranking of the individual members can also be examined and ways in which behaviour may be changed can be explored.

Developing a shared norm of conduct Each of the team's rankings is shared with other teams within the total group of students and any differences are discussed. It may be necessary to form new teams if the differences persist, until a shared norm exists.

Individual re-ranking of attitudes Each team member then re-ranks the alternatives, comparing this to the original ranking.

Critique of changes in attitudes This may be an optional part of the design and involves an exploration of how each member's attitudes have changed as a result of the discussion.

Critique of teamwork This is the same procedure as in the other designs.

Nurse education and synergogy

The four fundamental designs outlined above constitute the system of synergogy, but it is important to look at the role of the learning administrator. This role is very different from that normally seen in education, in that the administrator is neither facilitator nor subject expert. Their function is to carry out four key roles with regard to the organization of synergogy, one of which is to create the teams in which students will work. This requires decisions about the mix of abilities and experience of students, the numbers in any one team and other such aspects of team formation. Another function is to ensure that team interaction is effective, by intervening when procedural difficulties arise; these may be in-fighting, dominance by a single member and other counter-productive behaviours. The learning administrator is also responsible for providing support for individual students in a variety of situations, such as difficulties with materials, presentations, absenteeism and so on. He or she is also responsible for arranging meetings with specific subject-matter consultants, should this be felt to be beneficial for a team.

It is important at this point to address some of the drawbacks associated with its use. As with any type of medium for educational use, the planning and development can be time-consuming and expensive. Teachers may not feel at ease using a method that places responsibility upon the students, particularly one that may seem to reduce the skills of the teacher to those of an administrator of learning. Students themselves may not be happy with a method that makes them take responsibility for their own progress, particularly as it involves openness and honesty in a group setting.

REFERENCES

Bandura, A. (1977) *Social Learning Theory*, Prentice-Hall, New Jersey.

Hamachek, D. (1978) Humanistic Psychology: theoretical – philosophical framework and implications for teaching, in *Handbook on Teaching Educational Psychology*, (eds D. Treffinger, J. Kent Davis and R. Ripple), Academic Press, New York.

Knowles, M. (1990) *The Adult Learner: A Neglected Species*, 4th edn, Gulf Publishing, Houston.

Kramer, M. (1972) The concept of modelling as a teaching strategy. *Nursing Forum*, **XI**, 50–69.

Maslow, A. (1971) *The Farther Reaches of Human Nature*, Penguin, Harmondsworth.

Mouton, J. and Blake, R. (1984) *Synergogy: A New Strategy for Education, Training and Development*, Jossey Bass, San Francisco.

Pavlov, I. (1927) *Conditioned Reflexes*, Oxford University Press, Oxford.

Raichura, L. and Riley, M. (1985) Introducing nurse preceptors. *Nursing Times*, Nov 20.

Rogers, C. (1951) *Client Centred Therapy*, Houghton Mifflin, Boston.

Rogers, C. (1969) *Freedom to Learn*, Merrill, Ohio.

Rogers, C. (1983) *Freedom to Learn for the 80s*, Merrill, Ohio.

Watson, J. and Rayner, R. (1920) Conditioned emotional reactions. *Journal of Experimental Psychology*, **3**, 1–14.

Planning for teaching | 5

There are some activities in life that can be indulged in without prior planning, but teaching is seldom one of them. Professional teaching is an intentional enterprise with the aim of facilitating other people's learning. Of course, one person may unintentionally influence another's learning, as in observational learning, but I would prefer to use the term role-modelling for this. Professional teaching is characterized by an acceptance of responsibility for facilitating other people's learning through planned and purposeful educational interventions. A teacher may also use role-modelling to facilitate learning, but in this case it would be an intentional teaching strategy rather than an encounter with accidental, albeit beneficial, outcomes. This is not to say that teaching ignores the possibility of unplanned learning; indeed, there are powerful arguments to support the view that teaching must provide an atmosphere for students in which unpredictable or creative outcomes can emerge. However, even this example shows evidence of broad teaching intentions, namely, the provision of a climate in which unpredictable outcomes are encouraged.

Planning for teaching has to be viewed in context; the type of course, the year or level, the prior experience of the students, and the course aims and learning outcomes have all to be considered in the formulation of teaching plans. In addition, there are psychological, curriculum and organizational issues which will influence the planning process. These broader aspects are addressed in the appropriate chapters of this book; in this chapter, the focus is a range of issues, from subject-matter to organization, that arises when a teacher sets about planning a teaching session or a scheme of work for a series of sessions.

PLANNING THE SUBJECT MATTER OF A TEACHING SESSION

It must be acknowledged from the outset that subject-matter is not necessarily synonymous with content. The term subject-matter is normally attached to the various fields of knowledge that comprise the science and art of nursing, and in this sense it equates with the term content. However, some teaching sessions in nursing and health have as their content a variety of group processes and interactions which are not subject-matter *per se*, but which still require careful planning. This aspect is dealt with in Chapter 7 on small-group teaching.

It goes without saying that a teacher should possess a thorough understanding of the subject matter to be taught – in higher education the minimum benchmark for a lecturer is normally the possession of a first degree or equivalent. This level of knowledge does, in itself, present problems in the selection of subject matter for teaching. The more expert a teacher is, the more difficult it is to decide what must go in, and more importantly what has to be left out, of a teaching session. This may result in the inexperienced teacher cramming far too much information into sessions. The secret of successful teaching is to place severe limits on the amount of content in a given session by the judicious selection of the most important aspects of the topic, and the ruthless pruning of other, less crucial material. However, this is more easily said than done, but one way which can be helpful is the use of conceptual mapping.

Conceptual mapping uses diagrams to answer the following questions about selection of content in a teaching session:

- what *must* go in,
- what *should* go in, and
- what *could* go in.

These questions are in descending order of priority in terms of the importance for inclusion in a session, and conceptual mapping begins with the identification of the key concepts of the topic in question. This is done using the relevant literature and the teacher's personal knowledge and experience, and the key concepts are placed at the centre of the diagram. The next stage involves an analysis of the second-order concepts that are closely related to the key concepts, and any linkage between the concepts are identified and added to the map. Finally, any third-order concepts are identified. The result should be a fairly comprehensive concept map of the topic, from which the teacher can begin to make a selection for the session in question. An example of concept-mapping is shown in Figure 5.1.

At the level of the key concepts, selection is usually fairly straightforward; it is at the level of the second- and third-order concepts that the danger of over-inclusion of information is most likely to occur. There are

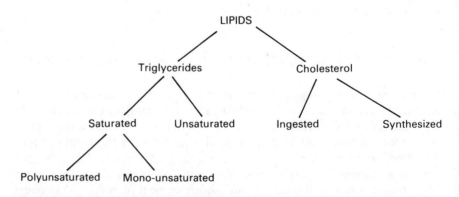

Fig. 5.1   An example of concept-mapping.

all kinds of fascinating facts and anecdotes attached to the key concepts of nursing and health, and as such these can be important elements in the maintenance of students' interest and motivation. Problems may arise when the teacher perceives that there are so many key concepts to include, leaving no time for these interesting, but non-essential aspects of the topic. This dilemma can be lessened if the aim of the session is taken into account. Provided sufficient book and periodical resources are available in the college, there should seldom be the need for the teacher to attempt to cover all aspects of a topic in detail. By the judicious use of references and further reading, the teacher can limit the number of concepts within the session, and in so doing will free up time for inclusion of anecdotes and other interesting facets of the topic.

Although the foregoing information has focused on the planning of a single teaching session, concept mapping is equally appropriate for planning a scheme of work for a series of sessions on a broad topic area. It can actually be easier to make a selection from a concept map if more than one session is available, as the time constraints may be less evident.

CHOOSING APPROPRIATE TEACHING STRATEGIES

There is a wide range of strategies available to the teacher, but evidence suggests an over-reliance on those involving the transmission of information, often combined with assessment methods that encourage the reproduction of facts. *Improving Student Learning Project* (CNAA 1992) identified ways in which teachers can encourage students to adopt a deep approach to learning as opposed to the superficial approach referred to above. A deep approach to learning involves a search for understanding, and there are four elements of courses which foster this:

1. *motivational context*: students experience a need to know, and are intrinsically motivated;
2. *active learning*: active involvement in learning is encouraged;
3. *interaction with others*: opportunities exist for exploratory discussion; and
4. *a well-structured knowledge base*: content is taught in integrated wholes and related to other knowledge.

The CNAA project identified several strategies which contain one or more of these elements.

- *Independent learning*: this involves the use of learning contracts that give the student a greater measure of control of the learning process.
- *Personal development*: student motivation and the involvement of feelings as well as intellect are key elements in this strategy.
- *Reflection*: this includes use of reflective diaries and journals, video and observers for skills learning.
- *Independent group work*: the emphasis here is on interactive group methods such as peer tutoring and group projects.
- *Learning by doing*: this is experiential learning and includes role play, gaming and work experience.

- *Learning skills*: these are not merely study skills *per se*, but a sense of purpose and awareness of task demands and flexibility.
- *Projects*: these involve activity and application of knowledge, and require a high level of student motivation.

The CNAA project makes the point that existing curricula need not necessarily be abandoned, but can be modified to include the above strategies. The starting point for selection of teaching and learning strategies is the broad purpose of the session(s). The strategies must be compatible with the aims of the session; lecturing is very commonly used as a vehicle for conveying subject matter to students, but there may well be more effective ways involving individualized instruction. If the intention of a session is to encourage discussion or debate about issues, student-centred activities should predominate; for skills teaching, demonstration followed by student practice is an appropriate strategy. A range of teaching strategies are discussed in detail in the appropriate chapters of this book. However, two general aspects of teaching strategies are included here; explaining and questioning.

PLANNING AN EXPLANATION

When teaching subject-matter to students, teachers are involved in giving explanations a great deal of the time. Brown and Armstrong (1984) define explaining as 'an attempt to provide understanding of a problem to others', and identify three types of explanation:

1. *interpretive*, i.e. answers the question 'What?'
2. *descriptive*, i.e. answers the question 'How?'
3. *reason-giving*, i.e. answers the question 'Why?'

When planning an explanation, Brown and Armstrong suggest that initially, the teacher should analyse the topic into its main parts or 'keys' and then establish any links between these, including any rules that might be involved. The particular type of explanation required is identified and incorporated into the lesson plan. Brown and Armstrong found that better explanations had more keys and a greater variety of cognitive levels of keys, so that the teachers in the study placed more varied demands on the pupils, particularly higher levels of cognitive demand. Better explanations also involved the use of examples, visual aids and rhetorical questions and were more appropriately structured and stimulating.

Brown (1978) offers the following sequence for planning an explanation.

Step 1 Decide precisely what is to be explained, in the form of a question, e.g. what, why, how?

Step 2 Identify any hidden variables. These might be prerequisite concepts which, although not immediately obvious in the problem, will influence understanding of the explanation. For example, a hidden variable in the question 'How does oxygen from the air reach the tissues?' would be the concept of diffusion of a gas.

Step 3   State the key points.

Step 4   Design the 'keys'. This involves taking each of the key points and writing each one as a simple statement. Each statement should have one or two examples to illustrate it and also elaborations or qualifications, as appropriate. It is useful to include a restatement or extension of the main point, using different words.

Step 5   Write a summary of the key points, to be used at the end of the explanation.

Step 6   Write the introduction to the explanation. Brown suggests that this is left until last so that a motivating and interesting introduction can be devised, which is appropriate to the sequence. Such devices as a provocative question or an interesting anecdote can be used to capture attention. A valuable opener in nurse education is to refer to the audience asking such questions as 'Has anyone nursed a patient with this sort of problem?'

Table 5.1 shows a planning sequence for an explanation, with the problem stated in the form of a question in Step 1. Step 2 shows the attempt to identify hidden variables by stating the relationship between the parts of the question. It can be seen that the explanation needs more than the four points made here, because there is a hidden variable namely the fact that

Table 5.1   Planning sequence for an explanation

Step 1   How do gallstones cause jaundice?

Step 2   Common bile duct conveys bile from liver to intestine via gall bladder.
Obstruction to bile flow causes jaundice.
Gallstones block the common bile duct.
Gallstones cause jaundice.

Hidden variable = gallstones do not always cause jaundice. Thus, the explanation must make clear in what circumstances gallstones cause jaundice.

Step 3   Secretion of bile; storage and passage of bile; formation of gallstones; migration and impaction of gallstone; results of obstruction to flow of bile.

Step 4   (a) Bile is secreted by hepatocytes and conveyed to the gall bladder via the hepatic duct and cystic duct.
(b) Bile is stored and concentrated in the gall bladder, from whence it is ejected by muscular contraction, and conveyed by peristalsis into small intestine via cystic duct and common bile duct.
(c) In some people, gallstones form from precipitation of bile constituents, for example cholesterol, in gall bladder.
(d) Small gallstones may be ejected during contraction of the gall bladder, passing by peristalsis into the common bile duct, where they may impact in the lumen.
(e) This impaction may cause obstruction to the flow of bile, with a resultant rise in back-pressure to the liver.
(f) This back-pressure will eventually cause reversal of flow of bile into the bloodstream, raising the serum bilirubin and discolouring the skin and mucous membranes, i.e. jaundice.

---

gallstones do not always cause jaundice. Step 3 is a list of the key points of the explanation, and these are expressed in Step 4 as statements or keys. Each of these keys would need to have some examples to illustrate the point and also elaboration or qualifications. For instance, in statement (c) the teacher would probably give examples of the kind of people who are likely to suffer from gallstones, possibly including the aphorism 'fair, fat, forty and flatulent'. Having designed the explanation, all that remains is for the teacher to incorporate it into the teaching plan, taking care to provide a motivating introduction.

USING QUESTIONS IN TEACHING

The use of questioning is an integral part of teaching, and a question can be defined as 'any statement intended to evoke a verbal response' (Brown and Edmondson, 1984).

It is useful to distinguish between two major types of questions: educational and management questions. Educational questions are those directly concerned with the educational outcomes of the student, such as subject-matter, feelings and opinions, whereas management questions are used to organize or control the classroom environment. Examples of the latter might be questions that are really commands, such as 'Would you please stop talking during my lecture?', or 'Would someone like to open a window?' This section focuses on educational questions.

Purposes of educational questioning

The purposes of educational questioning can be grouped under four main headings.

1. *Social purposes*: to promote active involvement of the students during a lesson; to encourage closer relationships between teachers and students; to elicit any special interests or experience from the students.
2. *Motivational purposes*: to develop the student's interest and motivation, e.g. 'How do you think that this problem might be overcome?'; to focus attention upon an aspect of the session; to provide a change of stimulus.
3. *Cognitive purposes*: to encourage the students to think at varying levels of complexity, and in a logical, analytical way.
4. *Assessment purposes*: to assess the previous knowledge or skill of a student; to assess the student's ability to use the higher levels of cognitive functioning such as analysis, synthesis and evaluation; to provide the teacher with feedback on the learning taking place during the course of a lecture.

These four categories emphasize the wide-ranging uses of questioning, but in practice, it seems that most teachers use mainly factual and closed questions (Delamont, 1983).

Classification of questions

There are many different ways of classifying questions, none of which is entirely satisfactory because questions depend very much on the context in which they are asked. However, there are several systems that may be used and three of these, Bloom's, Brown and Edmonson's, and Kerry's, are outlined below.

Bloom's taxonomy classification

In Chapter 12 (p. 275) the work of Benjamin Bloom (1956) is discussed in connection with educational objectives. The taxonomy of educational objectives can be used to formulate questions at different intellectual levels. Bloom classified intellectual or cognitive functions into a hierarchy of levels of increasing complexity, from simple recall of facts to evaluation and judgement of ideas. The most basic level is called 'knowledge' and questions aimed at this level will ask the student to recall a definition or term, state a fact, or identify certain things. The next level is 'comprehension', and the teacher can test this level by asking questions that require the student to restate meanings in his or her own words or to predict consequences or effects.

The third level is 'application', which requires the student to apply rules, methods and principles to specific situations. In a first aid lecture, for example, the teacher may have already given the rule for casualties, which states that they should be given nothing by mouth. Later in the lecture the teacher may give a specific example of a casualty with a fractured femur and ask the question, 'How would you deal with the casualty's request for a drink?'

'Analysis', the fourth level, requires questions to be phrased in such a way as to make the student break down concepts or situations into their component parts, whereas the fifth level, 'synthesis' asks the student to do the opposite, i.e. to build up a whole from a series of constituent parts. For example, a question such as 'From what we have done so far, can you tell us what the main areas of your nursing-care plan would be?' is an example of a synthesis-level question. The highest level of intellectual functioning, according to Bloom, is that of 'evaluation', and consists of questions that ascertain from the students their judgements about the best or most effective arguments or courses of action.

Brown and Edmondson's types of questions

Brown and Edmondson (1984) classify questions into two broad categories: 'cognitive', and 'speculative, affective and management'. Cognitive-level questions are arranged in a way similar to Bloom's above, with five subcategories:

1. *data recall* – includes recall of knowledge, tasks, naming, and classifying;

2. *simple deductions* from data – comparing, describing, and interpreting;
3. *providing reasons*, causes or motives that have not been taught in the lecture;
4. *problem-solving*; and
5. *evaluating*.

Speculative, affective and management questions comprise such aspects as speculation, intuitive guesses, expression of emotions, class control, attention and checking understanding.

Kerry's classification

Kerry (1980) has devised a ten-item classification of questions:

1. *data-recall* questions – facts are recalled but not used;
2. *naming* questions – things are named;
3. *observation* questions – these are what the student observes;
4. *control* questions – part of classroom management;
5. *pseudo-questions* – the teacher seems to give the impression that a range of answers will be acceptable, but in reality his or her mind is made up;
6. *speculative or hypothesis-generating* questions – these invite the student to speculate about a hypothetical situation;
7. *reasoning* questions – these ask for reasons as to why things occur;
8. *personal response* questions – these ask how the student feels about an issue;
9. *discriminatory* questions – these look for the points for and against an issue; and
10. *problem-solving* questions – which are geared to finding out about things.

The various classification systems outlined above are not exhaustive and there are other types of questions that have been identified. Probing questions encourage the student to develop his or her first answer, and prompting questions give students hints about the direction they might take. Convergent questions are those that narrow down to a specific answer, whereas divergent questions open out a number of possibilities.

Making questioning more effective

Questioning is often a rather haphazard affair, with questions being thrown out without too much thought as to their purpose. There are a number of criteria that apply to the formulation of good questions. The question should be short so that it can be remembered by the students whilst they are working out their answers, and it should be stated in language that can easily be understood. The question must also be appropriate to the level of the student, as it is unfair to expect an answer to questions that are at too high a level for his or her particular stage of education. On the other hand, the teacher must try to include questions that require more than simple recall of factual material, by posing questions containing problems that need a thought-out solution.

Needless to say, a question should never be ambiguous, and should contain only a single question. For example, it is confusing for a student to be asked a question like 'What are the main points in the pre-operative care of this patient, and why are they important?' Another example of a poor question is 'Are models of nursing useful in planning patient/client care?' The student need simply say 'Yes' or 'No' to answer the question and the teacher will then need to probe further to elicit the actual 'answer' required.

A useful tip for improving questioning technique is to write out the questions beforehand, and include them on the lesson plan. This ensures that the questions have received some careful thought before being included and so the teacher is less likely to ask poor questions. It is good teaching technique to explain to the students that, whenever a question is posed during a lesson, each of them is to think about the answer and that then one of them will be selected by name to answer it. This is sometimes referred to as the 'pose, pause, pounce' technique, and is useful in that it ensures that each student thinks about the question, just in case it is he or she who is selected. This method is superior to the overhead type of question technique, where the question is posed and students volunteer the answer, because any given student may well decide not to answer the question, leaving the bright members of the audience to vie for the privilege.

The teacher's response to the answers given by students is very important, as the act of questioning is highly threatening from the student's point of view. Teachers often seem unaware of the power they possess in a lecture; their responses can have a devastating effect on the individual student. Individuals can be made to feel humiliated by a thoughtless response from the teacher, so sensitivity is needed when dealing with this aspect. Correct answers must be reinforced adequately and this should also include the correct parts of a partially correct answer. An incorrect answer should not be left, but should be followed by a rephrased version at a lower level. A partially correct answer can usefully be referred to another student for further elaboration.

One problem that requires careful handling is that of the students who do not answer at all. It is tempting to try to relieve their discomfort by moving on to another person, but it is well worth rephrasing the question at a lower level of difficulty so that the reluctant students gains a little success if he or she answers. If the rephrased question still evokes no response, then the best strategy may well be to leave such students for the moment and then to see them privately after the lecture in order to attempt to find a solution to their difficulty.

The most common failing of questioning is that the response called for is at a low level of intellectual functioning, such as simple factual recall of information. It is therefore necessary for the teacher to plan for the inclusion of questions that test the higher intellectual functions.

THE SCHEME OF WORK

In Colleges and Departments of Nursing and Midwifery, teachers are normally responsible for the delivery of a specific area of the curriculum, such as a module or unit of study, being of a defined size and duration, and consisting of a series of sessions centred around a common theme or topic area. It may be difficult to maintain the overall continuity and coherence of a module if the teacher plans each session individually, so it is preferable to use a scheme of work that encompasses the entire module.

A scheme of work is a document that gives an overview of the key components of each teaching session within the module, and this would normally include the title, goals or learning outcomes, sequence of content, teaching and learning activities, assessment, and media resources. Table 5.2 shows an example of a scheme of work for a course

Table 5.2   Example of a scheme of work

Session	Outcomes	Content	Teaching methods	Assessment
Introduction to research	• Understand nature of knowledge	Mutual knowledge, formal knowledge, informed consent, confidentiality	• Lecture • Issue-centred groups • Resource material	Multiple-choice test
Types of research	• Understand principles of experimental research • Describe the nature of experimental research	Experimental research, non-experimental research	• Lecture/discussion • Carousel exercise	Nil
Action research	• Understand nature of action research • Discuss potential projects in own field	Principles: exploratory, practical, problem-centred	• Problem-centred groups • Case-study material	Quality of feedback from group work
Basic statistics	• Awareness of uses and limitations • Understanding of basic statistics	Uses and abuses, basic concepts, centrality, variability, correlation, probability, sampling	• Activity workshop • Handout material	Monitoring of activities
Research critique	• Understanding of principles of a critique • Undertake an elementary critique	Guidelines, academic fraud	• Lecture/discussion • Practical exercise	Assessment of critiques
Writing a research proposal	• Identify sources of funding • Write a draft proposal	Sources of funding: DOH, NHS, HEA, etc. Guidelines	• Lecture/discussion • Workshop on writing a proposal	Assessment of draft proposal Essay assignment on course outcomes

entitled 'Teaching research and enquiry skills for staff development of community practitioners'. By considering each of these components for a given session in relation to the others within the scheme, the teacher can ensure integration and coherence of the whole module. The scheme of work is a useful tool for checking on other important aspects of the module, such as whether or not there is sufficient variety of teaching and learning activities across the module, and the amount of assessment within the module as a whole.

THE TEACHING PLAN

It is interesting to watch how teachers and other public speakers use notes; these are often written on very small cards secreted in the palm of the hand, to which furtive glances are directed from time to time when a prompt is required. From this behaviour we might conclude that generally, people feel they should be able to speak without notes, their use being somewhat akin to cheating! However, it is the needs of the audience, not his own prestige, that should be at the forefront of the teacher's mind, and a teaching plan can help to minimize the chances of omitting some vital part of the session and ensure that all the necessary factors have been considered.

Teaching plans need to be distinguished from a closely related concept, that of the teacher's subject-matter notes. Subject-matter notes are used to provide a reminder to the teacher of the actual details of the subject matter during a session and eliminate the possibility of forgetting some crucial aspect. It is quite possible for a teacher to present a teaching session without having teacher's notes, depending on the type of subject-matter and the degree of expertise of the teacher. Indeed, many teachers do not use subject-matter notes *per se*, but put the key headings on overhead-projector transparencies, using these as prompts to their memory of the subject-matter. It is tempting for a newly qualified teacher to write down every word of what he or she plans to say, but this may well result in their notes being read aloud rather than delivered, and it is also easier for the teacher to lose their place! If anxious not to omit any detail, it is still possible to include all the major headings and subheadings, with suitable indicators of examples, etc., without writing the whole plan in prose form. Figure 5.2 gives a proforma for a teaching plan which will suit any type of teaching situation. It fits neatly into an A4 sheet and contains spaces for all the essential details on one side, with room for the actual sequence of delivery on the reverse. Most of the form is self-explanatory, but the following should be noted.

The column headed 'sequence' is for the main headings only, as finer detail should be contained in the teacher's notes, as should the questions that one is planning to ask. (I always use bright colours for the main headings, and write the notes in a much larger script than the normal writing style so that they are easily visible from a waist-height table or desk top when standing up.)

TITLE .... DATE ....

TEACHING METHOD .... TIME ....

VENUE ....

GROUP DETAILS

(a) Number of Learners:

(b) Type of Course:

(c) Educational Level:

(d) Previous Experience:

ROOM ARRANGEMENTS	LEARNING RESOURCES

EVALUATION FORMAT

(a) During Lesson: (b) End of Lesson:

AIMS AND OBJECTIVES

CHALKBOARD PLAN

TIME	SEQUENCE	ACTIVITY	
		TEACHER	LEARNERS

SELF-EVALUATION OF LESSON:

Fig. 5.2 Format for a teaching plan.

The Herbartian principles are useful as a general approach when considering the sequencing of the session; they state that teaching should proceed from the simple to the complex, from the concrete to the abstract and from the known to the unknown.

The 'activity' column is a useful indicator of the amount of interaction and activity during a lesson and should also include any use of learning resources as well as teacher talk. Although a 'time' column is included, the timing is meant to be an approximate guide only and the plan must be sufficiently flexible to allow for unplanned events.

Space is allowed also for the teacher's immediate reactions at the end of the session, so that key aspects are recorded whilst fresh in his or her mind, which can then form the basis for later reflection.

ORGANIZING THE TEACHING ENVIRONMENT

As the poet Robert Burns said: 'the best-laid schemes o' mice an' men gang aft agley', and this is particularly appropriate in the context of organizing the teaching environment. All a teacher's careful planning can be undone if he or she neglects the environment within which the session takes place.

It is always good practice wherever possible to prepare the room in advance of the students arrival, but this assumes that the previous teacher vacates on time. In reality sessions often overrun, but even so the incoming teacher should take a few minutes to check their lesson materials and set up any media resources before commencing the actual teaching. The problem may be compounded if the seating arrangements need to be changed, as this can be a time-consuming exercise. However, it can be accomplished more quickly if the students are asked to move their own desks and chairs.

It is useful to switch on the classroom lights, even if the daylight is adequate, since this can have the effect of focusing students' attention; the overhead projector is designed to operate in normal lighting and is therefore not affected. Sunlight, however, can bleach out the image on the screen if shining directly onto it, so window blinds or blackout curtains need to be closed if this occurs.

Institutions vary in the quality of their resources so teachers should be aware that their carefully prepared teaching plans may be ruined if vital media fail to arrive. Overhead projectors may not be available in every classroom; they may have to be projected onto an adjacent wall if a screen is not available; video replay facilities may not arrive when ordered, and do not always work when they do arrive.

Finally, one of the most frustrating situations a teacher can face is that, having prepared the classroom in advance, it transpires that another class has booked the room. Tense negotiations with the other teacher usually follow, taking up valuable time from the lesson and often resulting in a mass move to another room. In these situations, the interpersonal skills of the teachers are severely put to the test, but such events are all part and parcel of the work of teaching.

REFERENCES

Bloom, B. (1956) *Taxonomy of Educational Objectives: The Classification of Educational Goals, Handbook One: Cognitive Domain*, McKay, New York.

Brown, G. (1978) *Lecturing and Explaining*, Methuen, London.

Brown, G. and Armstrong, S. (1984) Explaining and explanation, in *Classroom Teaching Skills*, (ed. E. Wragg) Croom Helm, London.

Brown, G. and Edmondson, R. (1984) Asking questions, in *Classroom Teaching Skills* (ed. E. Wragg), Croom Helm, London.

CNAA (1992) *Improving Student Learning Project*, Oxford Centre for Staff Development, Oxford.

Delamont, S. (1983) *Interaction in the Classroom*, Methuen, London.

Kerry, T. (1980) *Effective Questioning*, Nottingham University School of Education, Nottingham.

Lecturing | 6

Lecturing is well-established as a teaching strategy in nurse education but there has been considerable variability in its use amongst the specialisms. Mental illness nursing, for example, tended to have very small student cohorts, perhaps ten or less in some cases and this helped to foster the development of small-group experiential techniques in preference to lectures. In contrast, group sizes in general nursing were typically larger, with lectures forming a fairly substantial component of the curriculum. However, with the advent of Project 2000 courses for first-level registration in nursing, the situation has changed quite dramatically. The partnership with HE has exposed nurse teachers to a new culture in which the availability of resources largely determines the approach to teaching. In this new culture, nurse teachers find themselves having to lecture to groups of students as large as a hundred or more in a common foundation programme, a daunting task for those teachers who have had little or no experience of the technique.

I have recently heard it said by nurse teacher colleagues that 'Project 2000 signals the death of experiential learning!' This quote indicates a real fear among nurse teachers that they will be forced into a lecture mode of teaching with which they have little, if any, empathy. However, two quotations might prove to be of comfort to nurse teachers in this situation: 'Variety is the spice of life', and 'necessity is the mother of invention'. Lectures do have the potential to provide a refreshing contrast to an unvarying and eventually indigestible menu of small-group work and experiential learning. The latter quote suggests that if large group lectures are inevitable in the new system, then nurse teachers will need to find ways of lecturing that ensure students' interest and motivation.

CAUSES AND EFFECTS OF LARGE STUDENT GROUPS

Higher education (HE) is having adapt to teaching large groups due to a number of factors: government policy, modularization and CAT (credit accumulation and transfer) schemes.

Government policy The Government is committed to increasing the number of students in HE up to the year 2000. Also, FE and HE institutions have been granted corporate status which in turn has led to a new financial realism. When giving a lecture to 150 students, the staff–student ratio (SSR) is 1:150; this helps to resource small group and laboratory teaching where the ratio may need to be as low as 1:8.

Modularization   Within the last decade there has been a major shift towards modularization of courses in HE. A module is a self-contained unit of learning, and individual courses comprise a number of modules. The attraction of modularization is the efficiency that can be gained. For example, an introductory module on psychology could be used for a great many courses in a variety of disciplines such as nursing, social science, humanties, etc. Such foundation courses are taught to very large groups, often several hundred students, and thereby create a favourable SSR.

Credit accumulation and transfer (CAT) schemes   These are a continuation of the concept of modularization, and in addition to the advantages outlined above, CAT schemes allow even greater freedom of choice for students to attend modules or units from the entire university credit framework, depending upon the nature of the pathway undertaken.

The increase in group sizes produces a range of difficulties, including a reduction in student participation in sessions, problems with acoustics in lecture rooms, less books in libraries and reduced access to facilities such as CDROM and OPAC catalogue. The 'Teaching More Students' project (Polytechnics and Colleges Funding Council, 1992) has identified a number of alternative approaches to resourcing of courses.

1. Teach some years more cheaply than others. For example, the first year of a Project 2000 course might be taught using large group methods so that the third year could focus on more expensive individual strategies.
2. Invest heavily in the early development of independent learning so that students can learn for themselves more cheaply later on.
3. Drop some goals to save others. For example, a course could reduce the length of its placements and thereby save resources to maintain one-to-one tutorial contact.
4. Use cheaper assessment methods such as multiple-choice tests, self-assessment, and peer assessment.
5. Use peer-tutoring to save on teaching staff resources. For example, post-registration students could act as tutor to pre-registration students, in a way similar to mentorship.
6. Use resource-based learning.

THE NATURE OF LECTURES

The term 'lecture' is applied to a particular type of educational encounter in which a teacher transmits information to a number of students, with the teacher doing most of the talking and the students mainly listening or writing. Walters and Marks (1981) suggest there are three kinds of lecture, the 'ideal' (or 'pure'), the 'classical' and the 'experiential', and it is the last two that apply more usefully to nurse education.

The 'ideal' lecture The hallmark of the ideal lecture is its voluntary nature; participants attend the lecture of their own volition and this implies commitment on their part. The role of the lecturer is to persuade the audience by virtue of the beliefs and values that are shared by both parties. The commonest example of the ideal lecture is the political lecture.

The 'classical' lecture In public-education systems, attendance at lectures is seen as being largely compulsory. This element of coercion tends towards a performance-centred focus, with students mainly concerned with attaining good grades. Because of this, the classical lecture tends to be very much more specific in its subject-matter.

The 'experiential' lecture This form of lecture is used prior to experiential learning activities and is intended to give participants basic concepts and explanations about the issue in question. For example, a nurse teacher may plan to teach students about self-awareness, and may begin with an experiential lecture that provides a theoretical framework for the various activities that follow. Such a framework could consist of the various components of the 'self', the formation of the self-picture, and a review of the methods of gaining greater self-awareness.

There are a number of designs for the sequencing of the subject-matter within a lecture; the 'classical' design is perhaps the most common, where the lecture is composed of a number of main headings, each having one or more subdivisions. Other designs include the 'comparative', which compares two concepts such as osteoarthrosis and rheumatoid arthritis, and the 'problem-solving' design, which poses a problem and its possible solutions, e.g. the stigma of epilepsy.

THE USES AND SHORTCOMINGS OF LECTURES

One of the great defenders of the use of lectures for transmission of knowledge is Ausubel (Ausebel *et al.*, 1978), whose work is described in Chapter 3 (p. 65). He maintains that it is simply wasteful to ask students to discover everything for themselves, when the transmission mode has been used successfully over generations to transmit the culture of a society. Evidence from the literature on the educational use of lectures is summarized below.

1. *Purposes*: lectures are as effective as other methods for conveying information, but less effective for the promotion of thinking skills and the changing of attitudes.
2. *Compulsory attendance*: students who absent themselves from lectures do less well in examinations and tests.

3. *Time of day*: morning lectures seem superior to afternoon lectures for the recall of information, but this may not apply to the 'evening-type' of learner, whose maximum physiological alertness occurs between 15.00 hours and midnight.
4. *Length*: attention declines considerably after some 20 minutes, with a reduction in the amount of information assimilated and noted.
5. *Recall*: recall on information from lectures is relatively inefficient, falling to something around 20% recall after one week.
6. *Delivery*: speed of delivery is closely related to the level of difficulty of the material, and evidence suggests that there is a critical level of difficulty and speed, beyond which the material is delivered with a loss of efficiency.

One common criticism of the lecture method is that the information could have been obtained from textbooks just as easily, yet this shows a lack of understanding of the purpose of lectures. Indeed, if they are used only to convey information readily available in other forms such as books, then they are likely to be simplistic or inaccurate due to time constraints. However, used thoughtfully, lectures can complement textbooks by providing:

- up-to-date research information that has not yet reached the textbooks;
- a synthesis of viewpoints from a wide variety of sources;
- clearer explanations of issues and phenomena, with the possibility of demonstration;
- personal involvement of the students by means of activities during the lecture; and
- the potential to motivate and inspire students to further study.

However, over-reliance on lectures may lead to dependence on the part of the students, who expect all the information to be handed to them 'on a plate'. All too often lectures are long, tedious and poorly organized, whereas with careful planning and practice they can be an effective vehicle for motivating students.

The advantages and disadvantages of the lecture method are summarized in Table 6.1.

THE ART OF LECTURING

I firmly believe that lecturing is analogous to acting, each requiring careful scripting, polished presentational skills, and a certain personal charisma for effective performance. This theatrical performance element may not be present in other forms of teaching and can provide a source of stimulation and job satisfaction for those teachers who enjoy the challenge. The requirements of good lecturing are creativity, well-developed verbal-exposition skills, clarity of ideas, an ability to make a subject interesting, enthusiasm and self-confidence. Verbal exposition is the term

Table 6.1 Advantages and disadvantages of the lecture method

Advantages	Disadvantages
Efficiency, i.e. one teacher can communicate with a large number of students.	Students attention may wane.
A well-presented lecture may increase student motivation.	Students are largely passive.
New knowledge may be presented which is not yet in textbooks.	Lectures do not cater for individual student's needs.
Teachers can integrate the subject matter better than students.	Pace of lecture does not suit all students.
Good for introducing a new topic.	Teacher's bias may be evident.
Useful for giving a framework upon which students can build.	Students obtain material 'second-hand' rather than from primary sources.

given to the kinds of talking in which the teacher engages during a lecture, or indeed in any other type of teaching, with the exception of individualized instruction. This 'teacher-talk' can be subdivided into a number of modes, the commonest ones being the stating of facts, the defining and classifying of material, asking and answering questions, giving explanations, comparing and contrasting information and evaluating material.

Figure 6.1 gives guidelines for planning and delivering lectures, and uses an acrostic arrangement under the headings 'before', 'during' and 'after'. (In an acrostic, the initial letters of each of the horizontal statements combine vertically to make another word.) This device can also be used as an organizing principle for lecturing on a given topic – any topic, provided you have the ingenuity to think up appropriate words!

Before the lecture

Believe in yourself By assuming the role of lecturer, one is, in a sense, claiming to have superior knowledge in comparison to the audience and this may lead to the feeling of vulnerability when facing them. Self-belief is a vital characteristic for successful lecturing; the teacher has an extensive knowledge and experience base which underpins their lectures, and this should provide the confidence to approach the lecture, and the audience, in a positive manner.

Explaining Explanations are a central activity in most lectures and great care must be taken in their preparation. Explaining is discussed in detail in Chapter 5.

Focus on selected aspects When planning the lecture it is important to be selective about what to put into it, the temptation being to cram in everything the teacher knows about a topic. Chapter 5 deals with this aspect of planning in more detail.

Overlearn your material It almost goes without saying that the teacher must know the subject matter of the lecture 'inside-out' if credibility is to

Believe in yourself
Explaining
Focus on selected aspects
Overlearn your material
Rehearse
Excitement/anxiety

Delivery
Unusual
Recap
Involve your audience
Notetaking
Get out of time

Average/mean Performance
Focus on well-done/less well-done
Tape the lecture and review
Experience other people's lectures
Retain a sense of proportion

Fig. 6.1   The art of lecturing.

be maintained. Students very soon see through any attempts to 'waffle' by a teacher who does not know a particular point or answer. No teacher can know everything about a subject and it can increase stature if a lack of knowledge is admitted. Needless to say, the teacher who constantly has to say, 'I'm sorry, I don't know,' has an inadequate background knowledge which requires attention. If the lecture has been prepared some time in advance, or if it has been given previously, the teacher needs to spend time going over the material again to ensure he or she has remembered it.

Rehearse   The analogy with acting emerges again here, with the advice that the teacher should spend time rehearsing various elements of the lecture until he or she is satisfied with the likely impact and timing. A videotape or audiotape recorder is invaluable for providing feedback on these aspects.

Excitement/anxiety   Lecturing to a large audience is often the main anxiety experienced by those new to teaching and it largely stems from the fear of making a fool of oneself by 'drying up' or forgetting what to say. The opening of the lecture is often the most nerve-racking part for the inexperienced teacher, but it is common to find that teachers still experience initial nervousness even after years of teaching. Actors often claim that this initial state of high arousal is beneficial, in that it puts an 'edge' on their performance. However, it is useful to distinguish between arousal and anxiety; arousal applies to the state of wakefulness or alertness of the individual, while anxiety applies to a state of arousal above that required for the optimum level of performance. Anxiety, therefore, reduces the performance effectiveness of an individual. What the lecturer is aiming at is a level of arousal sufficient to bring out the best in the performance without tipping over the edge into anxiety, which would reduce his or her effectiveness.

During the lecture

Delivery   On first entering the lecture room, it is important that the teacher takes a couple of minutes to organize the area, check the over head projector, etc. Very often the students have been sitting in the room prior to the teacher's entry, having already received a previous lecture and there is a temptation to commence the lecture straight away. So often lecturers begin their session and after a few minutes turn on the overhead projector only to find it is projecting onto the wall or somewhere other than the screen. It is important to spend a moment or two organizing the area, and to let the audience know so they can feel free to talk to their friends until everything is ready. This should ensure that the lecturer feels confident that all is well prior to commencing the lecture.

The introduction to the lecture is very important in gaining the students' interest and attention, so it is well worth attempting to provide a motivating opening. This could involve asking the audience whether anyone has had experience related to the topic, thus making the session relevant to them. It is also good practice to write out on the chalkboard a plan or outline of the sequence of the lecture, so that students may follow each section without losing track of the explanation.

The aim of a lecture is to communicate certain things to the audience and the main medium for this communication is the lecturer's voice. There are three components of the vocal apparatus:

1. *vocal cords* which vibrate as the breath passes between them;
2. *resonators* – the hollow spaces of the mouth, nose and pharynx; and
3. *speech organs* consisting of the tongue, palate, alveolar ridge, teeth, jaw and lips.

Volume or loudness is dependent on the force of the breath striking the vocal cords. Pitch is determined by the length, thickness and tension of the vocal cords, the first two factors being influenced by the size of the larynx. For instance, the small larynx of a child has short vocal cords, which give the voice a high pitch. Adult males, on the other hand, possess large larynxes with long cords, producing a low pitch, i.e. a deep voice. Nervous tension will produce a note of higher pitch and this is often detectable in persons who are anxious. Tone is the result of the air vibrating in the resonating spaces.

One of the most important aspects of speech in the lecture setting is audibility. This relies particularly on the careful use of consonants, which ensures clarity, and on the ability of the teacher to project his or her voice. It is good technique to stand up straight and speak from the lungs rather than the throat, ensuring that the lungs are well-inflated with each breath. Careful observation of the facial expressions and other non-verbal communication will provide feedback as to whether the rear row of the audience is hearing what is being said.

Expressiveness is another important aspect of speech, as it helps maintain the listeners' interest by providing variety. Variations in intonation are produced by changing the pitch of the voice and also by variations of the volume and rhythm. The use of stress to emphasize important words can make the voice more interesting and the speed of delivery needs to be at a pace suitable for the students to absorb the material and to write notes. Pausing is a strategy that new teachers need to develop; the tendency is to regard any periods of silence as undesirable, although pauses are a necessity during speech, since they provide the punctuation that makes the words meaningful. It can be useful to take a sip of water periodically, as a way of forcing oneself to pause.

One of the major problems that can cause loss of attention during lectures is the speed of delivery; this is often difficult to judge when inexperienced and the commonest error is going too fast when nervous. It is helpful for new teachers to keep a card on the desk or lectern with the words 'SLOW DOWN' written on it, which serves to catch their eye from time to time and remind them to think about the speed of delivery.

The aim of any lecture should be to provide an atmosphere of psychological safety in which the students feel free to volunteer comments or questions. If the teacher conveys the impression of warmth and acceptance towards the group, this, combined with a sense of humour, will go a long way towards establishing the rapport that is so essential to learning. Evidence suggests that interest and enthusiasm of the teacher are characteristics that are particularly valued by students, and this can be indicated by emphasis and tone of voice, and also by the use of non-verbal signals. It is difficult to overstate the fundamental importance of non-verbal communication during lectures. Students emit a variety of non-verbal cues and the teacher can gain valuable feedback on his or her performance by observing their facial expressions, which can convey feelings of surprise, puzzlement or astonishment. The teacher also emits non-verbal signals, so it is important to be aware of the role of such signals. Gesture can play a useful part in explaining concepts, especially those with spatial relationships, but other gestures may prove distracting, such as fiddling with chalk. Head nodding can be a reinforcer of behaviour and if a learner is talking to the teacher and the teacher nods frequently, this can encourage the learner to continue talking. When lecturing it is also important to engage the students in eye contact periodically, as this indicates interest and confidence. However, it should be noted that the length of time for eye contact should not exceed ten seconds, as this may provoke anxiety. Honesty is a quality which is not often mentioned in connection with verbal exposition and in this context it implies the willingness of the teacher to admit that he or she does not know the answer to something.

Unusual The inclusion of unusual or novel stimuli can be a powerful strategy for maintaining students' arousal and attention during a lecture. Such stimuli could be pictures, music, poems and activities which have an element of surprise or novelty.

Recap Recapitulation or repetition should be used frequently, so that the learner is exposed to the information on more than one occasion. Provision could also be made for this at the end of the lecture if time allows, and will help to retain the information for a longer period of time.

Involve your audience Adult students are never very happy just sitting listening to lectures; what they like to have is some personal involvement in them. There is a wide variety of strategies for involving students in lectures, even when faced with a large number of students. One effective way is to use buzz groups, in which students form groups of four to six by swivelling around to face the ones behind them, without moving their seats. These small buzz groups then spend a couple of minutes discussing some aspect of the topic and then feedback is invited.

The use of incomplete handouts is another way of ensuring student participation; the handout contains only key headings or diagrams and the student is required to fill in the details gleaned from the presentation. A quiz or test given at the end of the lecture may also serve to focus students' attention on the material presented!

Notetaking This is an important activity for students during lectures, and is discussed in detail in Chapter 16 (p.385).

Get out on time It is quite common to find that lectures over-run their allotted time, and in my book this is a cardinal offence! Students find it difficult enough to maintain attention during the normal span of a lecture, and over-running simply compounds the problem. There are also knock-on effects on the students' next class or lunch break, and it delays access by other groups to the lecture room. One of the causes of over-running is an over-ambitious lecture plan for the time available. These lecture plans seem to exert a powerful influence over teachers, who slavishly follow them until the bitter end, often regardless of the time or circumstances. From the teacher's perspective, the lecture plan contains important material that must be covered by the end of the lecture, even if this results in running late to do so. On the other hand, the students' perception is quite different, in that the important aspects of their college day are more likely to be the coffee and lunch breaks when they meet with their friends and peers. The teacher should aim to finish five minutes before the official end of the lecture, to give students and themselves a break before starting their next session.

After the lecture

Average/mean performance Teachers often worry unduly if a lecture does not go as well as they would like, but it is important to see it in the context of their average performance. Some lectures go very well, others we would rather forget; it is not helpful to spend time worrying about a less than satisfying one-off performance. The teacher should aim for a good overall standard of performance, but realize that there will inevitably be minor variations from day to day.

Focus on well-done/less well-done When evaluating a lecture it is helpful to try to focus on those aspects that were well-done, and those that were less well-done. By adopting this system the teacher will hopefully avoid distorting the evaluation by agonizing over a single unsatisfactory episode.

Tape the lecture and review Evaluation of a lecture can be much more effective if the teacher can videotape one from time to time. It is a salutary experience to watch yourself performing as a lecturer, but by and large it is an encouraging activity that can boost confidence considerably.

Experience other people's lectures Giving lectures can be quite an exciting experience for teachers, but it is easy to forget what it is like from the audience's point of view. It is helpful for teachers to attend lectures from time to time just to remind themselves what it feels like to sit in a lecture, especially if it is not particularly interesting or well-presented. Also tips and ideas may well be picked up that can be used in later lectures!

Retain a sense of proportion The problem with the lecturing/acting analogy is that teachers may feel they have to produce virtuoso performances in every lecture. Clearly, some teachers have a flair for lecturing, while others are merely competent; the important thing is to be yourself. A sense of proportion is a great asset in lecturing; if the teacher attempts to incorporate every good point of style gained from observation of colleagues, then there will be little room left for the most important quality that the teacher possesses, namely individuality.

VARIANTS OF THE LECTURE

The standard format for the lecture is capable of many adaptations to suit the purposes of the teacher and three such variants will be discussed: demonstrations, team teaching and dialogue.

The demonstration

A demonstration can be defined as a visualized explanation of facts, concepts and procedures. The purposes of demonstration can be broadly classified into:

- those designed to show the learner how to perform certain psycho-motor skills; and
- those designed to show the learner why certain things occur.

In the former, the learner must reproduce exactly the behaviour that is demonstrated, whilst in the latter the behaviour is intended only as a strategy to aid the learner's understanding of a concept or principle. Each of these is now examined in turn.

Demonstrating a psychomotor skill

In Chapter 3 the theory of skills acquisition was discussed, so we will bear these principles in mind when planning a demonstration. The following checklists identify 16 key points to consider before, during and after the demonstration.

Before the demonstration

1. Formulate the learning outcomes.
2. Perform a skills analysis and determine the sequence.
3. Assess entry behaviours of students, and determine prerequisites.
4. Formulate the teaching plan, with particular reference to:
   (a) ensuring optimum visibility; and
   (b) preparation of all materials.

It is crucial to formulate the objectives and prerequisites before commencing the lesson plan, just as in preparing any kind of lesson. As we saw in Chapter 3, the skills analysis will provide a detailed breakdown of the types of behaviour that constitute the total skill and these must then be set out in the correct sequence. This is a very important step, as it is not always appreciated that the learner must not only remember the techniques for each sub-skill, but also the correct sequence of these.

During the demonstration

5. State the learning outcomes to the students.
6. Motivate them by explaining why the skill is important.
7. Demonstrate the total skill at normal speed.
8. Write the sequence of part-skills on the chalkboard or overhead projector, as a checklist for the step-by-step demonstration.
9. Demonstrate each part-skill slowly, in the correct sequence.
10. Obtain feedback by questioning and observation of non-verbal behaviour.
11. Avoid the use of negative examples and variations in technique.

It is good practice actually to put the sub-skills on the chalkboard in the correct sequence, so this can serve as a guide when the learner is practising the skill. Whatever the purpose of the demonstration, it is imperative that each learner can see what is going on, and this implies very careful arrangement of the room and the lighting. Provision of seating is often considered unnecessary when giving a demonstration, but the students should be comfortable, so that they can give maximum concentration to the demonstration.

If closed-circuit television is available, it can provide a valuable addition to the demonstration, in that the camera can be placed so that it 'shoots' over the shoulder of the teacher, giving a 'demonstrator's-eye view' of the skill.

A full-speed total demonstration of the skill, at the commencement of the demonstration gives the learner an overall 'Gestalt' of the form of the total skill. If the teacher has not demonstrated the skill in class before, or not for some time perhaps, then he or she is well-advised to practise the skill a day or so before the class is due. This will have benefits not only from the point of view of the skill itself, but also from the timing. Some teachers like to teach a skill using examples of how not to do it, and others like to include one or two variations of the technique. A common example of this is aseptic technique, which has permissible variations within a framework of principles. However, when teaching a new skill, most authorities would agree that learning is facilitated by teaching only one method of performing the skill and omitting any negative examples. This will minimize the effects of psychological interference that would otherwise arise due to the similarity between the original material and the variations or negative examples. Of course, once the learner has become proficient in the skill, then interference from other techniques is unimportant.

After the demonstration

12. Provide immediate supervised practice, with adequate time allowance.
13. Provide verbal, rather than physical, guidance.
14. Make the environment psychologically safe by providing a friendly atmosphere and constructive criticism.
15. Remember that initial interest may wane, so provide motivation and encouragement.
16. Remember that students will acquire the skill at different rates, so individualize the planning to cater for the fast and slow learner.

The single most important aspect of the demonstration of a psychomotor skill is the provision of immediate practice for the students. A demonstration can only provide information about the cognitive and affective aspects and the psychomotor components must be learned through the students' own muscles, by practice. It is often tempting, when teaching a skill in a clinical setting, to take over from the student in order to 'show' how to do it. Of course, this is quite valid if the student is unsure of the correct technique, but generally speaking, he or she must be allowed to learn the skill by doing it themselves. It is thus that students receive the proprioceptive feedback from their own muscles and joints, which in turn modify their performance. No amount of 'showing' by the teacher will provide the necessary kinaesthetic feedback, without which, no skill can be learned. Learning a skill can be frustrating and tiring, so it is essential that the atmosphere is friendly and relaxed. Testiness on the part of the teacher will only lead to tension in the students and this in turn will lead to poor performance and increase in errors. This is why it is so important to allow sufficient time for practice and to bear in mind that not all students will master a skill at the same rate. In this kind of situation, competition between students can be quite counter-productive, so the teacher needs to emphasize that individuals differ in their rates of learning and that it does not matter if some people acquire a particular skill more quickly than others. What is important is that every student actually acquires the skill, not the speed of acquisition.

Demonstrating a principle or concept

Let us take as an example the concept of osmosis, a fundamental concept in medical science, which is readily demonstrated by a simple experiment using two glass beakers, each containing a piece of raw potato. The first jar is filled with plain water and the second with water containing a tablespoonful of salt. After several hours the potato in the beaker of salt water is seen to be shrivelled and dried up, whilst the potato in the first one remains much the same. If teaching the concept of osmosis in a deductive fashion, then the teacher would first explain and define the term and give examples from human physiology. The demonstration could then follow, as a further example. In the inductive method, however, the demonstration would be presented first and the students put into groups to decide how the findings could be explained. Hopefully, they would arrive at a definition of the phenomenon of osmosis having explored the possibilities.

Team teaching

Team teaching is defined by Shaplin and Olds (1964) as 'instructional organization in which two or more teachers are given responsibility, working together, for all or a significant part of the instruction of the same group of students'. There is often a measure of confusion with regard to the exact meaning of the term and many people claim to be using team teaching when the nurse teachers simply work in one or two teams within a college. However, within these teams, the individual teacher plans and delivers the teaching of a particular area, such as orthopaedic nursing, whilst another does likewise for paediatric nursing and so on. There is not necessarily a sharing of planning or of delivery, each one doing the preparation and teaching of his or her own area. In team teaching, on the other hand, the team actually plans each session together and also does the teaching together for a particular group of students. The methods of teaching are decided by the team and the lecture method can be employed to good effect here.

Organization of team teaching

For team teaching to be a viable proposition, there are some necessary prerequisites. At least two teachers who share a common interest in trying out new ideas are required. They should be people who do not feel threatened by a close working relationship with their colleagues and should be prepared to have their ideas criticized or questioned. It is probably wise to introduce team teaching into just one area of a given module initially, taking care to evaluate the effectiveness before enlarging the use of it. The key to successful team teaching lies in two areas, the interpersonal relationships of the team members and the quality of the planning. If these two aspects are good, then the presentation of the lessons will be very effective. There is considerable planning required for team teaching and this in turn makes large demands on the time of the teachers involved. Each lesson in the team-teaching situation must be planned by every member of the team, as each will normally be involved in its presentation. Without this careful, co-operative planning, the sessions will lack polish and convey an impression of disorganization to the students. During the planning stage such issues as the learning outcomes, teaching methods and evaluation are aired within the team and each member may question and argue the merits of a particular approach. It may not be necessary to have a leader in a teaching team, as then each member is free to be as creative as he or she wants to be. The actual lecture plan is best done in the form of a script to ensure that each team member knows exactly which area and at what time their contribution occurs, although experienced team teachers learn to 'freewheel' very much with each other.

Implementing team teaching

Team teaching can be a very exciting experience for students, provided that the team can create the right level of relaxation and confidence with each other. During ordinary lectures some students soon lose their concentration and attention wanders; team teaching can provide the necessary change of stimulus that will maintain their interest, particularly if the interchange between teachers is relatively frequent. When it works well, team teaching can provide much more stimulation and variety than an ordinary lecture, because each teacher can act as critic or evaluator of the other's points of view. Obviously, this needs great psychological safety if threat is to be avoided, but here again, the quality of interpersonal relationships between team members is the crucial factor for success.

Team teaching does, of course, increase the resource requirements, since there are two or more teachers occupied in doing what one teacher might normally undertake. This extra resource demand needs to be carefully evaluated, but not dismissed out of hand as being impractical; the use of team teaching may make more effective use of time, thereby reducing the total amount of teaching time required in a particular course component. In addition, team teaching can also act as valuable staff development, in that teachers are in a position to work together and evaluate their teaching in a way that cannot happen in the ordinary course of events. It still seems rare for teachers to sit-in on other colleagues' lectures, so it might be that team teaching has hidden extras that help to compensate for the additional resource demands.

Dialogue

This is a very unusual variant of the lecture. The principle of dialogue is that two teachers or colleagues either in nursing, or with health-related interests, sit together in a lecture-type situation with an audience. The two participants agree in advance what the topic for discussion will be and they then spend the time in the lecture engaging in a dialogue about the issues in question. This type of activity is very familiar to television audiences, since it is a common technique for raising people's awareness of particular issues. Two leading personalities from some walk of life engage in dialogue about an issue and there may or may not be a chairperson.

This technique of dialogue can be very useful for value-laden issues and can involve such personnel as a chaplain, a service manager and indeed, any two persons with views on a particular issue. The audience is not normally involved in the dialogue, but are privy to the thinking and argument of the two participants. Since lectures are not very useful for generating changes in attitude or for dealing with issues involving the affective domain, it would seem that dialogue could be a useful way of raising students' awareness and feelings about issues in nursing and health care.

REFERENCES

Ausubel, D., Novak, J. and Hanesian, H. (1978) *Educational Psychology; A Cognitive View*, Holt, Rinehart and Winston, New York.
Brown, G. and Edmondson, R. (1984) Asking questions, in *Classroom Teaching Skills*, (ed. E. Wragg), Croom Helm, London.
Polytechnics and Colleges Funding Council (1992) *The Teaching More Students Project*, Oxford Centre for Staff Development, Oxford.
Shaplin, J. and Olds, H. (1964) *Team Teaching*, Harper and Row, New York.
Walters, G. and Marks, S. (1981) *Experiential Learning and Change: Theory, Development and Practice*, Wiley, Chichester.

7 Small-group teaching and experiential learning

For many educationalists, small-group teaching is the essence of education, providing them with the opportunity for more intimate and rewarding engagements with students than is possible in lectures. The term small-group teaching covers a very wide range of strategies and techniques and is one of the main ways in which students learn from and through experience. Although experiential learning is not confined to a single teaching or learning method, small-group strategies do provide a major vehicle for many aspects of it. This chapter explores the nature and implementation of educational small groups, and of experiential learning. In addition, experiential learning is discussed in Chapter 8 in the context of practice-based learning, Chapters 10 and 12 in the context of accreditation of prior learning, Chapter 17 in the context of biological science, and Chapter 18 in the context of interpersonal communication skills.

Small-group teaching

The concept of a 'small group' is not simply defined by the numbers of students involved, rather, it is the purpose that defines a 'small group' in education. Broadly speaking, the function of an educational 'small group' is to put the student at the centre of things; to allow opportunities for face-to-face interaction with other group members in order to exchange ideas and feelings, to be challenged by other people's viewpoints – in short, to expand the student's universe of awareness.

Clearly, the size of the group will have an effect on the processes occurring within it, particularly with regard to the amount of face-to-face interaction with other group members. With numbers greater than about 25, this becomes impossible and subgroups have to be formed in order to allow for it.

Group size has another important bearing on education: the larger the group, the less time each individual member will have available for contribution. Let us take a typical one-hour group session; if there are 30 students, each will have a maximum possible contribution time of two minutes: with a group of only ten students, the individual contribution time becomes six minutes. If we assume that not all students contribute to the same extent, it becomes quite probable that certain students will gain at the expense of others; it is interesting to note that none of the above timings include any input from the tutor and the more the tutor becomes involved, the less time there is for student participation.

Experiential learning

The term 'experiential learning' is used in a number of ways in education; some apply it specifically to the learning of 'interpersonal skills', whilst others see it as pertaining to 'field placements' away from the educational institution. Burnard (1991) describes a study in which nurse tutors were interviewed about their perceptions of experiential learning and experiential learning methods. The range of definitions given by respondents was quite wide-ranging, and included

- tautological definitions (experiential learning is learning from experience),
- all-encompassing definitions (any activity could be experiential),
- time-related definitions (learning from the past and the present),
- practical definitions (learning from clinical placements),
- personally focused definitions (gaining awareness), and
- contrast-with-tradition definitions (less cognitive input).

Although the study used a very small sample, the results graphically illustrate the wide range of perceptions that these nurse tutors have about the concept.

This chapter aims to broaden the definition considerably to encompass a wide variety of educational applications in nursing. At its simplest, experiential learning is learning that results from experience, but since almost everything in life constitutes experience, this becomes an impossibly global notion. Essentially, experiential learning is learning by doing, rather than by listening to other people or reading about it. This active involvement of the student is one of the key characteristics of this form of learning, together with student-centredness, a degree of interaction, some measure of autonomy and flexibility and a high degree of relevance.

It is useful to distinguish between learning *from* experience and learning *through* experience (Burnard, 1990). The former involves utilizing past experiences to gain new insights, whereas the latter consists of deliberately planned experiences to facilitate learning. In other words, both 'there and then' and 'here and now' experiences can be useful learning stimuli.

In Burnard's study (1991), one of the respondents suggested that for him experiential learning was more like doing therapy, and this view is supported by Rogers (1983) and Heron (1986). It is important, however, that nurse teachers are fully aware of the problems associated with the blending of teaching and therapy. The primary objective of an educational group is the learning of particular aspects of curriculum, whereas the purpose of a therapeutic group is helping group members to 'heal' themselves in a therapeutic setting. Although it is important for students to understand the working of therapeutic groups, the teacher must be careful to avoid running educational groups as therapeutic groups, since there are ethical and moral implications such as informed consent of students.

The psychological underpinning of small-group work and experiential learning lies mainly in the work of David Kolb and Carl Rogers as outlined in Chapters 3 (p. 83) and 4 (p. 101).

FUNDAMENTAL GROUP PROCESSES

Whatever the nature of the group, there are a number of fundamental processes that are identifiable and a knowledge of these will help the nurse teacher to understand certain events that occur in educational small groups. Reference has already been made to social factors that influence learning in Chapter 2 (p. 28) and these should be borne in mind when considering group dynamics.

Social roles

In any given group, there are many social positions called social roles; the family has roles called 'father' and 'mother', nurse education has roles called 'teacher' and 'student' and the individual 'in his time plays many parts'. A number of roles are played concurrently, as with a post-registration student who is also a ward manager; others are played sequentially as with the roles of child, adolescent, adult and elderly person.

It is useful to differentiate between ascribed roles and achieved roles in society; the former are roles that cannot be altered without difficulty, such as sex roles and social class and the latter are roles that are achieved by the individual's own volition, such as the roles of husband, engineer and so on. Primary roles are those that are always played, i.e. sex roles and social class; secondary roles are linked to economic awareness and employment and tertiary roles are occasional ones such as 'captain of the local netball team'.

Group norms

Group norms are defined as required or expected behaviours and beliefs of group members, which may be covert or overt. Covert or implicit norms are usually typified by the phrase 'it just isn't done', whereas overt norms are usually formulated as explicit rules of behaviour. In nursing, there are explicit rules about the way in which uniform is worn, but in clinical settings, there may be implicit norms such as, 'The Ward Manager likes it done this way.' It could be argued that norms are simply roles that are applied to all group members rather than to different concepts.

Both roles and norms may be considered as either imposed or emergent. Imposed roles are those that arise from outside the group, such as the appointment of a new Principal in a College of Nursing; emergent roles are those arising from within a group, such as the election of a chairperson. Norms may also arise from outside the group as when a nurse teacher lays down the rules for conduct in a small-group session. Alternatively, the group may itself develop norms for behaviour and these are often termed group rules.

Group conformity and decision-making

The notion of group conformity has attracted considerable attention by researchers over the years and there are a number of classic experiments in this area of social psychology.

Sherif (1935) used an optical illusion known as the 'autokinetic effect' to study conformity in groups; this effect occurs when a stationary point of light is viewed against a dark background and appears to move. Subjects were asked to judge the amount of movement of the point of light in two experimental conditions; one group made individual estimates and then came together as a group and the other group did this in the opposite way by making a group decision first and then making individual estimates. In both conditions, subject's individual judgements were influenced by the group norm for the amount of movement.

Asch (1956) studied conformity by using experiments that required subjects to judge the lengths of lines in comparison to a line of standard length. Subjects were seated in front of a screen and shown the standard line alongside three comparison lines and they had to say out loud which line was equal to the standard one. In reality, only one of the subjects was genuine, the remainder being confederates of the experimenter and these confederates all gave responses that were obviously wrong. About one-third of the genuine subjects gave judgements that were wrong, despite the evidence of their own eyes.

These two studies show that group pressure is a powerful agent for conformity, although one could argue that the Asch study shows that two-thirds of the subjects did not conform to group norms. It could also be said that the Asch experiment dealt with physical judgements, whereas normal social interaction is concerned very much more with social judgements, where there is no objective criteria for judgement.

It is useful to ask why subjects conform to a majority judgement; the prevailing notion has been that subjects fear rejection by the group if they deviate from the group norms, whereas conformity leads to rewards. This notion has been criticized as being too simplistic by Eiser (1980). He cites several studies that indicate that a consistent minority can influence the majority of a group to alter its position. Eiser argues that individuals may want to differentiate themselves in a group and that in certain circumstances, such innovation may be valued by the group if it leads to useful new directions.

Another phenomenon of group decision-making is that known as the 'risky shift'; groups who have to make decisions that involve risks tend to take riskier decisions as a group than when making individual decisions (Wallach and Kogan, 1965). This is explained by the notion of diffusion of responsibility, where individual responsibility for failure is diffused throughout the group, resulting in a feeling of less personal responsibility.

Diffusion of responsibility was also investigated by Latane and Darley (1968) who studied bystander intervention. Subjects were given questions to fill in purporting to be a consumer survey and were seated in a room either alone or with someone else. A simulated emergency was enacted in an adjoining room and the time subjects took to respond to this was measured. There were four experimental conditions in this study, the subject being either alone, with a friend, with a stranger or with a confederate of the experimenter. Results showed that subjects were much more likely to respond when alone than when with someone else, particularly a stranger. Again, responsibility for intervention is said to be diffused between two people and this has the effect of inhibiting social behaviour. Diffusion of responsibility may also explain the phenomenon called 'social loafing', where the output of individuals may reduce when he or she is part of a group, particularly if the individual contributions cannot be easily measured, as in clapping or pushing a car.

Social facilitation and inhibition

The presence of others can be either inhibiting or facilitating, depending upon the nature of the task. 'Audience effects' is the term given to the effects on an individual's performance of having other people observing it, whereas 'coaction effects' are those that result from other people actually performing alongside the individual in question. Coaction effects are very much in evidence in athletics, where pacemakers help athletes to increase their performance.

Bond and Titus (1983), reviewing a large number of studies on social facilitation, consider that task complexity is the main determinant of social facilitation. The presence of others has a facilitating effect on both speed and accuracy of performance with simple tasks, but decreases them when the task is complex.

Tajfel (1978) suggests that an individual's commitment to a group depends upon the contribution it makes to his or her sense of positive social identity. If it fails to provide this, the individual has several courses of action; he or she may leave the group, but this may not be possible if there are pressing reasons for remaining, such as employment or important values associated with membership. Alternatively, he or she may remain as a group member but try to improve the status of the group by some means, or he or she may attempt to justify the undesirable features of the group to make them acceptable. An example might be useful here to help in understanding Tajfel's notion. Let us take a trained nurse who entered nursing some years ago because he or she always wanted to be a nurse. Lately, this nurse may have felt that nursing had lost a lot of its standing as a desirable social role in comparison with other professions such as teaching or social work. One option is to leave nursing, but in the present climate of unemployment this may not be wise.

Instead, the nurse may mount a campaign to make nurses more autonomous from medical staff. Alternatively, he or she may attempt to justify the fall in status by attributing it to the growth of materialism in society and the lack of personal commitment to caring in young people nowadays.

Communication and interaction in groups

The study of communication and interaction in groups has tended to fall into two distinct types of approach – those in which the pattern of communication is under the control of the experimenter and those in which the natural pattern occurring during group interaction is observed. The former studies involve small numbers of subjects who work on a task, each of whom has an item of information necessary for successful completion of the task in question. Hence, subjects must pool their information and these experimental studies seek to explain which patterns of communication facilitate completion of the task (Bavelas, 1948; Leavitt, 1951; Mulder, 1960). Subjects were organized into four different patterns of communication (Figure 7.1) and could only communicate directly with those subjects with whom they were connected.

It can be seen that in each pattern there are differences in the number of other people that any particular subject has to go through in order to communicate with other members. In the chain, for example, subject number one has to relay their message through three people if he or she wishes to communicate with subject number five. In the circle, subject number one can communicate directly with both number five and number two; in the 'Y' pattern and the wheel, subject number three occupies a key position, which is often identified as leader. The speed of problem-solving was faster in the 'Y' pattern and the wheel, but as the really interesting role was performed largely by subject number three, peripheral members experienced less enjoyment than subjects in the circle. These findings are based on experimental groups set up specifically for the purpose, but a number of researchers have investigated groups interacting in a natural group setting, the best-known example being that of Bales (1950). He observed groups working in committees and classified the contributions of individual members into twelve main categories, as shown in Table 7.1.

These contributions are divided into two major areas, those concerned with the task in question and those termed social-emotional reactions, the latter being either positive or negative. Bales' system provides a method for analysing the working of a group in a systematic way.

Lawrence (1986) suggests that small groups develop through the following processes:

forming,
storming,
norming,
performing, and
informing.

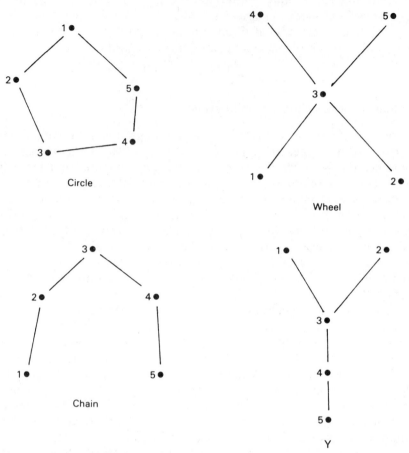

Fig. 7.1 Patterns of communication.

The first stage refers to individual commitments to the group, whilst storming refers to the stage of conflict and hostility within the group. This is followed by the stage of norming, in which the emphasis is on interaction and harmonious relationships. The performing stage is concerned with pursuance of the goals of the group and this is followed by informing, which involves the development of systems for communicating with other groups.

AIMS AND PURPOSES OF EDUCATIONAL SMALL GROUPS

There are many aims or purposes of small-group teaching in education; the main ones are outlined in Table 7.2.

It can be seen that the use of small-group teaching has benefits not only in terms of academic learning, but in the development of social skills and confidence in the presence of other people. In nursing, these social skills are vital to the proper functioning of the practitioner and the expressive skills that small-group work generates can make a significant contribution

Table 7.1 Bales' interaction process analysis

Reactions	Task area	Problems
Attempted answers	4. Gives suggestions, direction, implying autonomy for others. 5. Gives opinion, evaluation, analysis, expresses feeling, wish. 6. Gives orientation, information, repetition, confirmation.	Control, evaluation, orientation.
Questions	7. Asks for orientation, information, repetition, confirmation. 8. Asks for opinion, evaluation, analysis, expression of feeling. 9. Asks for suggestion, direction, possible ways of action.	Orientation, evaluation, control.
	Social-emotional area	
Positive	1. Shows solidarity, raises others' status, gives help, reward. 2. Shows tension release, jokes, laughs, shows satisfaction. 3. Agrees, shows passive acceptance, understands, concurs, complies.	Reintegration, tension-management, decision
Negative	10. Disagrees, shows passive rejection, formality, withholds help. 11. Shows tension, asks for help, withdraws out of field. 12. Shows antagonism, deflates others' status, defends or asserts self.	Decision, tension-reduction, reintegration.

to the political dimension of the profession by ensuring that nurses can argue effectively from their unique perspective.

REFLECTION IN SMALL-GROUP AND EXPERIENTIAL LEARNING

One of the most useful strategies for learning in small groups or experiential learning is reflection, and the teacher can assist the student in this process by using a model devised to promote reflection (Boud, Keogh and Walker, 1985). The model consists of a series of stages through which the student nurse should progress, having completed an experience. For example, the student may have completed a blanket bath on an elderly patient and some time later, takes time to reflect on this using the following stages.

Stage 1: Returning to the experience   During this first stage the student is encouraged to simply 'replay' the whole experience over again, describing what happened but not judging it.

Stage 2: Attending to feelings   The aim of this stage is to put students in touch with their own feelings about the experience. They should try to

Table 7.2 Aims and purposes of educational small groups

Area	Examples
Intellectual	Trying out ideas for size
	Clearing up misunderstandings
	Clarifying issues
	Follow-up of key lectures
	Development of critical, logical thinking
	Solving problems
	Examining evidence and assumptions
	Applying theory to practice
Affective	Self-evaluation
	Personal development and confidence
	Tolerance of ambiguity
	Motivation
	Attitude change
Social	Awareness of other people's strengths and weaknesses
	Sensitivity to others
	Identification with a group
	Group cohesion
	Ability to listen to others
	Tolerance of opposing viewpoints
	Independence
	Closer teacher–student relationships
Expressive	Developing power of expression
	Developing public-speaking skills
	Ability to formulate an argument
	Ability to engage in debate
Experiential	Participating in experiential activities
	Reflecting upon experiences
	Analysing the implications of the experience

utilize any positive feelings they may have about it, such as the pleasure felt at being complimented by the patient. Some feelings can actually form barriers to learning, so these need to be removed by such means as laughing about an embarrassing incident during the blanket bath or by expressing feelings to another person. This removal of obstructing feelings is vital if learning is to take place.

Stage 3: Re-evaluating the experience This final stage consists of a number of substages, which in essence involve the students in associating the experience with their existing ideas and feelings about blanket bathing and in testing for consistency between them.

This model of reflection needs to be practised until the students feels comfortable with each stage and this is best accomplished by sharing the reflections with other.

PLANNING AND IMPLEMENTATION

Steinaker and Bell (1979) describe an experiential taxonomy (Table 7.3) that can be used for all kinds of small-group teaching and learning. Their

Table 7.3 The experiential taxonomy

Taxonomic level	Description
1.0 Exposure	Consciousness of an experience
2.0 Participation	Deciding to become part of an experience
3.0 Identification	Union of the learner with what is to be learned
4.0 Internalization	Experience continues to influence lifestyle
5.0 Dissemination	Attempt to influence others

Source: Steinaker and Bell (1979).

Table 7.4 Nursing applications of experiential taxonomy

Taxonomic level	Nursing applications
1.0 Exposure	(i) I see an injection given. (ii) I hear about the nursing process.
2.0 Participation	(i) I administer an injection. (ii) I attempt to use nursing process.
3.0 Identification	(i) I become competent in giving injections. (ii) I become adept at nursing process.
4.0 Internalization	(i) Giving injections is now part of my life. (ii) Nursing process is now part of my life.
5.0 Dissemination	(i) I teach other students to give injections. (ii) I show other students how to use nursing process.

taxonomy can be used for a single lesson or for a complete curriculum unit. Table 7.4 shows two applications to nursing for each of the main categories.

The physical environment

As with all learning settings, the physical environment should be as pleasant and comfortable as the facilities allow. It is useful if particular rooms are designated as discussion rooms so that students associate them with democratic participation and equality. The main aspect of the physical environment, though, is the arrangement of seating (and desks if used). Some people feel that small-group methods are best when students are seated without desks, as this lends an air of informality to the group. Certain students, however, prefer to have a surface upon which they can jot down key thoughts, especially when the group is working on a specific task that requires writing. A good rule of thumb is to ensure that whether desks are used or not, every group member has the same facility, including the tutor. It is common to see a group of students sitting in a circle without desks, with a tutor firmly ensconced behind one; this inequality may serve to highlight the differences in status between tutor and students to the detriment of group effectiveness. There is a variety of arrangements for seating during group work, some of the common ones being illustrated in Figure 7.2.

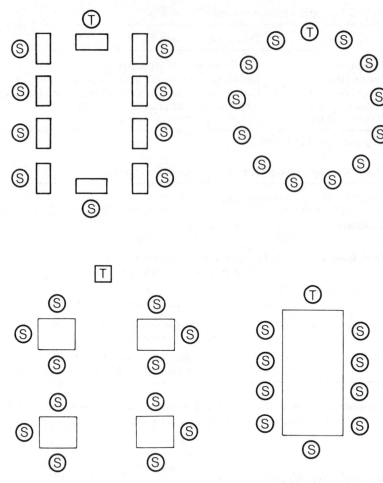

Fig. 7.2 Seating patterns for small-group teaching. S = student; T = teacher.

- The 'U' arrangement is useful for tutor-led discussion, as each member can be seen clearly and, equally, the students can see any material the teacher may want to show to them.
- The circle, with or without desks conveys a sense of equality amongst all members of the group; it is particularly intimate when chairs alone are used and even a group of 15 can create a feeling of close personal contact.
- The idea of a number of 'horseshoes', each consisting of a table around which three students are seated, can provide a very effective way of breaking larger groups into subgroups. The seating arrangement ensures that each student can see the tutor during plenary periods, but each 'horseshoe' can work independently with its members on some aspect of a topic or problem. This arrangement can also capitalize on shortage of space, where a large circle is not feasible.
- The 'committee' arrangement is a useful one for small groupwork that has more formal purposes, providing a large surface, in the form of a

central table, around which each member is seated. Although each member can engage in eye contact with the rest of the group, the shape of the table can make a big difference to the pattern of interaction. A rectangular table has a natural 'head' at either end, and students occupying these may be seen as the leader or chairperson, whereas a round table has no such natural positions of power. A rectangular table has corners and students occupying these seats tend to make the least contribution to discussions; people generally interact most with those sitting diametrically opposite, again this being more obvious in a rectangle than a circle.

One of the common errors that inexperienced teachers make is to rearrange seating in the classroom without adequate explanation to the group. Students of all ages tend to be quite sensitive about their personal seat and usually sit in the same place for all sessions. If they suddenly find that the seating arrangements have been altered they may become resentful; indeed, many an unwitting student tutor has entered a class-room only to find that their carefully-planned seating arrangement has been returned to its normal state by the students. Such, then, is the emotive nature of seating positions that the tutor must ensure full and adequate explanation as to why he or she is wishing to rearrange it. A few minutes spent in explaining one's philosophy of teaching and the import-ance of the students' contributions can save a great deal of trouble later on by giving students rational, sincere reasons for such a rearrangement. Students are usually tolerant of such innovations, provided they have been consulted before it is implemented. If a group is particularly resistant to rearrangement, it may be wise to leave the seating as it is, but to use a small-group activity early in the lesson that requires students to interact with others. This will encourage natural pairing and movement, which can be capitalized on for the remainder of the session.

Psychological environment

The ideal environment for small-group and experiential learning is that which is termed a 'learning community'. This is characterized by a climate of acceptance, support and trust, where each member of the team acknowledges that he or she is still learning and where the needs of students are recognized. This notion of a learning community can apply to both the college and the clinical or commnity area and contains an implicit value judgement that students are equal to trained staff in all respects other than those of age and experience. In a learning-community approach, opportunities for learning are made available and professional growth is encouraged by graded responsibility. A large element of negotiation is typical of this approach, where students can determine what they want to learn and the means by which this will be achieved and evaluated.

The establishment of trust among group members is fundamental to successful small-group and experiential learning. The length of time the small group is likely to be together is an important factor. For example, small-group techniques may be used on a study day, and in this short timescale it would be impossible to develop group identity. On a course or pathway, on the other hand, small groups may well remain together for months or years, and it is therefore crucial that the group is given the time and opportunity to foster interpersonal relationships and trust. This means that the tutor must avoid the temptation of setting the group tasks and issues too early. Taking time to facilitate group cohesion will pay dividends later on when the group is able to work effectively without interpersonal conflict and competition.

Techniques for fostering relationships in small groups

There are a great many ways in which small groups can be made aware of individual members. One technique is a pairs exercise which aims for maximum interaction.

Group members are asked to form pairs, choosing someone they do not know. Each member spends two minutes introducing himself to the other. After this, group members are asked to find another partner whom they do not know, and spend two minutes each on explaining what they hope to gain from the group membership. This pairing continues until all the group has met each other, using topics such as 'My feelings about small-group work', 'Problems in my current job', etc.

In another example, group members are asked to form pairs, and each member must choose a character from literature, theatre, films or television whom they would most like to be. They must explain the reason for their choice, taking up to two minutes to do this.

When members of a small group trust each other, they are able to contribute without fear of being ridiculed if their suggestion seems wrong; indeed, such suggestions may be seen as creative rather than stupid and may lead the group into a new direction. Students need to be able to try out their ideas, and this can only be encouraged in an atmosphere of psychological safety. Where there is trust in a group, each student is free to concentrate his or her energies on learning, rather than wasting them on building up defensive barriers against attacks from other group members. Trust may be developed using techniques which involve the group members in such activities as being led around the room blindfold. Other examples are given in Chapter 13. Yet another important way in which trust can be developed is the use of group evaluation at the end of each session. The group is asked to allow five minutes at the end for some spontaneous evaluation of the group's performance.

Participation of the tutor

There are many roles that the tutor can adopt in small-group work; he or she may function as the leader, taking the major responsibility for the conduct of the group, or alternatively, adopt varying degrees of involvement, such as facilitator, resource person and group trainer.

The presence of the tutor is more likely to influence a very small group, but be less obtrusive in a larger group. Indeed, the tutor may decide to leave the group entirely on their own during group work, but being available close by, but out of sight, should the group feel they need assistance. If the tutor decides to be involved in the group, there is always the danger that they will see the tutor as the leader, even if the position has been made clear that the tutor's function is as facilitator only. The tutor's role is invested with authority and it is difficult for students to overcome this barrier. Compare the interaction of a group of student nurses talking in the local pub and their contributions in a small-group learning session. It is obvious that lack of knowledge or interest is not the main factor for the poor response so commonly found in group work; rather, it is the climate of the situation that determines how well students involve themselves in discussions. Presumably, in the local pub there is no danger of humiliation from other people, since it is generally accepted that individuals have the right to express their opinions, however unusual these might be. In addition, the group in the pub are usually friends and a degree of trust is present, which adds to the climate of psychological safety. If this atmosphere can be captured during group work in the college of nursing, then there would be fewer problems of participation. Very often it is the tutor's own anxiety that stifles the spontaneous flow of ideas and opinions; the tutor must learn to trust the group to control their own discussion to a large extent, even if he or she is acting as their leader. If the tutor leads the group, then it is vital that he or she avoids evaluating the members, since they may become hesitant about giving their own opinions. Many of the dissatisfactions that are experienced with the use of small groups stem from the fact that they have not been properly organized. Because a small group is informal does not mean that it can be conducted in an off-the-cuff manner, and it is sensible to indicate to the students the goals to be achieved and the roles they must assume during the discussion. Each member must be prepared to contribute something to the group, and the importance of this should be explained at the first meeting. The teacher must be aware of attempts to participate by members and, if these are unsuccessful, should assist. A careful watch of non-verbal communication will provide good feedback as to how the students are feeling, and will also reveal such non-productive behaviour as opting out, dominating and seeking sympathy. It is possible to identify four styles that the tutor might adopt during smallgroup teaching (Royal College of General Practitioners, 1986): authoritarian, Socratic, heuristic and the counselling style.

The authoritarian style This style is one in which the tutor is seen as the authority – telling the students what is important and asking questions, largely to clarify whether they understand. There is no place for dissent or argument; the tutor's view is the correct one.

The Socratic style This ancient style relies on a question-and-answer technique, with the tutor asking questions and the student answering

Table 7.5 Role of the teacher in experiential learning

Taxonomic level	Role of teacher
1.0 Exposure	Motivator
2.0 Participation	Catalyst
3.0 Identification	Moderator
4.0 Internalization	Sustainer
5.0 Dissemination	Critic and evaluator

them. The tutor's questions are not random, but are used to elicit what the student knows, with each answer acting as a stimulus for the next question. The tutor only supplies information when it is apparent that the student does not know the answer. This technique is really intended for individual students, but it is a style that many tutors adopt during small-group work, with the answers being supplied by the group as a whole rather than by a single individual.

The heuristic style   This style acknowledges that both tutor and students have areas of shared knowledge and ignorance and that both parties also have areas of knowledge that the other lacks. This style puts the student in a position of responsibility for finding out information.

The counselling style   This focuses on the student's feelings about the material to be learned and about their interaction with the tutor. The goal is for the students to understand their own behaviour and this is accomplished by the use of reflective questions and other counselling techniques.

In the experiential taxonomy referred to earlier, the role of the teacher changes as the student ascends the hierarchy of levels, as shown in Table 7.5.

SOME COMMON DIFFICULTIES

The teacher may find that difficulties arise from time to time in a small group and these require sensitive handling. It is usually better to deal with them as they arise, but occasionally it may be necessary to have a private word with a group member after the session has finished. A common problem in small-group discussion is that of all the members talking at once, which leads to a chaotic situation where no progress is made. The teacher should exert firm, friendly control to bring the session to order and a sense of humour is invaluable in keeping the atmosphere informal, while at the same time maintaining order. Very often there is a vocal member of a group who tends to monopolize the session and it is important not to 'squash' them, as motivation can easily be lost. Ignoring the contributions may lead to extinction of the response, but it usually makes the student feel hurt and resentful. Possibly the best solution is to remind them gently that other group members need a chance to air their views also.

A similar problem is that of the student who attempts to engage the tutor in a dialogue, to the exclusion of the rest of the group. This often arises when a student wishes to show that he or she has a particular piece of knowledge or expertise that the other students do not. Again, sensitive handling is required and a particularly useful strategy is to deliberately open out the dialogue to the rest of the group by using such statements as, 'You are raising some interesting points here, would anyone else like to comment or react to any of them?'

Group discussions can become very heated, especially when debating an issue that is emotionally charged, such as abortion. However, conflict is not always undesirable, as productive conflict can be an effective aid to learning. It is useful to reassure the group that disagreement is quite in order, but that it should be the opinion of another group member that is questioned and not that person as an individual. Each group member is respected, but his or her opinions are open to challenge and disagreement. Occasionally, the teacher may be confronted with an emotional outburst by a group member and one of the most dramatic of all gestures is that of a student walking out of the group. It is always difficult to know how best to handle such a situation. Resisting the temptation to follow the individual, the tutor should stay with the group and attempt to help them to realize that such behaviour (flight, rather than fight) is one way that people have of coping with anxiety or anger; it is important to convey to the group that this is not a major disaster. However, it is extremely important for the welfare of the group as a whole that the tutor make contact with the distressed student before the next group meeting to discuss the incident with a view to deciding how best to raise it with the group. Whilst every student has the right to behave in this way when under stress, the tutor cannot ignore the effects of such behaviour on the rest of the group. It might be that at the next meeting the student concerned with the incident should be invited to make a statement to the group about their feelings at the time and thus use the incident as a positive learning experience for all concerned.

Another common problem in small groups is that of the student who is unwilling to participate. Arguably, every individual has the 'right to remain silent' but this obviates the whole purpose of an educational small group. However, the tutor must acknowledge that students will differ in the degree of confidence they possess for making public contributions and this may be due to a variety of factors including basic personality, lack of knowledge, feelings of lack of personal worth or inadequate preparation. On the other hand, it may be the tutor's own style that is inhibiting a student; if the climate of the group is not conducive to psychological safety, then it is unlikely that students will risk contributing to discussion, lest they be humiliated or made to feel inadequate in some way. The previous background and experience of students will also influence their desire to contribute to group discussions; in certain cultures, the teacher is seen very much as an expert who is not to be questioned and this may be difficult to overcome. Childhood experience of college teachers who humiliated students may have left scars that ensure that the student is never again put in such a position. Some of these factors may be impossible to change, although the tutor can do a great deal to ensure that the group members are valued and respected. Students can be invited into the discussion by gentle questioning, particularly in areas that rely upon student opinion rather than hard fact, since there is no likelihood of giving an incorrect answer. It may well be that such reticent students require more specific help in the building up of confidence in public, by a systematic programme of interaction that begins in pairs and gradually builds up to larger numbers, but such provision has obvious resource implications for the college or department of nursing.

BASIC CLASSIFICATION OF SMALL-GROUP TEACHING

The classification of small-group teaching presents a major conceptual problem, in that there is a bewildering array of possible types. It is useful to distinguish between these basic types of small group and the various techniques that might be used with each. For example, role-playing is really a technique that can be used in many types of small group, so it is not included here as a basic type of group. On the other hand, 'syndicate work' seems to have a very specific function and is structured in a particular way, and is thus seen as a basic type of group. The following section explores a number of basic types of small groups in education, and the various techniques that might be used as part of these basic types of group.

Tutorial groups

This is perhaps the commonest type of group to be found in colleges of nursing, yet it can take many different kinds of form. It is often used synonymously with the term 'seminar': it can also mean a one-to-one encounter with a student, an encounter with three or four students and a tutor, or can be synonymous with a controlled discussion. Clearly, the purpose of the tutorial group will largely determine its organization; a one-to-one tutorial is usually related to individual student progress and comments upon specific aspects of the student's work. The same kind of function can be achieved with three or four students together, although this may inhibit some individuals from speaking as freely as they might if they were alone.

The term 'tutorial group' is often used for convenience to describe the collection of personal tutees for whom a tutor has responsibility, and there may be a great many different purposes for such a group.

Seminar groups

A seminar group is mainly concerned with academic matters rather than with individual students and commonly involves the reading of an essay or paper by one group member, followed by a discussion by the total group on the topic. The teacher may decide to be the leader, or may delegate leadership to the group. It can be a motivating strategy in nursing, where a student presents a paper on some aspect of nursing and then participates in a discussion with the group. The presentation of a seminar by the student can be counted as an assignment for continuous assessment purposes and this may serve as a motivating factor in ensuring a good-quality seminar.

Controlled-discussion groups

In this form of discussion group the teacher assumes leadership and the purpose is to clarify points raised during a lecture and to develop the ideas that it contained. Thus it can provide feedback to the teacher on the level of understanding achieved in a lecture and gives an opportunity for further explanation if the students have any difficultiess with regard to the subject-matter.

Free-discussion groups

In contrast to the controlled discussion, this type of discussion is under the control of the group members and the teacher acts merely as an observer and resource person. The topics and direction are decided by the group. This can be a useful method in nursing for developing autonomy in the students, by giving them responsibility for their own learning. In addition, the fact that the topic has been chosen by the students may increase the motivation of the group.

Issue-centred or subject-centred groups

An issue-centred group has as its focus an issue that has no right or wrong answer, and which is usually controversial or provocative. Topics such as 'Is nursing a profession?' or 'Should resuscitation be carried out on the terminally ill?' provide an opportunity for students' opinions to be questioned and attitudes to be changed. It also provides a forum for public presentation of an individual student's own beliefs and values and gives practice in the efficient presentation of arguments.

Step-by-step discussion groups

This involves a prepared sequence of material designed by the tutor and consisting of key questions or issues that are to be used to draw out the students' own knowledge about the topic. It utilizes inductive technique rather than didactic presentation.

Problem-solving groups

In this form of small-group discussion the students are given a problem to solve and are usually provided with certain sources of information from which to draw their solutions. The problem may be something that requires a single correct answer, or may involve a number of correct answers, the students being required to decide which one is most appropriate to the situation. There are eight steps in the systematic approach to problem-solving (Barker *et al.*, 1979) in small-group discussion.

1. Define the problem.
2. Limit the problem to allow coverage during the session.
3. Analyse the problem by collecting evidence and facts.
4. Establish criteria that any solutions must meet.
5. Suggest possible solutions.
6. Check solutions against criteria.
7. Implement the solution.
8. Evaluate the success of the solution.

The main purpose of problem-solving groups is to encourage critical thinking by the students and this method has had considerable success in the teaching of medicine at McMaster University in Canada. The nursing faculty there has also developed a problem-solving approach to nurse education, using real and simulated patients. A common strategy for problem-solving groups is to present a detailed case history of a patient and then to ask specific questions related to nursing or medical science. The students are required to define the problems and to devise nursing measures that will help to overcome these. I have had experience of using a problem-solving approach in a pre-registration nursing course. The students were not given any input in the usual subject areas, but instead were given two case histories of patients, one during the first three weeks and one for the last three weeks of the foundation module. Problem-solving groups were used to work on the solutions and the students had to identify the areas of knowledge that they needed to explore.

The use of problem-solving groups encourages critical thinking and is also motivating, as the solutions are provided by the group and not simply passively acquired during a lecture situation. Allen and Murrell (1978) offer further details of the above problem-solving situations.

LTD (learning-through-discussion) groups

LTD (learning through discussion) groups were described by Fawcett-Hill (1969) and are similar in some respects to the free group discussion outlined above. However, in an LTD group, the topic is decided by the teacher rather than the students. The teacher's role in LTD is that of resource person and group trainer only; they do not take part as a group member. The roles normally taken by a teacher or chairperson are seen to be the responsibility of each and every group member. Fawcett-Hill maintains that students have little preparation for involvement in small-group work and so need to have a plan by which to proceed. The purpose of this method is to enhance learning of course material by utilizing the skill of each group member.

Table 7.6 Example of a group cognitive map for anxiety in hospital patients

Step 1   Definitions
Anxiety, fear, phobia, stress, tension, psychoanalytic, id, ego, super-ego,
learning theory, limbic system, reticular activating system, coping mechanisms

Step 2   General statement of message
'Nurses can help prevent anxiety in patients by the use of thoughtful nursing
care and interaction.'

Step 3   Identification of major themes and sub-themes
1. Psychology of anxiety
     (a) Definition of terms
     (b) Theories of anxiety
     (c) Effects of anxiety
            physiological
            psychological
     (d) Measurement of anxiety
2. Nursing the patient in situations of anxiety
     (e) Admission to hospital
     (f) Prior to surgery
     (g) Dying

Step 4   Allocation of time
   Step   Time
   5   5 min
   6   5 min
   7   15 min
   8   20 min
   9   5 min

Step 5   Discussion of major themes and sub-themes

Step 6   Integration of material
e.g. relate to patients whom you have nursed with anxiety.

Step 7   Application of material
e.g. to next ward allocation, when dealing with pre-operative patients.

Step 8   Evaluation of author's (lecturer's) standpoint

Step 9   Evaluation of the group's performance

There are three parts to the LTD method, the group cognitive map,
group roles and skills and criteria for an effective group. The group
cognitive map is a plan that gives a rational sequence of steps for the
group to follow, thus minimizing the possibility of aimless discussion. An
example is given in Table 7.6.

The group will have been given some assignment to read prior to the
meeting and the cognitive map is designed to guide the group through
their discussion of it. Steps 1 to 3 of the cognitive map are concerned with

1. defining the terms and concepts of the assignment,
2. stating the main message, and
3. identifying the major themes and sub-themes.

Step 5 allows discussion of the main themes and sub-themes, from the
author's point of view, while step 6 attempts to integrate the material with
the student's past learning thus applying it to real life situations. Step 8

involves the personal opinions and feelings of the group members. Obviously, this method can be applied to discussion of a lecture, not just of reading.

The second part of the LTD method is group roles and member skills. In order for the group to be successful, each member must assume the following roles when appropriate: initiating the discussion, volunteering and requesting information and reactions, rephrasing and exemplifying points, confronting other members' contributions, clarifying and summarizing, timekeeping, spreading the participation by inviting members to comment, encouraging others to contribute by giving praise, etc., relieving tension by joking, evaluating and setting standards for the group's work. It often takes some time for these roles to be internalized in each group member, but once this has occurred the group will become truly efficient. There are a number of non-productive roles that Fawcett-Hill identifies, which must not be allowed to happen in the group. Behaviours such as aggression, withdrawing, fooling around, status-seeking, dominating, seeking sympathy, pushing a special interest and competing are all counter-productive to the aims of a group and each member is responsible for watching for these.

The third part of the method is the criteria for an effective group. Fawcett–Hill outlines the main criteria which must be present for a successful group.

- The climate must be warm, non-threatening and psychologically safe.
- Learning is approached as a co-operative venture.
- Learning is seen as the main reason for the group. Everyone participates and interacts.
- Leadership is distributed throughout the group.
- The sessions are enjoyable.
- Material is covered adequately and efficiently.
- Evaluation is an integral part of the function of the group.
- Members come prepared and attend regularly.

The LTD method can be a very powerful tool for small-group discussion, and the time spent training the students will be amply rewarded by the learning achieved. This kind of group work has implications far beyond the learning task being considered. The member roles and skills provide sound training for future committee work and stimulate the development of responsibility for one's own learning. An LTD group can function without the teacher even being present. It is better not to try to teach every small-group session by this method, as the constant use of any method will lead to boredom on the part of the student. My own experience of this method has convinced me that it provides an interesting form of learning for group members, and also encourages strong interpersonal relationships between them. Any teacher attempting this method for the first time should be aware that the group will feel initial frustration until the method has been internalized and should thus provide considerable support and encouragement in the early part of the group training.

Syndicate groups

This type of group is valuable for putting students in a position for discovery learning. The total class is given a major topic and then dividedinto small groups of about six members. Each of these small groups selects one aspect of the major topic and studies this over a period of two weeks or so. Contact with the teacher is maintained intermittently to report progress. When the work has been completed, each group reports its findings to the total group, after which the findings are assessed and interpreted by the teacher and a grade awarded.

Project groups

The project method can be defined as a unit of purposeful experience in which the educational needs and interests of the student determine the aims and objectives of the activity and guide its process to a conclusion. The main characteristics of the method are that the students are very much involved in the formulation of the aims and objectives of the project and that they are actively participating in the learning experience. Projects may be done by individuals, but more commonly they are undertaken by a small group of about six members. The main topics can be suggested by the teacher, or left completely to the student's imagination, but in both cases it is crucial for the teacher to ensure that the aims of the project are clarified, so that the students are in no doubt as to the purpose of such an exercise. The kinds of aims that a group project can foster are the ability to work co-operatively in groups, collection of information, development of confidence in decision-making and many others.

For the project method to be successful, it is necessary to have motivated students and this in turn requires subject-matter areas that are seen to be interesting and to contain scope for individuality and imagination. It is common for students to be required to undertake community-based projects such as a neighbourhood study, and this allows the students scope to be imaginative. For example, when doing a neighbourhood study, one of my small-groups decided to focus their project on access to local facilities by individuals confined to a wheelchair. One of the students sat in a borrowed wheelchair and two other students accompanied him to the local shopping centre. This was an example of experiential learning for the students, as it soon became apparant that it was extremely difficult to withdraw money from a cashpoint due to the position of the dispenser on the wall of the bank. Similarly, the students tried to gain access to a well-known tourist attraction, but found that it was impossible to do so in a wheelchair. The findings of the students were reported back to the rest of the group, and provided very thought-provoking discussion about life in a wheelchair.

The project method itself is not a new development, having its origins in the 1920s. The method was first described by John Dewey of Columbia University and further developed by his colleague W.H. Kilpatrick. Dewey's philosophy was that the process of educational thought was more important than the results of such thought, and he believed that a child would undergo mental growth if he actively participated in solving a problem that he saw as real. Use of the project method declined in the 1950s, but with the advent of the Nuffield Foundation Science Teaching Project and the personal topic in the Certificate of Secondary Education, interest in the method has revived. A number of advantages are claimed for the use of the project method, including greater interest for the student, development of resourcefulness and independence in learning and the opportunity for the student to use important skills such as the identification and analysis of problems and the exploration of solutions. On the other hand, this method has its critics, and the main disadvantages are the time-consuming nature of project work and the difficulty in evaluating the student's achievement.

When planning to use the project method for the first time, the teacher of nursing should ensure that the exercise is carefully organized. Groups may be allocated by the teacher, or selected by the students according to personal preference. The latter has the advantage of allowing them to work with friends, which may increase motivation and spur their efforts to succeed. As indicated earlier, it is important for the teacher to clarify the purpose of the project so that the enthusiasm and co-operation of the groups are obtained and it is equally necessary to allocate sufficient time for the work to be accomplished.

When the groups have chosen, or have been allocated, a specific subject area then they decide amongst themselves which objectives and methods of inquiry they will use. The teacher must not control the direction of approach, as this would stifle independence and enthusiasm. The progress of each group's project should be monitored by the teacher, but only to ensure that difficulties are being overcome and that the most efficient techniques of data collection are being used. The channels for obtaining information from personnel in the hospital or community must be clearly understood by the group. It is important to check that personnel who are likely to be approached by students are willing to spend time talking to them. The form of presentation of the projects should be decided before the students commence their work. All projects should be written up regardless of the form of presentation and the teacher can negotiate with the group as to whether the projects are presented to the total group, or simply submitted to the teacher in written form. My own preference is for a presentation to the total group, as this is seen as the culmination of the students' work and reinforces their feelings of accomplishment and success. Assessment of project work is often considered difficult, owing to the subjectivity of the work, but it is possible to develop a more objective assessment scheme. The National Association of Teachers in Further and Higher Education (NATFHE, 1976) have produced an assessment scheme for project work, which involves awarding marks or grades for the following aspects:

- comprehension of the task and the establishment of project objectives;
- collection, selection and collation of information;
- design and application of experimental procedures;

- collation and analysis of results; and
- presentation of the final project.

Hirst and Biggs (1969) assessed mathematics projects under four headings: exposition, use of literature, originality and scope of topic.

Small-group projects, then give students the opportunity for more intensive study of a topic, challenging them to seek more widely for resources and giving experience in the skills of problem-solving and decision-making, all of which are important for the changing role of the nurse.

Experiential learning groups

These groups are characterized by the use of experiential techniques to develop greater expertise in a variety of fields, for example, interpersonal communication skills (discussed in Chapter 18) and research and enquiry skills (discussed in Chapter 19). There are other applications of experiential learning that may not at first be obvious. For example, 'health promotion' is seen as an increasingly important aspect of the role of nurse and midwife, and forms a component of curricula at pre-registration and post-registration level. It is commonly taught as an 'academic' topic by lectures and discussion, but there is an excellent approach devised by the Health Education Authority and called the 'Look After Your Heart' (LAYH) project, which is targeted at the general public. However, it offers the potential for experiential involvement for students and teachers when teaching health promotion. The programme has three main components:

1. *Exercise and health* This involves dynamic exercises that are graded according to the level of fitness of the participants, and safety is ensured by regular pulse-rate monitoring and perceived exertion monitoring. The exercises are varied, and utilize group support for motivation and enjoyment. They are not time-consuming, and can take as little as half an hour, three times a week.
2. *Stress and relaxation* This involves both information about the nature and management of stress, and also a basic relaxation programme of ten lessons covering all muscle groups.
3. *Healthy eating and other health topics* This involves information about healthy eating, energy balance and weight loss, heart disease, cancer, and uses and abuses of drugs.

The LAYH programme can be readily incorporated into nursing curricula as part of a module on health promotion, and is a very good strategy for encouraging students and staff to participate in exercise and relaxation. Rather than simply being told about the value of exercise, students can undertake the actual exercise programme, and should see the benefits on their fitness levels quite early on in the programme. Similarly, undertaking relaxation on a regular basis is not something many students will have experienced, and this in itself can be a valuable way of learning. By using an experiential approach such as LAYH, the learning of health promotion principles becomes much more personally relevant to the student.

Table 7.7 Categories of techniques for small-group teaching

Category	Techniques
1. Techniques to maximize group members' interaction with each other	Snowball groups; square-root or crossover groups; buzz groups
2. Techniques to generate creative solutions	Brainstorming; synectics
3. Techniques to generate data	Carousel exercise
4. Techniques to develop group members' self-awareness and empathy	Role-play; simulation; gaming; case-study
5. Techniques to develop group members' presentational ability	Debate; seminar; peer-tutoring; microteaching; square-root technique
6. Techniques for applying knowledge and skills to real-life	Role-play; simulation; case-study; brainstorming
7. Techniques to develop group members' awareness of group processes	Fishbowl technique; peer review; group-interaction analysis

Synergogy groups

Synergogy utilizes the notion of synergy, i.e. that the sum of the work of a group of individuals is greater than that of any individual alone. The central concept is teamwork, and the synergogy system involves the use of peer-tutoring and teamwork for the achievement of specific outcomes. The system is described in detail in Chapter 4 (p. 107).

TECHNIQUES USED

So far we have identified some twelve basic types of small group in education, each having fairly specific purposes or functions. Within any one of these twelve basic types, there are a number of techniques that might be employed to help group members to achieve the purpose of the small group. Again, it is useful to categorize them according to their main purpose, although some techniques have a wide range of application (Table 7.7) and to give an outline of each of the techniques mentioned in the Table.

'Snowball' groups

As the name implies, this technique involves group members in subgroups of ever-increasing size until the total group is involved together. It begins with each individual group member working on a problem and then sharing this information in pairs. Each pair then joins with another pair for further work on the problem and then these tetrads join with each other to form groups of eight. Work continues in this fashion until the

Table 7.8 Square-root technique for a total group of 16 members

Group A	Group B	Group C	Group D
A1	B1	C1	D1
A2	B2	C2	D2
A3	B3	C3	D3
A4	B4	C4	D4

entire group comes together to share its ideas in a plenary session. The work can become progressively more detailed as the 'snowball' grows and this technique is useful for getting every member of the group involved in participation.

'Square-root' or 'crossover' groups

This technique is extremely useful in a number of ways, the starting point being the number of students in the total group. The tutor takes this total number and forms a series of horseshoe-shaped groups, each containing the number of students that equals the square root of the total group. Thus, if there are 16 students, each horseshoe group will contain four students; if there are 25 students, each horseshoe group will contain five students.

Each student is then given a card with a letter and a number on it, which determines the group in which each student starts, as shown in Figure 7.3 for a group of 16. After an appropriate amount of time spent in discussion of an issue or problem, the groups disband and reform according to their numbers, i.e. all the number ones form a group, as do all the number twos, number threes and number fours. This means that each contains only one member of the original group, thus giving the maximum exchange of ideas. At the commencement of the new groups, each member is required to give a summary of what their previous group's findings were and this also helps to break the ice in the new group.

'Buzz' groups

Buzz groups consist of from two to six members and are most frequently used to provide student involvement during a lecture or other teacher-centred session. For example, during a lecture on post-operative nursing care, the large class can be asked to form 'buzz' groups to discuss the complications of surgery for three or four minutes. The group leaders then feed back their contributions to the total group. It is often a good idea simply to ask the first row to turn and face the second and the third to turn and face the fourth and so on. These rows can then be segmented into groups of six students and this system minimizes the reorganization of the room. Buzz groups can be used more than once in any given lecture, and provide the students with social activity and involvement, helping to maintain their level of arousal during the lecture. It is often a useful way to begin a session to ask them to form buzz groups and write down everything they know about a subject, for example, the structure of the heart. This can be fed into the main group and forms the basis of the lecture.

'Brainstorming'

This is another effective method of obtaining creative solutions to a problem (Osborne, 1962). The idea is for each member to generate as many ideas as they can about the problem in question. The emphasis is on free expression of ideas, and no criticism is permitted, however unlikely the suggestions. De Bono (1986) suggest that there are three main features of a brainstorming session: 'cross-stimulation', 'suspended judgement' and a 'formal setting'. Cross-stimulation refers to the effects of other people's ideas on an individual and the fact that these ideas may interact with existing ones to produce creative solutions. As the name implies, suspended judgement means that no criticism of suggestions is allowed, however silly the ideas may seem. It is important that the leader or chairperson be on the lookout for any evaluative comments and stop them immediately. It is not vital to produce entirely new or novel ideas; indeed, it may be that an old idea is the best solution to a difficulty in certain situations.

A formal setting is important so that participants can feel that there is something special about the group and thus be less inhibited about saying things that might seem ridiculous. The organization of a brainstorming group involves a leader or chairperson and someone to make notes of the ideas as they arise; it is helpful to use audiotape recording to ensure that no ideas are lost. The brainstorming activity can take any amount of time up to a maximum of about 30–40 minutes, and frequently lasts only some 5–10 minutes.

The activity itself is only a means to an end, so there has to be an evaluation session in order to see what the next steps should be. This evaluation should take place some little time after the brainstorming session itself, and involves the sifting out of all the useful ideas into three categories – those ideas that are of immediate use, those that need further exploration and those that represent new approaches.

Synectics

Synectics is a system of problem-solving that aims to produce creative solutions by making people view problems in new ways. Creative ideas are seen as involving the making of new connections between ideas, and one way of facilitating this is the use of the 'SES Box Steps' method (SES Associates, 1986). This method is based on the assumption that all problems contain a paradox or contradiction that can only be solved if new connections can be made. It uses the notions of analogy and metaphor to create these new connections and there are four distinct steps in the process:

1. identify the paradox, which is the essence of the problem;
2. develop an analogy or metaphor to provide a creative, different viewpoint;
3. identify the unique activity associated with the metaphor or analogy; and
4. apply equivalent thinking, in which the unique activity is transferred to the current problem, resulting in a new idea for its solution.

An example will be useful to help understanding of this series of stages. Consider the following problems. A health visitor wishes to put on classes in health education for mothers of young children, but despite much advertising there is a very poor turnout.

Step 1: Paradox
Health education classes tend to interfere with the informal social interaction such as visiting friends or attending coffee mornings with other mothers and young children.

Step 2: Analogy
Tupperware parties are well attended by mothers and young children, and have become established on a national basis.

Step 3: Unique activity
The Tupperware salesperson combines business with a social setting, including company and refreshments.

Step 4: Equivalent thinking
The health visitor must combine the business of health education with an opportunity for social interaction. This means she must organize her classes as social events by providing refreshments and an atmosphere of informality.

The 'carousel' exercise

This is an excellent and novel way of generating data from a group of students and also for the development of interviewing skills. The first step is for the tutor to identify a series of topics or sub-topics that will be the focus of the session. The group is then divided into two, half of whom will be interviewers and the other half who will be respondents. Each interviewer is given a sheet of paper that is blank apart from a question that is written across the top of the page. The desks are arranged in a circle, with the interviewers seated on the inside facing out and the respondents seated on the outside facing in (Figure 7.3).

This arrangement ensures that there is a pair of students sitting opposite one another and separated by a desk. At a given signal from the tutor, each interviewer proceeds to ask their respondent to answer the question at the top of their sheet of paper and to answer it as fully as possible. Each interviewer has a different question and five minutes is allowed for each interview, after which time the tutor signals 'all change' and the outer circle of interviewees moves round to the next seat on each person's right. The inner circle of interviewers remain in the same position throughout the exercise and every five minutes, a new respondent arrives opposite

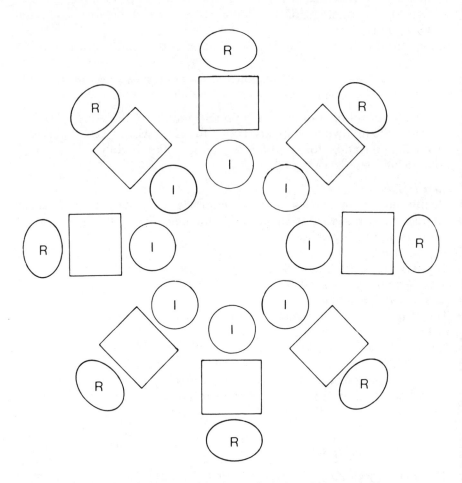

Fig. 7.3 Carousel exercise – arrangement of seating. R = respondent, I = interviewer.

each of them. They proceed to ask their question to each respondent as they appear, recording the various answers on the same sheet of paper.

Eventually, all the outer circle will have been interviewed by each of the interviewers and the latter will have a sheet of different responses to their question. This data can then be analysed to reveal the opinions of those group members who were in the outer circle. It is desirable to then exchange the roles, so that the outer group become the interviewers and vice versa, thus generating twice as much data for analysis.

Simulations

A simulation is an imitation of some facet of life, usually in a simplified form. It aims to put students in a position where they can experience some aspect of real life by becoming involved in activities that are closely related to it. Airline pilots spend time working in flight simulators, which are identical to the flight deck of an aircraft and in which the pilots can gain simulated experience of handling emergencies that cannot (for safety and/or expense reasons) be gained in any other way. For example, they are able to practise emergency procedures for such things as sudden depressurization, failure of engines, etc., and this experience should transfer to the real-life setting, if it is ever required. The notion of 'transfer of learning' underpins all aspects of simulation, the aim being to use the simulated experience to help the student to learn how to cope with the real thing.

In nursing, a commonly used simulation is that of the cardiac-arrest procedure or 'crash-call'. The tutor organizes the simulation by providing an authentic environment that simulates a ward setting, with a 'patient' in a bed, a locker, charts, etc. Certain staff or students are designated roles such as anaesthetist, sister, relatives and nurses and the whole scenario of what happens when a patient has a cardiac arrest is enacted. The scenario can be used to give student nurses an insight into how the procedure operates and in this instance, would serve a demonstration. Alternatively, students can be asked to take the part of the student who discovers a patient with a cardiac arrest and to imitate the procedures required following such detection. By this means it is possible to give the student experience of a situation, without the associated anxiety of learning it initially in the real-life setting. It is always debatable whether or not there is 'transfer of learning' to the real-life setting, but at the very least, the student will have had an opportunity to internalize the sequence of procedures required and to appreciate the urgency of the whole situation. One of the important hallmarks of a simulation is that the students are not required to act out any kind of script; they are expected to behave and react in any way they feel is appropriate. In other words, a simulation involves the students in 'being themselves, and dealing with situations using their normal, everyday behaviour. Whatever the scenario of the simulation may be, the students are expected to be themselves and to deal with the situations presented.

One of the most valuable areas in which simulation can be used is that of first aid. Although this topic has some theoretical basis, the main emphasis is on practical techniques, so it is important to teach first aid in a way that helps students to cope with real-life situations. I prefer to use the first part of each session introducing the concepts in question and then demonstrating the techniques required. I then invite volunteers to join in with a simulation, in which they are required to give first-aid treatment to a 'casualty', and the simulation should be as realistic as possible within the limitations of the college setting. With a little imagination and dramatic flair it is quite possible to create a scenario that simulates to a reasonable extent a first-aid emergency such as a head injury, a fracture, poisoning and the like. The aim is to create a simulation that is as near as possible to the real-life situation that the student will encounter, so that the established behaviours and procedures can be transferred easily to the new setting.

The term 'simulation' is closely related to the concepts of role-play and gaming; indeed, many simulations will involve an element of role-playing by other people, even though the student in question remains themselves. For example, a tutor may wish to do a simulation involving the admission of a mentally disturbed patient to the admission ward. A student is first identified who will be the admitting nurse, whilst another student or tutor will undertake the role of the disturbed patient. In this scenario, one nurse will be acting out the role of a disturbed patient, i.e. he or she will indulge in role-play; the other nurse, however, will simply behave and react in the way they feel appropriate in order to carry out the admission, i.e. they remains themselves throughout the simulation.

When carrying out simulations, it is important that the tutor should give full briefing beforehand and allow sufficient time for an adequate debriefing at the end. These aspects are discussed in the next section on role-play.

Role-play

Role-play is derived largely from the work of Moreno on psychodrama, and utilizes acting and imagination to create insights into the student's own behaviour, beliefs and values and those of other people. Students are required to take on someone else's identity and to act as they think that person would behave. Although some scripting is essential to delineate the role, this should be kept to a minimum so that the student can act out the role in their own way. Role-play can be an excellent way of creating empathy with other people's points of view, particularly if the student is given a role that is opposite to the position or viewpoint currently held. This counter-attitudinal role-play forces the students to consider issues and feelings from the other person's point of view and can help them to gain insight into why that person's behaviour is occurring. One of the important points about role-play is that the student, after some initial self-consciousness about the role in question, then quickly settles down to project their own character and values into the role. It is this identification with the role that forms the basis for subsequent debriefing and experiential learning. Role-play can be used for almost any social situation and is the method *par excellence* for exploring interpersonal communication skills. Some examples of brief role scripts are given in Table 7.9 and a checklist for organizing role-play is given in Table 7.10.

As mentioned earlier, a vital part of the process of role-playing is that of briefing and debriefing of participants. Briefing is an important preliminary process prior to many kinds of small-group activity and is particularly pertinent to role-playing situations. Briefing involves giving prior guidelines about rules, intentions and goals, and is designed to ensure that participants benefit from the subsequent activities. It is not necessary to declare the outcomes beforehand, particularly if this might 'give the game away'; many role-play activities are designed to allow students to discover things for themselves, so it is important not to pre-empt this.

One of the essential rules of role-play is that no member of the group

Table 7.9 Examples of role-play scripts in nursing

Role-Play Number 1

Nurse
You are a post-graduate nurse working in the Burns Unit.
   You are nursing a young woman who has had severe burns to the face; she is called Sally and is aged 17. She asks to talk to you. You go over to her bed.

Sally
You are a 17-year-old and have experienced severe facial burns. Although the pain is now much easier, you are desperately worried about the long-term effects on your appearance. You don't have a steady boyfriend, but do enjoy going out with boys. You decide to talk to the staff nurse.

Role-Play Number Two

Nurse
You are a post-graduate student nurse working in the plastic surgery children's ward.
   A toddler has been admitted for repair of hare-lip and cleft palate, accompanied by his mother. The child is called Gary Turner and has a severe deformity. His mother asks to speak to you after the admission formalities are completed.

Mother of Gary
You have arrived at the hospital with your toddler son Gary, who is being admitted for repair of hare-lip and cleft palate. The deformity is quite severe and you are wondering how successful the operation will be. You decide to ask the staff nurse about the operation after she has finished the admission formalities.

Table 7.10 Checklist for organizing role-play

A. *Before the Role-Play*
 1. Organize the room to allow for free interaction.
 2. Write out the role briefs for each participant.
 3. Write out instructions for process-observers.
 4. Do warm-up exercises.
 5. Do a briefing session, outlining purpose, rules, etc.
 6. Invite or select participants.

B. *During the Role-Play*
 7. Enact the role-play.

C. *After the Role-Play*
 8. Facilitate group discussion and evaluation.
 9. Re-enact the role-play if required.
10. Facilitate group discussion and re-evaluation if re-enacted.
11. Explore the implications and applications arising out of role-play.
12. Encourage actors to de-role.
13. Summarize the original aims and purposes of the role-play.
14. Organize group thanks to the actors.

should be allowed to be a passive observer; any students who are not directly engaged in one of the acting roles should be given the job of 'process observers'. This implies that they are actively observing the role-play, including the verbal and non-verbal signals emitted by the actors. Such 'process observation' is a crucial part of the feedback and debriefing session that follows the role-play.

Debriefing occurs after the activities have been concluded and can be seen as having three stages:

1. a description of what occurred;
2. sharing of participants' feelings about the activity; and
3. the examination of the implications of the activity for future work.

The first stage simply asks participants and observers to describe what occurred during the role-play; this is followed by a sharing of group members' feelings about the activity and it is important to have an atmosphere of mutual trust for this stage. The final stage involves the application of what has been discussed to the real world of nursing and where the insights gained can be shared with other students. The actors may receive much useful feedback from the observers about their personal skills of communication and the group as a whole can benefit from the range of ideas and values generated by the role-play. Since a great deal of emotion can be generated during role-play, it is important that the participants are encouraged to de-role at the end, so as to establish contact with reality again. This can be done by simply having students say out loud that they are out of role and that they are their normal selves again.

Gaming

Gaming is the third of these closely related concepts of simulation and role-play; gaming differs from simulation by the fact that it has very precise sets of rules and is usually competitive in nature. Unlike simulation, games have no scenario, being complete in themselves and participants behave as their normal selves. Educational games are simply extensions of recreational games such as board-games, card-games and quizzes and the aim is to create a method of learning that is both enjoyable and beneficial.

Case-studies

Case-studies are textual descriptions of specific situations that may either be genuine or fictional and that provide a trigger for the discussion of issues and the examination of real-life events. Case-studies differ from simulations in that they offer the student a cognitive view of the event rather than an experiential one. However, it is possible to use a case-study as the basis for a simulation or role-play, with students taking the parts of the characters involved. Case-studies usually entail making decisions about particular courses of action or, alternatively, making judgements about decisions contained within the case-study. Case-studies can be used to very good effect in bringing theoretical issues closer to the real world of nursing; for example, students may be given a case-study of the nursing care of a patient and asked to evaluate the care given in the light of their own knowledge and skills. In some instances, it is useful to use fictional studies to abstract the typical features of issues or problems, but generally speaking, it is better to use real-life examples, since these are based on actual nursing practice. Writing a good case-study is time-consuming and difficult and Davis (1955) suggests three basic questions that need to be addressed when planning a case-study.

1. What is the major issue or problem? This needs to be clearly stated along with any subordinate problems related to it.
2. What facts does the student need? It is important to include all relevant data required to deal with the problem or issue, but not to overload the case-study with superfluous material.
3. How should the material be presented? This involves deciding on the sequence of the material, such as background to the case, significant facts, use of the past or present tense and inclusion of statistics. The writer must avoid putting in personal opinions, keeping only to factual material.

One of the great uses of case-studies is to integrate information from a wide range of topics in nursing; in order to solve a nursing-care problem in a case-study the students will need to integrate their knowledge of biological and behavioural science, nursing science and other areas. When using the case-study method the tutor must be very familiar with every detail of the case, so that he or she can be of greatest use to the group during the discussion. The tutor needs to be particularly careful that the group does not skim over the case-study too quickly, thereby missing many of the important aspects. It is very useful to jot down an evaluation of how the session went, so that this is available for reference when the same case-study is used again.

The 'fishbowl' technique

This technique is very useful for process observation of group behaviour. The total group is divided into two and one of these subgroups arranges itself into a circle for discussion and interaction. The other subgroup arranges itself outside the first circle concentrically and can then observe the inner group as though it were in a fishbowl. After the inner group has completed its interaction, the outer group can give feedback and evaluation about the group processes.

Debate

Although commonly thought of as a large-group technique, debate can be used to good effect in small-group teaching. Debate is a formal way of examining issues that can be very exciting to the participants as well as the audience and it has the added advantage of not only raising the students' awareness of issues and values, but also giving them the opportunity to formulate an argument and present it in a public arena.

Debate is quite easy to set up; the tutor can choose a number of issues, or the group may come up with its own list. Four students are required to present their view, two speaking for the motion and two against it. Following the presentations, the issue is opened up to the audience to contribute and then a vote is taken on whether the motion is carried or defeated. Debate is particularly useful for topical, emotive issues and can serve to make students examine their beliefs and values about such issues.

Peer-tutoring and peer-review

Peer-tutoring involves two students working as a co-operative pair, with one taking the role of tutor. Reciprocal peer-tutoring involves the exchanging of the tutor/student roles between the two participants.

Peer-review consists of evaluation of groups or individual group members by the small group in question. Details of peer-review techniques can be found in Chapter 11 (p. 254).

Microteaching

Microteaching is a small-group activity that has many uses in nurse education. Essentially, microteaching consists of a cycle of events as those outlined in Figure 7.4. It can be seen that the cycle consists of the performance of some microskill, i.e. some aspect of a social or psycho-motor skill such as asking questions, which is recorded on videotape. This recording is then played back to the small group; the performer firstly evaluates their own performance and then the group members contribute their evaluation. The performer then replans the performance using the feedback gained during the analysis. The performance is then repeated, incorporating the changes suggested in the analysis and this is also videotaped. The video is then replayed, further analysis takes place and the cycle is repeated as often as is required until the performance is satisfactory. Microteaching can be a very potent tool for the acquisition of skills, but it does need a fair amount of time in order to allow students the chance to teach and re-teach several times.

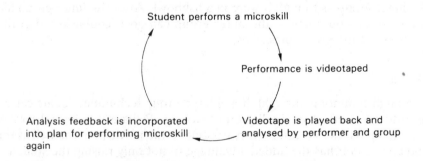

Fig. 7.4 The microteaching cycle.

Field visits

A well-established technique in nurse education, field visits can provide insight when extending students' experience of nursing. Visits can be clinical (to a hospice or specialist centre) or non-clinical (to museums or public utilities). Within the Project 2000 courses for initial registration, it is common to find that students are required to undertake field visits as part of a neighbourhood study e.g. to the local government offices, sports centres, supermarkets, etc. Briefing and debriefing are important if the maximum learning value is to be gained from the visit. Figure 7.5 gives an algorithm for planning such a visit.

Exercises

Exercises are particularly common in experiential learning, and consist of structured sequences in which students are actively involved, often containing written instructions. Exercises consist of dyadic, triadic or small-group activities, usually ending in a discussion of participants' feelings about the exercise.

Body movements

Also extensively used in experiential learning, physical contact may or may not be involved in this kind of experience, but is common in the various forms of 'warm-up' exercises prior to interpersonal skills sessions. Relaxation comes under this heading also.

Guided imagery and meditation

These experiential techniques are useful for gaining greater self-awareness. Guided imagery involves the use of fantasy by the student under the guidance of the teacher. The student sits comfortably with eyes closed while the teacher verbally guides them through some kind of guided fantasy pertinent to nursing. Meditation is also carried out in a relaxed environment with eyes closed and there are many techniques for this. One of them consists of simply attending to one's thoughts as they pass through the mind.

Instrumentation

A variety of instruments are used to facilitate activities, the commonest being questionnaires and inventories that direct the student to self-exploration.

REFERENCES

Allen, H. and Murrell, J. (1978) *Nurse Training: An Enterprise in Curriculum Development*, McDonald and Evans, Plymouth.

Asch, S. (1956) Studies in independence and conformity: a minority of

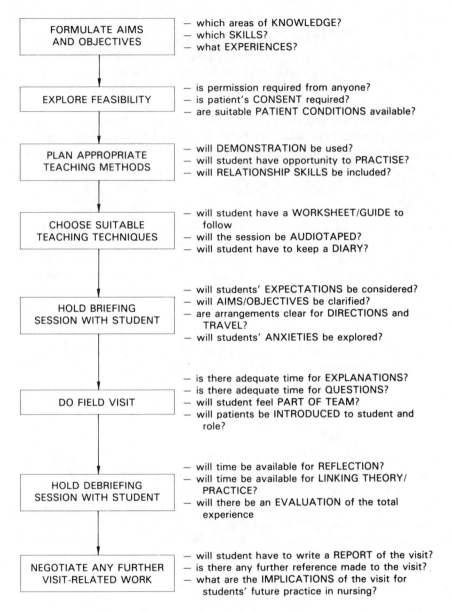

Fig. 7.5 Algorithm for planning field visits in nursing.

one against a unanimous majority. *Psychological Monographs*, **70**(9), 416

Bales, R. (1950) *Interaction Process Analysis: A Method for the Study of Small Groups*. Addison-Wesley, Cambridge, Mass.

Barker, L., Cegela, D., Kibler, R. and Wahlers, K. (1979) *Groups in Process*. Prentice-Hall, New Jersey.

Bavelas, A. (1948) A mathematical model for group structures. *Applied Anthropology*, **7**, 16–3.

Bond, C. and Titus, L. (1983) Social facilitation: a metaanalysis of 241 studies. *Psychological Bulletin*, **94**, 265–92.

Boud, D., Keogh, R. and Walker, D. (1985) *Reflection: Turning Experience into Learning*, Kogan Page, London.

Burnard, P. (1990) *Learning Human Skills*, 2nd edn, Heinemann, London.

Burnard, P. (1991) Defining experiential learning: nurse tutors' perceptions. *Nurse Education Today*, **12**, 29–36.

Davis, R. (1955) Some suggestions for writing a business case, in *Teach Thinking by Discussion*, (ed. D. Bligh), SRHE/NFER-Nelson, Guildford.

De Bono, E. (1986) Brainstorming, in *Teach Thinking by Discussion*, (ed. D. Bligh), SRHE/NFER-Nelson, Guildford.

Eiser, J. (1980) *Cognitive Social Psychology*, McGraw Hill, London.

Fawcett-Hill, W. (1969) *Learning Thru Discussion*, Sage, California.

Heron, J. (1986) Six category intervention analysis, Human Potential Research Project, University of Surrey.

Hirst, K. and Biggs, N. (1969) Undergraduate projects in mathematics. *Educational Studies and Mathematics*, **1** (3), 252–61.

Latane, B. and Darley, J. (1968) Group inhibition of bystander intervention in emergencies. *Journal of Personality and Social Psychology*, **10**, 215–21.

Lawrence, G. (1986) Social procedures of task-orientated groups, in *Teach Thinking by Discussion*, (ed. D. Bligh), SRHE/NFER-Nelson, Guildford.

Leavitt, H. (1951) Some effects of certain communication patterns on group performance. *Journal of Abnormal Social Psychology*, **46**, 38–50.

Mulder, M. (1960) Communication structure, decision structure and group performance. *Sociometry*, **23**, 1–14.

NATFHE (1976) Student projects. *NATFHE Journal*, February.

Osborne, A. (1962) *Applied Imagination*, Scribner, New York.

Rogers, C. (1983) *Freedom to Learn for the 80s*, Merrill, Ohio.

Royal College of General Practitioners (1986) Tutorial Styles, in *Teaching Thinking by Discussion*, (ed. D. Bligh), SRHE/NFER-Nelson, Guildford.

SES Associates (1986) The SES box method for creative problem-solving, in *Teaching Thinking by Discussion*, (ed. D. Bligh), SRHE/NFER-Nelson, Guildford.

Sherif, M. (1935) *The Psychology of Social Norms*, Harper, New York.

Steinaker, N. and Bell, M. (1979) *The Experiential Taxonomy: A New Approach to Teaching and Learning*, Academic Press, New York.

Tajfel, H. (1978) *Differentiation between Social Groups: Studies in the Social Psychology of Intergroup Relations*, Academic Press, London.

Wallach, M. and Kogan, N. (1965) The role of information, discussion and consensus in group risk taking. *Journal of Experimental Social Psychology*, **1**, 1–19.

8 Teaching and learning in practice placements

The placement of students in practice settings, under appropriate professional supervision, is a fundamental educational strategy in nursing and midwifery education. Most students, and many professionals, would argue that learning gained from placement experience is much more meaningful and relevant than that gained in the lecture room, and theoretical support for this can be found in the writings of learning theorists such as Carl Rogers, Malcolm Knowles, David Kolb and Donald Schon. The term 'practice placement' covers a wide variety of settings, including hospital wards and departments, community health centres, GP surgeries, schools, nurseries, day centres, residential homes, and industry.

Although practice placement is much more common in pre-registration programmes, many post-registration courses or pathways contain requirements for professional practice. Fish and Purr (1991), however, argue that the profession has not addressed the role and purpose of clinical practice in continuing education programmes. Their findings indicate that there is still a predominant view of practice as being 'application of theory', with little appreciation of the 'bottom-up' approach to theory generation; they also found an emphasis on narrow training outcomes such as attainment of competencies. They concluded that supernumerary status led to far more learning than if the student were a full member of the working team, as the former allowed greater opportunities for thinking and reflection on practice.

Practice placements may be undertaken in a new placement or in the case of continuing education programmes, in the student's own practice setting. An example of the latter is the enrolled nurse conversion programme, where the student's placement may be their own practice setting. In principle, there should be no difference between these, but in the latter example there is the danger that qualified staff will forget that the enrolled nurse is now a student as well as a colleague, and who therefore requires specific support in relation to their conversion course.

It is important at this point to differentiate between experience and learning in practice placements; it is sometimes assumed that exposure to an experience is synonymous with learning from that experience, and while some learning probably does happen in this way it is not the kind of professional learning that comes from systematic analysis and reflection upon experience. The latter requires an environment conducive to learning and appropriate support from skilled practitioners and educationalists.

This chapter explores the Benner adaptation of the Dreyfus model of skill acquisition in nursing, the requirements for a satisfactory learning environment in practice placements, placement audit, concepts and roles of supervision, mentorship and preceptorship, staff development for support roles, and stress and burn-out.

BENNER'S MODEL OF SKILL ACQUISITION IN CLINICAL NURSING PRACTICE

Patricia Benner's book *From Novice to Expert* (1984) has become one of the most frequently quoted research studies in nurse education. Benner conducted paired interviews with beginners and experienced nurses about significant nursing situations they had experienced in common, in order to identify any characteristic differences between their descriptions of the same situation. Additionally, she carried out interviews, critical incident technique, and participant observation with a sample of experienced nurses, new graduates, and senior students, to ascertain the characteristics of performance at different stages of skill acquisition. Using an adaptation of the five-stage model of skill acquisition developed by Dreyfus and Dreyfus (1980), she described the characteristics of performance at five different levels of nursing skill: novice, advanced beginner, competent, proficient, and expert. During her passage through these stages, the student relies less upon abstract rules to govern practice, and more on past experience. Nursing situations begin to be seen as a unified whole within which only certain aspects are relevant, and the nurse becomes personally involved in situations rather than a detached observer. It is important to note that Benner uses the term skill in its widest sense to mean all aspects of nursing practice, and not simply psychomotor skill performance.

Stage 1: novice   This level is characterized by rule-governed behaviour, as the novice has no experience of the situation upon which to draw, and this applies to both students in training and to experienced nurses who move into an unfamiliar clinical area. Adherence to principles and rules, however, does not help the nurse to decide what is relevant in a nursing situation, and may thus lead to unsuccessful performance.

Stage 2: advanced beginner   Unlike principles and rules, aspects are over-all characteristics of a situation that can only be identified by experience of that situation. For example, the skills of interviewing a patient are developed by experience of interviewing previous patients, and the advanced beginner is one who has had sufficient prior experience of a situation to deliver marginally acceptable performance. Advanced beginners need adequate support from supervisors, mentors and colleagues in the practice setting.

Stage 3: competent   This stage is characterized by conscious, deliberate planning based upon analysis and careful deliberation of situations. The competent nurse is able to identify priorities and manage their own work, and Benner suggests that the competent nurse can benefit at this stage from learning activities that centre on decision-making, planning and co-ordinating patient care.

Stage 4: proficient   Unlike the competent nurse, the proficient nurse is able to perceive situations holistically and therefore can home in directly on the most relevant aspects of a problem. According to Benner, proficient performance is based upon the use of maxims, and is normally found in nurses who have worked within a specific area of nursing for several years. Inductive teaching strategies, such as case-studies, are most useful for nurses at this stage.

Stage 5: expert   This stage is characterized by a deep understanding and intuitive grasp of the total situation; the expert nurse develops a feel for situations and a vision of the possibilities in a given situation. Benner suggests that critical incident technique is a useful way of attempting to evaluate expert practice, but considers that not all nurses are capable of becoming experts.

THE LEARNING ENVIRONMENT IN HOSPITAL PLACEMENTS

The qualified staff are a key factor influencing the learning environment in hospital placements, the role of ward manager being particularly influential. Not only do they have control of the management of the area, but also serve as role-models for nursing practice. The leadership style and personality of the ward manager are important determinants of an effective learning environment (Orton, 1981; Fretwell, 1983; Ogier, 1982, 1986; Pembrey, 1980).

Characteristics of a good clinical learning environment

The following summarizes the main perceptions of students in these research studies with regard to the characteristics of a good clinical learning environment.

A humanistic approach to students

Qualified staff should ensure that students are treated with kindness and understanding and should try to show interest in them as people. They should be approachable and helpful to students, providing support as necessary, and be very much aware that they are students rather than simply pairs of extra hands. They should foster the students' self-esteem.

Team spirit

Qualified staff should work as a team and strive to make the student feel a part of that team. They should create a good atmosphere by their relationships within the team.

Management style

This should be efficient and yet flexible in order to produce good quality care. Teaching should have its place in the overall organization and students should be given responsibility and encouraged to use initiative. Nursing practice should be compatible with that taught in the College of Nursing and Midwifery.

Teaching and learning support

Qualified staff should be willing to act as supervisors, mentors, preceptors, assessors, and counsellors as appropriate, and these aspects are discussed later in this chapter. Opportunities should be given for students to ask questions, attend medical staff rounds, observe new procedures and have access to patients/clients records. Non-nursing professionals such as doctors, physiotherapists, dieticians and chaplains can also contribute to the learning environment provided they are made to feel part of the total team. It is important for the ward manager to spend a little time with new non-nursing colleagues in order to explain the ethos of the ward or department in relation to learning, thus encouraging them to see themselves as a resource for student learning.

It is not always appreciated that students themselves are very much a part of the learning environment and not merely the passive recipients of its influences. An effective environment will encourage the students to take responsibility for their own learning and to actively seek out opportunities for this. Critical thinking and judgement are fostered in an atmosphere where the student can question and dissent without feeling guilty or disloyal. An important part of the learning process is experimentation, in which the student can try to apply concepts and principles in different ways; this implies that the student will need to adopt different approaches to patients and to be innovative. There must of necessity be an element of calculated risk in this, and it is the responsibility of staff to ensure that the risk of danger to the patient is minimized. Reilly and Oermann (1985) suggest that teachers may set unrealistic demands on students by expecting them to do everything perfectly, whereas mistakes are an inseparable part of the learning process. Teachers and students should work together to examine the reasons for failures so as to learn by such mistakes.

There may be other students at different levels of training in a clinical area and this peer support can be invaluable. By planning for two students to work together, there can be substantial benefits for both, provided they take time to discuss approaches and decisions and their underlying rationale.

Helping the students to be self-directing in their learning is of the utmost importance. Knowles (1986) suggests that a learning need is the gap between where the student is now, and where he or she wants to be in regard to a particular set of competences. The student should be helped to become aware of his or her learning needs in order to become self-directing, and initial pre-placement discussions are invaluable as a way of establishing a preliminary learning contract.

THE LEARNING ENVIRONMENT IN COMMUNITY PLACEMENTS

So far we have discussed learning environments with reference to hospital settings, but the environment is equally important when students are in community placements. Prior preparation in advance of a student placement is vital to ensure that the student gains the most from it. It is good practice to establish empathy with the student many weeks before the actual placement, for example, by the mentor giving the student his or her work and home telephone numbers in order to discuss expectations, and also 'housekeeping' issues such as transport arrangements etc.

The physical environment is clearly very different from that of a hospital, particularly when it involves domiciliary visits to patients in their own homes. Nursing staff are guests in this situation, with no right of entry and consequently, much of the teaching will occur by observation, with discussion following later after leaving the patient's home. Much of this discussion takes place in the practitioner's car in a one-to-one setting, calling for very good interpersonal skills on the part of the teacher. The practitioner needs to put the student at ease and treat him or her as an equal. The effects of a strained relationship are much more difficult to cope with when there are only two people involved. Clinics and post-natal groups provide another community learning environment for students. When running a well-baby clinic the mentor can combine tutorials for both student and parent, since the information is common to both. In community placements, media resources are much more scarce than in hospital settings, and hence the mentor places greater reliance on discussion and role modelling strategies.

PRACTICE PLACEMENT AUDIT

Auditing of practice placements forms a significant component of an institution's quality assurance system and helpful guidelines on educational audit have been produced by the English National Board for Nursing, Midwifery and Health Visiting (ENB, 1993). Practice placement audit focuses on six categories.

1. *Student learning experience/evaluation* This includes provision for orientation, appropriate and accessible learning opportunities, adequate length of placement, ethos, appropriate care model, staff commitment, and mentorship system.
2. *Academic staff perspective* This includes commitment to relationships with placement staff, maintenance of clinical competence, integration

of theory and practice, monitoring of placement evaluation, and staff development of unit staff.

3. *Service provider unit staff perspective*   This includes a commitment to individualized care, team approach, multidisciplinary teamwork, communication with the College, commitment to PREPP by service managers, and appraisal system.
4. *RHA purchaser/other purchaser requirements*   This includes identifiable and agreed standards, and quality assurance mechanisms.
5. *Environment*   This includes adequate physical environment to deliver quality care, to facilitate development of competencies, to provide teaching and learning opportunities, space and equipment, and health and safety requirements.
6. *Quality assurance mechanisms*   This includes congruence of curriculum and placement, unit staff preparation, monitoring and annual review mechanisms, system for ensuring clinical knowledge base of academic staff, and adequate supervision of students.

ROLE OF THE LECTURER-PRACTITIONER OR LINK-TEACHER

Until quite recently there were two types of nurse teacher: the nurse tutor, whose primary responsibility lay in classroom teaching, and the clinical teacher, whose primary responsibility was teaching in practice placement settings. These roles have now been unified under the title of lecturer/practitioner, a qualified teacher who has retained clinical competence and whose responsibilities include teaching, supervision and assessment of students. The lecturer/practitioner role, however, requires a re-orientation of teaching staff towards practice, and this is not likely to happen in a short timescale. Many institutions are attempting to bridge the gap between education and service by the use of link-teachers, whose role is to establish relationships with a small number of clinical areas for the purposes of liaison, trouble-shooting and staff development. The latter is primarily aimed at qualified staff in clinical areas, who will be acting as supervisors, mentors and preceptors to students undertaking practice placements. The link-teacher model may be criticized on the grounds that it could be seen as an abdication of direct teaching and assessment responsibility by the College of Nursing and Midwifery. This is not to decry the important teaching and supervisory roles of practice-based staff, but to question whether they should be the sole providers of such support, given that practice placements may constitute up to one half of a student's programme of study. In the light of the dual impact of educational contracting and skill-mix, it is unlikely that service providers would be happy with a system in which they contract with colleges for educational provision, only to find that they are responsible for providing a considerable proportion of the teaching, supervision and assessment that forms part of the contract.

Teaching on a one-to-one basis demands skills quite different from those used in the classroom setting; both teacher and student are more exposed to each other and the encounter takes place in the presence of other staff, patients and visitors. The need to appear competent and credible to all these groups, including the student, can add considerable pressure on the teacher, making it more difficult to allow the student to make decisions or to try out new approaches. On the other hand, there can be great personal satisfaction in helping to provide good quality nursing care whilst at the same time facilitating the growth of nursing skills in the student. Gerrish (1992) identifies three key roles for teachers in practice settings:

1. *Educational support for practice-based staff* This includes advice about dealing with supernumerary students on pre-registration programmes, and support for staff acting as mentors to students.
2. *Tutoring students* This includes facilitating the development of students' autonomy as students, and their skills with regard to reflective practice.
3. *Facilitating good practice* This includes awareness of current practice, providing a resource to unit staff, promotion of research-mindedness, and fostering a critical approach to practice.

Gerrish suggests that teaching in practice placements requires a commitment by the teacher, collaboration between education and service staff, and staff development for teachers on their new role in relation to practice.

PLACEMENT SUPPORT SYSTEMS FOR STUDENTS AND STAFF

There is a triad of terms used to describe practice placement support systems for students, supervision, mentorship and preceptorship. Within the literature, however, there is no consensus of opinion regarding definitions and some writers subsume all three concepts under umbrella terms such as 'practice facilitation'. For example, Butterworth and Faugier (1992) employ the term 'clinical supervision' to encompass mentorship, preceptorship, supervision of qualified practice, peer review, and maintenance of standards. Within the literature, the terms mentor and preceptor have been used largely to describe support systems for pre-registration nurses and midwives, but there is growing interest in the application of these in post-registration programmes. The UKCC Post-Registration Education and Practice (PREP) final proposals require all newly qualified nurses to complete a period of some four months under the guidance of a mentor, known as a preceptor, to ensure they do not assume too much responsibility, too soon or inappropriately.

Supervision

This is the least well-defined of the three terms and also the least developed in nursing, which has had to adapt models of supervision from other disciplines such as social work and psychotherapy (Faugier, 1992). In social work, supervision is defined as 'planned, regular periods of time that student and supervisor spend together discussing the student's work in the placement and reviewing the learning progress' (Ford and Jones, 1987). The English National Board for Nursing, Midwifery and Health Visiting (ENB, 1993) define a supervisor as 'an appropriately qualified and experienced first-level nurse/midwife/health visitor who has received preparation for ensuring that relevant experience is provided for students to enable learning outcomes to be achieved and for facilitating the students' developing competence in the practice of nursing/midwifery/ health visiting by overseeing this practice. The role of the supervisor is a formal one and is normally included in the individual's managerial responsibilities.'

According to Faugier (1992), the role of the supervisor is to facilitate personal and professional growth in the supervisee, and to provide support for the latter's development of autonomy. She proposes a 'growth and support' model comprising the following elements:

1. Generosity of time and spirit
2. Rewarding supervisee's abilities
3. Openness
4. Willingness to learn
5. Being thoughtful and thought-provoking
6. Humanity
7. Sensitivity
8. Uncompromising rigour and standards
9. Awareness of personal supervisory style
10. Adoption of a practical focus
11. Awareness of differences in orientation between supervisor and supervisee
12. Maintenance of distinction between supervisory and therapeutic relationship
13. Trust

In their evaluation of practice-based learning in continuing professional education in nursing, midwifery and health visiting, Fish and Purr (1991) found that supervisors had heavy workloads and their role was not well-defined. They tended to lack status and demonstrated a striking lack of confidence about their teaching and facilitating roles.

Mentorship

Mentorship is perceived as an important concept by the nursing and midwifery professions, as evidenced by the considerable number of papers published in the area. These are not confined solely to journals, and significant papers on mentorship have been produced by the recently by the English, Welsh and Scottish National Boards for Nursing, Midwifery and Health Visiting. The English National Board (1993), for example, defines a mentor as 'an appropriately qualified and experienced first-level nurse/midwife/health visitor who, by example and facilitation, guides, assists and supports the student in learning new skills, adopting new behaviour and acquiring new attitudes'. Morle (1990) argues that the term mentorship is not defined sufficiently to be a useful concept, preferring to use the term preceptor to describe the assigning of a student to a role model and resource person in the clinical setting. Armitage and Burnard (1991) suggest that mentorship is primarily about a close, personal relationship with the student, whereas preceptorship is more concerned with the teaching, learning and role-modelling aspects of the relationship. Mentorship is seen by many writers as being a long-term relationship that extends throughout a student's programme, whereas others limit the concept to a relationship within a specific placement. In some systems, students are encouraged to choose their own mentors, and in others the mentor is assigned to the student. The former is preferable if possible, since it increases the likelihood of compatibility between mentor and student, an important factor in the relationship.

One of the controversial issues in mentoring is whether or not a mentor should also act as an assessor in relation to their students. Anforth (1992) argues that the role of mentor is incompatible with that of assessor, since it presents a moral dilemma between the guidance and counselling role and the judgmental assessment role. However, I find it difficult to understand why there should be a dilemma between these two aspects, since assessment should constitute an important teaching and learning strategy and not simply a punitive testing of achievement. If the mentor has an open, honest and friendly relationship with the student, assessment can provide a rich source of feedback and dialogue to further the student's development. At this point I should nail my colours to the mast with regard to mentorship: I use the term mentor to describe a qualified and experienced member of the practice-placement staff who enters into a formal arrangement to provide educational and personal support to a student throughout the period of the placement. This support may involve a range of functions including teaching, supervision, guidance, counselling, assessment and evaluation. However, the mentor is not the only member of the practice-placement staff who carries out these functions, and other staff will undertake these according to the needs of the student and the practice area.

Maggs (1994), in a discussion of research issues in relation to mentorship, acknowledges the need for more research, and also highlights the danger of researchers being compromised by associating too closely with the policies of funding bodies.

Preceptorship

From the foregoing discussion it is apparent that there is much overlap in the literature between the concepts of mentor and preceptor. Burke (1994) sees preceptors and students as having a short-lived, functional relationship for a specific purpose in a practice setting. Given my definition of mentorship above, I see preceptorship as a specific teaching and learning strategy rather than as a generic support system for students. My definition of a preceptor, therefore, is 'an experienced nurse, midwife or health visitor within a practice placement who acts as a role model and resource for a student who is attached to him or her for a specific time-span or experience'. Preceptorship utilizes the principle of learning by 'sitting next to Nelly' but in a more systematic and planned way. A student is attached to the preceptor for a relatively long period of time such as a day or a week, and 'shadows' the preceptor throughout. The student's role is to observe the various interactions and decisions that the preceptor is involved with in the course of his or her work, and then time is made available for the student and preceptor to meet privately to discuss the events that have occurred. During these meetings, there is two-way dialogue about the various approaches adopted and the decisions made by the preceptor; and the student can ascertain the basis for such decisions. Clearly the person chosen to be the preceptor needs to have the confidence and interpersonal skills to be questioned about why one course of action was taken rather than another, and the system needs an equally confident student who will not be overawed by the power differential. In management training, the preceptorship is often conducted in an institution other than the one in which the trainee works, and this has the advantage of avoiding a 'boss' relationship between preceptor and student.

Preceptorship offers not only benefits to the students, but also to the preceptors, since the system helps the preceptors to clarify their reasons for making particular decisions or taking certain courses of action.

STAFF DEVELOPMENT FOR SUPERVISION, MENTORSHIP AND PRECEPTORSHIP

The careful selection of practice-placement staff for these important roles is crucial, and Burke (1994) suggests that personal characteristics, clinical expertise, teaching skill, and motivation are important. Courses of preparation may take the form of recognized courses such as Teaching and Assessing in Clinical Practice (ENB 997 and 998), City and Guilds of London Course 7307, and the University of Greenwich/Nursing Times Open Learning unit Teaching and Learning in Practice. On the other hand, they may be specifically designed in-house courses of preparation, and these need careful joint planning between education and service, and also ongoing monitoring and quality assurance. Fish and Purr (1991) found that training for supervisors in post-registration education was infrequent and insufficient, lacking in current knowledge of theory and practice, and in debriefing and reflection from practice. The latter are quite new concepts in nursing and midwifery, and practice-placement staff will need preparation to help them approach students in a different way from that used in direct teaching. Encouraging student autonomy means a 'hands-off' approach which some experienced practitioners may find uncomfortable. There is also the potential for perceived threat on the part of practitioners who qualified some time ago, when supporting DipHE or undergraduate students. This may result in barriers arising between mentor and student, to the detriment of learning.

One very useful strategy for staff development is networking between practice-placement support staff. Networking can be formal or informal, and functions in much the same way as self-help groups by providing mutual support and sharing of experiences. Jinks and Williams (1994) describe a study of the effectiveness of an educational strategy for community nurses in relation to teaching, assessing and mentoring of Project 2000 students. They found that half the sample felt their preparation had been adequate and this correlated with the taking of a formal course of teaching and assessing.

SPECIFIC TEACHING AND LEARNING STRATEGIES IN PRACTICE PLACEMENTS

Case-conferences

Ideally these should involve all members of the nursing team in discussion and evaluation of the nursing care of a particular patient. Medical staff have long used the case presentation method as a learning tool for students and qualified doctors, and the same principles apply to the use of nursing-care conferences. There is no standard format for such a conference, but it is usual for one nurse to present the patient's case and then for the whole team to be involved in the discussion. This helps the student to feel part of the nursing team as well as providing the skills in a public presentation of 'self'. Such conferences provide a useful holistic view of the patient and his or her problems, together with an opportunity to analyse critically the care that has been received, to the mutual benefit of both nurses and patients.

Ward report

Many trained nurses see the ward report as a valuable opportunity to do some teaching, since it involves the nursing team meeting together for a reasonable period of time during the day. If the report is made interactive, with each nurse explaining about their own patients, then it is more likely to be a useful learning experience. The ward manager or staff nurse often take time to ask questions about specific aspects of patients' conditions and care, and provided that the atmosphere is relaxed and informal, this can be a motivating way of learning. There are important trade-offs from a ward report in addition to the actual report itself, namely the fostering of team spirit and the development of public speaking ability and confidence in presenting information to peers.

Clinical rounds

Students can gain a great deal from accompanying a doctor or nurse on a clinical round. The former is useful for gaining insight into the role of the medical team in patient care, and it is interesting to listen to the discussion with regard to treatment. Students may find it valuable to accompany a nurse teacher on a similar round and to make comparisons of the needs of patients with similar conditions, and also to look at the difference in attitudes between such patients. Examples of pathology can be pointed out, for example oedema or inflammation, and the reasons discussed at the end of the round. Students should always carry a notebook to write down any queries or observations, but single sheets of paper must not be allowed, as they can easily be lost and other patients may read the confidential details.

Reflective practice diary

Reflective diaries or records are one of the key strategies in experiential learning and consist of brief written descriptions of situations that can be used as the basis for reflection later. The following examples are from the reflective diary of a health visitor who is undergoing training as a mentor.

Situation 1: student's first day on community placement

The first day of the student's placement was spent in discussion and negotiation of her learning contract in the light of my case load requirements. Since child protection is a major facet of my work, I made it clear to the student that this aspect must by law take priority over all other matters. Before commencing their community placement students are required to complete a Community Profile so that they have insight into the area. However, the student in question arrived at my office having completed a Community Profile on a completely different area to the one in which I work. This meant that the student had no information whatsoever about the area, so we had to negotiate a series of sessions in which I could explain the key aspects of the placement community. I also contacted her personal tutor in the College of Nursing to emphasize how important it is for the student to undertake a Community Profile which relates to their placement.

Situation 2: student's first visit to a client's home

One of the items on my student's learning contract was to visit a family with a new baby. By accompanying me on the visit, the student was able to see and understand exactly what a health visitor does in such a visit. During a prior briefing discussion I explained the official standard for a new-birth visit, and asked the student to pay particular attention during the visit to how I taught the mother to look after the baby, and to compare my performance with that of the official standard. I wanted her to focus particularly on my use of verbal and non-verbal communication with the family, since interpersonal relationships are fundamental to the health visitor role.

On arriving back at the surgery following the visit, we had a debriefing session in which I challenged the student by asking her to evaluate my performance against the official standards, and how she would now approach her next new-birth visit in the light of what she had learned.

Situation 3: developmental assessment in the clinic

At age 18 months infants come to the clinic for assessment of physical and behavioural development, and this involves a variety of tests, e.g. hearing, speech, vision, motor movements etc. I acted as a role model for the student, in that she was asked to observe and record carefully my relationships and involvement with the clients, with particular emphasis in this case on the practical aspects of testing. One of the objectives in the student's learning contract was to develop the skills of developmental assessment of infants, so I planned the learning environment with this goal in mind. During the clinic, the student was asked to observe me performing the developmental assessment on a number of infants, and was then encouraged to participate in the assessment of a number of infants. Once I was satisfied that she had grasped the essential points, I allowed her to conduct an assessment in partnership with me, but she was asked to take the lead, and to treat me as her student, showing me what to do. This was a very effective way of teaching, as it showed the student aspects which she needed to study further.

Critical incident technique

Critical incident technique (CIT) is a useful tool for identifying aspects of practice which the student felt were particularly positive or negative (Flanagan, 1954). These critical incidents can then be reflected upon and analysed to give new insights into practice. Critical incident technique was used by Benner (1984) in her study of acquisition of nursing skill, and she identified critical incidents as any of the following:

- those in which the nurse's intervention really made a difference in patient outcome;
- those that went unusually well;
- those in which there was a breakdown;
- those that were ordinary and typical;
- those that captured the essence of nursing; and
- those that were particularly demanding.

Subjects were asked to include the following information in their description of critical incidents:

- the context,
- a detailed description,
- why the incident was critical to the subject,
- what the subject's concerns were at the time,
- what they were thinking about during the incident,
- what they felt about it afterwards, and
- what they found most demanding about it.

Learning contracts

Learning contracts are an effective tool for developing student autonomy in practice placements. It is useful to meet with students prior to the placement to begin the initial contract negotiation, and this can be modified as required once the placement has commenced. The theory and components of a learning contract are discussed in Chapter 4 (p. 106).

ORGANIZATIONAL STRESS AND BURN-OUT

One of the key psychological factors that is influenced by the type of learning environment is the concept of stress and anxiety; anxiety is an unpleasant emotion that occurs in anticipation of threat or harm and results in increased general arousal. Each individual has an optimal level of arousal at which they perform at their best; under-arousal or over-arousal results in a deterioration in performance of learning tasks, particularly complex ones. Figure 8.1 shows the relationship between arousal level and performance

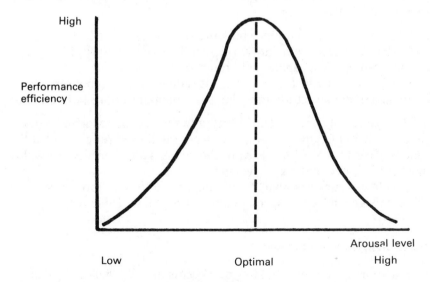

Fig. 8.1 Arousal level and performance.

It can be seen that arousal beyond the optimal level for a particular student will result in problems with learning and decision-making. It is quite likely that most practice placements are intrinsically stressful by nature of the human problems encountered there, such as patients in pain or dying. The pressure of work may also be stressful, particularly for student nurses who are still unsure of their practice, and there is a high element of risk involved in nursing patients in acute areas. All of these factors may combine to affect all but the most basic and well-learned responses, resulting in errors and negative experiences. Stress is a very difficult concept to define and one approach to stress is called 'person–environment fit theory' (Caplan, 1983), in which stress is defined as either demand exceeding the individual's capability, or capability exceeding the demand. Barnard (1985) points out that stress is a natural phenomenon that results in challenges of 'fight or flight', but that modern life-styles produce too much of the wrong sort of pressure. Duckworth (1985), on the other hand, finds the concept of organizational stress of little use, claiming that it distracts people from developing more useful theories and diverts attention away from awareness of the wide range of processes involved in psychological disturbance in organizations. He cites as examples of these disturbances such common behaviours as anger, jealousy and guilt, which would not be thought of as stress reactions. 'Burn-out' is another concept that is closely related to stress, and is characterized by emotional and physical exhaustion. It is a syndrome and as such, there will be wide variation in the range of symptoms that any individual will manifest.

Sources of organizational stress

Cooper and Marshall (1976) have identified five major sources of organizational stress:

1. factors intrinsic to the job – pressure of time and overload;
2. role-based stress – ambiguity, role-conflict, lack of clarity;
3. relationships – colleagues, subordinates, superiors;
4. career-development factors – fear of redundancy, promotion; and
5. organizational structure and climate – communication, politics, trust.

Another source of stress is the conflict between occupational and parental roles. Lewis and Cooper (1986), reviewing the literature, concluded that research is equivocal with regard to the stresses and benefits of employment versus home-making for women.

Hall (1976) suggests that there may be different job stressors at different stages in career development, as shown in Table 8.1.

Effects of stress and burn-out

The reaction of the individual to stress occurs in three well-defined stages termed 'the general adaptation syndrome' (Selye, 1956).

Table 8.1 Job stressors in relation to career development (Hall, 1976)

Stage in career	Needs	Stressors
1. Establishment	Safety Recognition	Relations with superiors Role ambiguity
2. Advancement	Moving up the ladder Mastering the organization.	Promotion Future development Work versus family
3. Maintenance	Levelling out Guiding others	Obsolescence Frustration about career

1. *The alarm reaction* This is a short-term reaction characterized by changes in physiology such as increased heart rate, respiration, endocrine activity and sympathetic-nervous-system activity.
2. *Resistance to stress*   In this stage the body processes return to normal and the individual adapts to the stress.
3. *Exhaustion* This rarely occurs in psychological stress, although it is common in extreme physical conditions such as severe exposure. Here, the individual has used up all the resources for coping, and death may occur.

This adaptation syndrome is non-specific, in that it occurs when the person encounters any form of stress, of whatever severity. There is growing evidence of a link between stress and heart disease, and a number of tools have been devised to measure the extent to which individuals are prone to stress-related disease. Examples are 'the social readjustment scale' (Holmes and Rahe, 1967) and 'the job stress check' (Cooper, 1981).

Burn-out is characterized by both physical and psychological symptoms. Physical symptoms are typically fatigue, exhaustion, headaches and gut disturbances, sleeplessness, dyspnoea and inability to fight off minor infections (McConnell, 1982). Psychological problems occurring with burn-out are dislike of work, irritability, working harder to accomplish less and less, disenchantment, rigidity in interpreting policies and absenteeism.

Coping with stress and burn-out

One helpful way of coping is to embark upon an anti-stress programme such as that of Barnard (1985), which has three main parts.

1. *Know your own personality* In order to best cope with stress, a degree of self-awareness is important; people with Type A personality tend to be hard-working, driving, competitive and aggressive, whereas Type B are more relaxed and placid and not very competitive. There is greater susceptibility to coronary heart disease in people with Type A personality, and although one cannot alter basic personality, it is important to realize this susceptibility and adjust the lifestyle accordingly.

2. *Choose an appropriate response to stress* This involves general guide-lines such as the avoidance of becoming overtired, ensuring adequate restful sleep, developing the ability to say no, acknowledging your limitations and being able to seek advice about stress.
3. *Your life in your hands* This involves the use of time management and relaxation.

Barnard (1985) cites Cooper's advice on time-management at work:

- arrange a period of time for organizing each day that cannot be interrupted;
- plan tasks in priority order;
- set realistic achievable deadlines;
- concentrate on one task at a time;
- avoid indecisiveness;
- consider each problem in depth;
- always take lunch outside of the office;
- do not neglect family time;
- develop a hobby that demands total concentration; and
- plan leisurely holidays.

There are a variety of relaxation techniques that can help reduce stress, such as physical-relaxation techniques and meditation. McConnell (1982) gives the following organizational strategies for helping staff to cope with stress:

- encourage staff to express feelings;
- support, encourage and reward risk-taking;
- provide recognition;
- work with knowledgeable and capable leaders;
- encourage sharing of needs and wants;
- invite staff to participate in decision-making;
- develop problem-solving skills; and
- include stress management in staff development programmes.

Social support from colleagues can help to reduce stress and there is some evidence that colleague support has a greater effect on stress reduction than family support (Glowinkowski and Cooper, 1985). It can be valuable if the ward, department or community group sets up peer-support groups to combat stress, where practitioners can discuss their reactions and feelings to organizational matters in a supportive atmosphere. A development of this is the notion of 'co-counselling', in which two people enter into a contract to give a stated amount of time to each other for the purpose of counselling.

REFERENCES

Anforth, P. (1992) Mentors, not assessors, *Nurse Education Today*, **12**, 299–302.

Armitage, P. and Burnard, P. (1991) Mentors or preceptors? Narrowing the theory–practice gap. *Nurse Education Today*, **11**, 225–29.

Barnard, C. (1985) *Your Healthy Heart*, MacDonald, London.

Benner, P. (1984) *From Novice to Expert: Excellence and Power in Clinical Nursing Practice*, Addison-Wesley, London.

Burke, L. (1994) Preceptorship and post-registration nurse education. *Nurse Education Today*, **14**, 60–6.

Butterworth, T. and Faugier, J. (1992) *Clinical Supervision and Mentorship in Nursing*, Chapman and Hall, London.

Caplan, R. (1983) Person–environment fit: past, present and future, in *Stress Research: Issues for the Eighties* (ed. C. Cooper), Wiley, Chichester.

Cooper, C. (1981) *The Stress Check*, Prentice-Hall, London.

Cooper, C. and Marshall, J. (1976) Occupational sources of stress. *Journal of Occupational Psychology*, **49**, 11–28.

Darling, L.A. (1984) What do nurses want in a mentor? *Journal of Nursing Administration*, Oct, **14**(10) 42–4.

Dreyfus, S. and Dreyfus, H. (1980) A five-stage model of the mental activities involved in directed skill acquisition. Unpublished report supported by the Air Force Office of Scientific Research, University of California, Berkley.

Duckworth, D. (1985) Is the 'organisational stress' construct a red herring? *Bulletin of the British Psychological Society*, **38**, 401–404.

English National Board for Nursing, Midwifery and Health Visiting, (1993) *Guidelines for Educational Audit*, ENB, London.

English National Board for Nursing, Midwifery and Health Visiting, (1993) *Regulations and Guidelines for the Approval of Institutions and Courses*, ENB, London.

Faugier, J. (1992) in Butterworth, T. and Faugier, J. (1992) *Clinical Supervision and Mentorship in Nursing*, Chapman and Hall, London.

Fish, D. and Purr, B. (1991) An evaluation of practice-based learning in continuing professional education in nursing, midwifery and health visiting. *Project Paper 4*, ENB, London.

Flanagan, J. (1954) The critical incident technique. *Psychological Bulletin*, **51**, 327–58.

Ford, K. and Jones, A. (1987) *Student Supervision*, Macmillan, London.

Fretwell, J. (1983) Creating a ward learning environment: the sister's role. *Nursing Times Occasional Papers*, **79** (21 and 22).

Gerrish, K. (1992) The nurse teacher's role in the practice setting. *Nurse Education Today*, **12**, 227–32.

Glowinkowski, S. and Cooper, C. (1985) Current issues in organisational stress research. *Bulletin of the British Psychological Society*, **38**, 401–404.

Hall, D. (1976) *Careers in Organisations*, Goodyear, New York.

Holmes, T. and Rahe, R. (1967) The social readjusment scale. *Journal of Psychosomatic Research*, **11**.

Jinks, A. and Williams, R. (1994) Evaluation of a community staff preparation strategy for the teaching, assessing and mentorship of Project 2000 Diploma students. *Nurse Education Today*, **14**, 44–51.

Knowles, M. (1986) *Contracting for Learning*, Jossey Bass, San Francisco.

Lewis, S. and Cooper, C. (1986) The stress of combining occupational and parental roles: a review of the literature. *Bulletin of the British Psychological Society*, **36**, 341–5.

Maggs, C. (1994) Mentorship in nursing and midwifery education: issues for research. *Nurse Education Today*, **14**, 22–9.

McConnell, E. (1982) *Burnout in the Nursing Profession*, Mosby, London.

Morle, K. (1990) Mentorship – is it a case of the emperors new clothes or a rose by any other name? *Nurse Education Today*, **10**, 66–9.

Ogier, M. (1982) *An Ideal Sister*. RCN, London.

Ogier, M. (1986) An 'ideal' sister – seven years on. *Nursing Times Occasional Papers*, **82** (2).

Orton, H. (1981) Ward learning climate and student nurse response. *Nursing Times Occasional Papers*, **77** (17).

Pembrey, S. (1980) *The Ward Sister – Key to Care*, RCN, London.

Reilly, D. and Oermann, M. (1985) *The Clinical Field: Its Use in Nursing Education*, Appleton Century Crofts, Norwalk.

Selye, H. (1956) *The Stress of Life*, McGraw Hill, New York.

Tutoring and counselling | 9

THE NATURE OF TUTORING

Until very recently nurse teachers were called 'nurse tutors', and it is interesting to speculate on the differences between teaching and tutoring. Teaching is commonly defined as an activity involving a presentational style of delivery to large groups, whereas tutoring involves activity in small groups or on an individual basis. However, tutoring is more than simply small-group teaching as there is also a pastoral element to the role, and this is usually referred to as counselling (Waterhouse, 1991). In Sixth Form Colleges, for example, a form tutor's role focuses on the personal dimension of a student's learning such as enjoyment of the course, and how they are coping generally with their studies. Subject teachers, on the other hand, focus primarily on their students' achievements in relation to their particular subject, although this does not exclude a personal interest in the students. The term tutor is used in another sense in the context of student-centred and resource-based learning, where the role of the tutor is to provide support and guidance for students in the management of self-directed learning.

The aim of the tutorial system is to forge a close relationship between tutor and student that will facilitate the student's learning and provide individual support and guidance, usually throughout the timespan of the student's programme. If learning outcomes are to be meaningfully achieved, then the tutor and the course member need to form a learning partnership in which each individual is recognized as having expertise and experience. The tutor will usually have much more of both within the particular specialist field of the course, but will still need to recognize that the student brings a variety of knowledge and experience to the relationship, which will vary according to whether the programme being undertaking is pre- or post-registration.

Characteristics of an effective tutor

Personal tutoring, like any other relationship, involves a number of qualities and values on the part of the tutor.

1. *Self-awareness* This is a fundamental requirement for helping others;

an insight into our own strengths and hang-ups allows us to be more effective when dealing with others.

2. *A climate of trust* This is essential to the relationship and can be engendered by appropriate self-disclosure by both parties, and a warm, open, honest approach toward each other.

3. *Respect for the student* The tutor must convey respect for the student's worth by treating him or her as an equal and by realizing that nursing is only a part of the student's life. There are many other competing activities involved, each of which is perceived as important by the student, so the tutor needs to take a realistic view of this potential conflict.

4. *Retaining individuality* In personal tutoring, it is important to be one's natural self; Bramley (1977) states 'some personal tutors still have not fully realized that their own personality is their principal tool in the tutoring job'.

5. *Credibility* Personal credibility is important as a basis for mutual respect, so the tutor needs to be seen as a good teacher as well as a sympathetic tutor.

Apart from teaching, the tutorial role comprises a wide range of elements including guidance (encouraging and supporting, informing and advising, liaising and representing, monitoring and coaching), negotiation of learning contracts, profiling, and counselling (Figure 9.1).

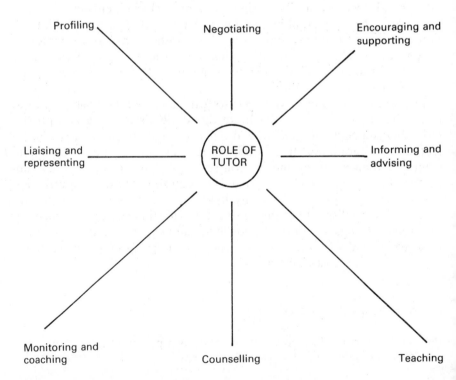

Fig. 9.1 The elements of tutoring.

GUIDANCE

Under this heading are subsumed a number of functions, all of which are concerned with helping the tutee to cope with the demands of the nurse education system. It is common practice in pre-registration programmes to allocate a personal tutor to each student for the duration of their course. With part-time post-registration programmes the tutorial provision often takes the form of a signing-up system on the notice-board during the day of attendance at the course. Tutees' will develop increasing expertise as they progress through their programme, so the tutor should change the focus of his or her role. In the early stages the main role is as a motivator and catalyst for ideas, whereas in the later stages it should shift to that of a constructive critic and evaluator.

Encouraging and supporting

It is invaluable for the student to have a personal tutor who can provide the necessary encouragement when things become difficult, as well as a friendly, sympathetic person to whom the student can unburden themselves. This element is no less important for mature post-registration students, since they often have difficulties with coursework and assessment if they have not been engaged in formal study for some considerable time. The relationship between the tutor and course member is paramount. The course member needs to be able to express views, opinions, and feelings in an atmosphere of psychological safety. However, the tutor should also expect to be challenged about his or her views and beliefs as the tutees grow in knowledge and confidence.

Informing and advising

The personal tutor is a valuable learning resource for tutees, particularly in relation to coursework and assessment. The tutor should ascribe to the course member appropriate independence and autonomy as a learner, so that critical thinking and enquiry is encouraged. Advising is one step beyond information-giving, in that the personal tutor is making suggestions or recommendations to the tutee believed to be in the tutee's best interests. One of the pitfalls of giving advice is that it removes the individual's autonomy to some extent. On the other hand, it is quite appropriate as a form of helping, provided that it is used thoughtfully. The sheer weight of experience often enables the tutor to see things more clearly than the tutee, although this is no guarantee of infallibility.

Liaising and representing

Tutors should undertake regular liaison visits to discuss their students' progress with practice-placement staff. This can often forestall problems and tensions and help to foster relationships with both student and placement colleagues. Liaison with other teachers is also necessary to ascertain how the tutee is functioning in his or her various groups and classes. Tutors are often called upon to furnish report of students' progress to funding bodies, and to support students' claims for study leave and funding for courses. It is sometimes necessary for the personal tutor to attend examination boards to provide information about factors affecting a tutee's performance.

Monitoring and coaching

Monitoring of student progress is a key responsibility of the tutor that can be achieved in a number of ways. Academic work can be monitored by noting the grades given for assignments, and clinical practice by direct observation, ward reports and informal feedback from both trained staff and student. Here again, self-assessment is an important tool to foster, so that the student can compare his or her own internal monitoring with that of the tutor and placement staff. Coaching is the term given to the remedial assistance provided by the tutor to help overcome specific learning difficulties. It is also used to refer to tutorial sessions for assessment examination revision and the marking of specimen examination answers.

NEGOTIATION OF LEARNING CONTRACTS

One of the basic tenets of adult education is that students should be actively involved in the educational process, including any decisions about the curriculum that affect them. In the past it was common for educationalists to prescribe the goals, methods of learning, and evaluation without involving the student in these decisions. The principles of adult education include negotiation of curriculum elements. By definition, to negotiate implies reaching mutual agreement or compromise, so the negotiation needs to be more than simply a token involvement of the student. One of the more effective ways of using negotiation is by drawing up a contract for learning which is then signed by both parties. A learning contract is not a substitute method of learning, its sole purpose is to give the student a degree of control over the goals, content, methods and evaluation of some aspects of the curriculum. The balance between the relative proportion of teacher-prescribed activities and negotiated ones will depend upon the nature of the student's programme and the ethos of the institution.

The experience of negotiating a contract puts the student in an active role with regard to learning, in marked contrast to the passive acquiescence in an entirely imposed curriculum. The autonomy conferred by contract learning tends to be a potent motivating force, and the negotiated work is perceived as being the student's own, rather than that imposed by

Student ....   Tutor ....

Goals/expected outcomes	Subject-matter	Learning experiences	Evaluation methods

Fig. 9.2 Example of a learning contract.

the teacher. It puts the responsibility for learning squarely with the student, an important factor for lifelong learning. Contracts can vary greatly in the amount of work required and in the time available for completion. They can be used effectively for just one day of a study module, for example, where students are told that a particular day is un-programmed to allow them to negotiate what they would like to do. Obviously, the contract for this kind of experience will be relatively limited, given that students have only a short time to spend on their chosen activities. However, this exercise can be a good way of introducing the notion of contract learning to a group before more ambitious use in the programme. Contracts need not only be about individual work; a group of students may negotiate to have a lecture or other form of input, the important thing being that they have chosen it. Figure 9.2 shows a learning contract; the headings chosen will depend on the teacher's preference. Each component of the contract is negotiated with the tutor and then signed by both parties. Negotiating a contract requires the student to have effective planning skills and good time-management skills.

It is quite feasible to negotiate for the grade if the contract is intended to form part of continuous assessment. In nurse education, the system of grading assessments seems to imply that all students are capable of achieving the highest grade in all areas, and anything less is seen as an indication of weakness. This takes no account of the interests of the student, nor of the fact that few individuals are good at everything. It seems sensible to allow a student to negotiate for a C grade in some parts of the course, and for B or A grades in others. Obviously, a C grade would be the minimum acceptable grade, but the choice of negotiating for a grade allows the student to concentrate efforts into his or her areas of interest. The criteria for contracts at different grades need to be standardized to ensure fairness in assessment. It is quite in order for the tutor to state some non-negotiable aspects of the contract such as an emphasis on health rather than disease and in this case the students would have to focus on this aspect, whilst allowing freedom in the choice of the other elements of the contract.

STUDENT PROFILING

The keeping of records is a key aspect of the role of personal tutor and has many serious implications. Accurate records are a necessary requirement for assessing student progress throughout a course and serve as legal documents in the event of disciplinary action. Profiling has arisen out of the move towards more involvement of students in their education, coupled with a desire to convey the widest possible picture of the student's abilities and interests. Student profiles are documents that record 'a wide range and diverse range of assessments of knowledge, skills and experiences' (Miller, 1982). Profiles are not methods of assessment, but rather a means of recording a wide range of assessments such as skills, attitudes, attainments and personal qualities (Hitchcock, 1990). Hence, profiles take a holistic view of the individual rather than the narrow view obtained only from examination results. Few people are good at everything; individuals have areas of greater and lesser expertise whatever their seniority, although professionals must always be judged as competent within their field. Thus, nurse teachers, whilst being basically competent in all areas of teaching, will naturally be better at some things than others. Many teachers are most at home in the lecture setting, while others prefer the small-group setting. If we accept this, then the idea of a single overall grade becomes meaningless. To state that a student maintained an average grade of B over a course means that the areas of greater or lesser expertise are being lost in the notion of average performance. It is surely better for all concerned to be able to read an account of the student's abilities and interests that bring out this range of achievement.

Purposes of profiling

Hitchcock (1990) gives several advantages of profiling which, although focused on the school sector, have relevance for nurse education.

1. *Greater student motivation*   This is largely due to the ethos of profiling which emphasizes co-operation and recognition of achievement. Students should have the opportunity to participate in their formulation, as in the case of self-assessment of progress.
2. *Improved relationships and communication*   Profiling requires one-to-one communication and encourages development of personal relationships between tutor and tutee. The student is asked to consider their progress over the last module, and to bring written comments to the meeting with the personal tutor, where both parties then discuss the student's progress from their respective points of view.
3. *Facilitation of guidance and counselling*   The process of profiling involves close interaction between tutor and tutee, and this can facilitate pastoral care where appropriate.
4. *Improve diagnosis of learning needs*   Profiling can lead to better diagnosis of learning needs when this is built in as part of the formal profiling process.

5. *Improved selection information for employers* Profiles are intended for public consumption and act as references for prospective employers and other interested parties.

Types of profiles

Hitchcock (1990) gives five categories of profiles.

1. *Student recording* These contain such things as personal achievements and self-assessments.
2. *Student/teacher negotiated records* These are compiled jointly by student and teacher.
3. *Criterion checklists* Student achievements are matched against predetermined criteria.
4. *Comment banks* Statements relevant to the student are selected from a prepared computer bank and structured in prose form.
5. *Grid-style profiles* A series of hierarchical statements are given, and the most appropriate one ticked to indicate the student's level of achievement.

Data Protection Act, 1984

When dealing with profiles, tutors need to be aware of the Data Protection Act, which applies only to computer-stored data; tutors must adhere to the main principles:

1. personal data shall be obtained and processed fairly and lawfully;
2. personal data shall be held for specified lawful purpose only;
3. personal data held for any purpose shall not be used in any manner incompatible with that purpose;
4. personal data shall be adequate, relevant and not excessive for the purpose for which it is held;
5. personal data shall not be kept longer than is necessary for the purpose;
6. an individual shall be entitled
   (a) to be informed of any data held by user,
   (b) to have access to such data, and
   (c) where appropriate, to have data corrected or erased; and
7. users must take appropriate security measures against unauthorized access/disclosure/alteration/accident, etc.

COUNSELLING

At the beginning of this chapter a range of elements that comprise tutoring were identified, and one of these was pastoral care or counselling. The term counselling is used in three senses (Nelson-Jones, 1993):

1. *To describe a helping relationship* This refers to the core qualities of

the counsellor, and includes emphathic understanding, respect for the client, and genuineness.

2. *As a set of activities and methods* These activities and methods include the empathic relationship with clients, and theoretical approaches such as psychoanalytical, behavioural, and rational-emotive.

3. *As a special area for providing services* The difference between psychological therapies and counselling lies in the type of clients. In counselling, the focus is on clients in non-medical settings who are less disturbed than those receiving psychological therapy in hospitals.

The British Association for Counselling suggest that the task of counselling is to give the client the opportunity to explore, discover and clarify ways of living more resourcefully and towards greater well-being. Inskipp (1986) sees counselling as providing help and support and an understanding listener for someone who is concerned or perplexed. Thus, counselling can be seen as a helping relationship that assists the client to become self-directing, and is very much based on Carl Rogers' notion of client-centred therapy as discussed in Chapter 4 (p. 101). It differs from the other forms of helping referred to earlier, since they rely on the expertise of the tutor; counselling assumes that the client has the necessary resources to deal with the problem. It is important at this point to distinguish between the process of counselling and the counselling skills themselves. I believe that a counselling relationship should be a conscious contract between two individuals, i.e. the client should decide whether or not he or she wishes to enter into such a relationship, having been informed about the nature of it. I am unhappy about the notion of a tutor counselling a student without the latter being aware of it. However, this does not mean that a tutor cannot use the skills of counselling to facilitate a relationship, since the basic skills are generic ones, which apply to all manner of relationships.

The process of counselling

There are a number of models of the counselling process, and two are described below:

The 'skilled helper' model (Egan, 1981)

This is a developmental model that is firmly based in the person-centred approach of Carl Rogers. It serves as a map to guide the helper through the helping process, and identifies the skills he will need at each stage. There are three stages in the model, but the counsellor may need to traffic back and forth between the stages during the interview.

Stage 1: Exploration In this first stage the role of the helper is to establish a warm, trusting, non-threatening relationship with the client to enable him to explore the problem from his own frame of reference. and to focus on specific concerns. It is important to communicate acceptance of the client for what he is, and also to convey attention. Active listening is more than simply listening to what the client is saying; it involves paraphrasing the client's words, reflecting back to the client what the counsellor thinks he is feeling, and making a summary of what the client has said in order to clarify understanding by both parties. The counsellor should help the client to focus on specific, concrete concerns using open and closed questions, and also on the client's strengths as well as weaknesses.

Stage 2: New understanding During this stage the counsellor helps the client to see himself and his concerns from alternative perspectives and to focus on ways in which the client might cope more effectively using his own strengths and resources. In addition to the Stage 1 skills the counsellor will use advanced empathy, which involves sharing hunches about the client in order to reveal hidden meanings and feelings. The client is helped to use alternative frames of reference for viewing his situation and concerns, and in this stage the use of confrontation by the counsellor helps the client to explore discrepancies and distortions in his perspective. Immediacy is used to bring what is happening between the client and the counsellor into the 'here-and-now'. Self-disclosure by the counsellor of her feelings or experiences should only be used if it will help the client to progress, otherwise it will remove the client-focus of the interview.

Stage 3: Action In this stage the counsellor's role is to help the client to consider the action he wants to take, in the form of concrete attainable goals, and the resources and skills he may require. The client may need to be helped with decision-making and problem-solving skills, and will require support and encouragement. Brainstorming may be helpful as a way of encouraging creative thinking, and role-play can help the client to practice new behaviours or skills.

The 'ideal' counselling model (Newsome, Thorne and Wyld, 1973)

There are ten stages in this model:

1. *Person comes for help* This may occur at the client's own volition or at the suggestion of a third party.
2. *Counsellor attempts to relate to client* This is the stage of establishing rapport in a non-threatening environment. The manner of the counsellor is crucial at this stage if the client is to feel psychologically safe.
3. *The helping situation is defined* Here there is clarification of the sort of help needed and the goals which might be aimed for. This gives the client the chance to see the goal and the progress being made towards it.
4. *Counsellor encourages client to express his or her concerns freely* This will only happen if the client perceives that the counsellor is interested.

5. *Counsellor accepts, recognizes and helps to clarify negative feelings* It is imperative that negative feelings are allowed free expression, even if the counsellor finds them difficult to cope with. It is necessary to work through such feelings before more positive ones can be considered.

6. *Counsellor accepts and recognizes positive feelings* This implies the counsellor is understanding the situation but making no judgmental evaluation.

7. *Development of insight* As the relationship progresses the client begins to feel less fearful and to experience insight into his or her problem.

8. *Establishing new goals* These may need to be formulated as the client's needs become more clear.

9. *Growth of confidence and ability to take decisions* By this stage the client may be making tentative decisions of their own volition, so the counsellor's role is one of support and reinforcement.

10. *No more need for help* This is the time when the relationship is ready to be terminated, and the client will often initiate this. However, the counsellor must be aware of the danger of breaking off too early.

Basic counselling skills

Regardless of the model employed, there are a number of basic skills involved as outlined in Table 9.1.

Table 9.1 Basic counselling skills

Skill	Description
Attending	Shows complete attention to client by non-verbal signals, i.e. eye-contact; relaxed open posture, leaning forward; sitting opposite client; close proximity without invading client's personal space.
Observing	Watching client's non-verbal behaviour for signs of stress or incongruity with what is being said.
Active listening	Concentrated listening, not only to the message, but also to the prosodic, paralinguistic and indexical features of speech (see Chapter 18).
Summarizing	Making a summary of what client has said helps to clarify understanding for both parties.
Reflecting	Paraphrasing client's words, or saying what counsellor thinks client is feeling.
Questioning	Need to avoid interrogation; use open questions rather than closed, to allow expansion by client.
Silence	Effective use of silence can encourage client to talk. Counsellor needs to control own anxiety about lengthy periods of silence.
Independence	Giving client responsibility for solving their own problem by appropriate questions.
'Concreting'	Assisting client to give concrete examples of how he or she is behaving or feeling.

As mentioned earlier, these skills are really generic skills for any type of social relationship, but there is a tendency towards mystification of these skills as a result of counselling training (Hopson, 1983). These skills may then be looked upon as being limited to a particular group, i.e. those who are trained counsellors, and thereby de-skilling others who could perform this valuable work. Nurse teachers need to be aware that counselling is only one form of helping and that other forms are also appropriate, otherwise they may feel afraid to give information or advice for fear of violating a 'counselling' role. Bramley (1977) puts this point succinctly: 'Tutors should be wary of submerging their own personalities beneath a welter of sympathetic grunts and long spells of silent listening.'

So far, this section has concentrated on the role of the counsellor in relation to the client or student, but no mention has been made of the counsellor's own needs. A counselling relationship can be very demanding and it is important that the tutor/counsellor has recourse to the same service – this is termed 'co-counselling' and involves the counsellor making a contract with another counsellor/tutor for an agreed amount of time together. The co-counsellor agrees to act in a counselling role and the tutor can then discuss feelings or problems about his or her own work with the clients, with the co-counsellor.

REFERENCES

Bramley, W. (1977) *Personal Tutoring in Higher Education*, Kogan Page, London.

Egan, G. (1981) *The Skilled Helper: A Model for Systematic Helping and Interpersonal Relating*, Brooks/Cole, Monterey.

Hitchcock, B. (1990) *Profiles and Profiling: A Practical Introduction*, Longman, Harlow.

Hopson, B. (1983) Counselling, in *Psychology and Medicine*, (ed. D. Griffiths), British Psychological Society, London.

Inskipp, F. (1986) *Counselling: The Trainer's Handbook*, National Extension College, Cambridge.

Miller, J. (1982) *Tutoring*, Further Education Curriculum Unit, London.

Nelson-Jones, R. (1993) *The Theory and Practice of Counselling Psychology*, Cassell, London.

Newsome, A., Thorne, B. and Wylde, K. (1973) *Student Counselling in Practice*, University of London Press, London.

Waterhouse, P. (1991) *Tutoring*, Network Educational Press, Stafford.

10 Media resources and information technology

Education has always been a labour-intensive profession whose main activities centre on face-to-face contact between teachers and students. Over the next decade this situation will undergo almost unbelievable change in the light of new educational technologies. The transmission of information by fibre optics, electronic mailing, and satellite is beginning to revolutionize traditional concepts of teaching, and it is envisaged that students will have their teaching and other communication delivered via interactive computer systems in their own homes, thus eliminating the need to travel to their college or university. Although these changes will take some time to develop and implement, information technology is already well established in education.

This chapter discusses the spectrum of information technology available for teachers, from the simple chalkboard to the highly complex computer-assisted learning.

THE IMPORTANCE OF AUDIO-VISUAL STIMULI

The sense of sight is the most important of all the senses in gathering information and combined with the sense of hearing, it provides almost all of the sensory perception of the world around us. It follows from this that audio-visual media have an important part to play in facilitating learning, since ideas can be conveyed far more easily using pictures rather than words. The old adage 'a picture is worth a thousand words' conveys the importance of sight in learning. It is often difficult for the teacher who can perceive a concept quite clearly, to realize that it may not be at all clear to the students who are listening to the explanation.

Another aspect of audio-visual stimuli is the fact that it is easier to remember something if one can picture it. Thus, the details of mortality rates for different diseases may be remembered better if the data are presented pictorially in a graph, using the slide or overhead projector.

The following sections deal with the various types of media, from the simple to the complex, but these descriptions are not intended to be substitutes for the instruction manuals of the various models. It would be quite unsafe to generalize with regard to the operation and maintenance of media, and so the reader must refer to the equipment available, and practise safely using the instruction manuals specific to it.

THE CHALKBOARD AND ITS VARIANTS

The chalkboard is the most familiar visual aid in the classroom, but, as in many other aspects of life, familiarity breeds contempt and chalkboard work is not always of the highest standard. The term 'chalkboard' is preferred to the older term 'blackboard', since many boards can now be obtained in colours such as green. The traditional wooden structure is giving way to glass or metal and a number of variations are now available. The main purpose of the chalkboard and its variants is to record, in semi-permanent form, the key points and explanations during a lesson. This enables the student to see as well as hear the points and to copy them down as a source of reference for the future. A checklist for the effective use of the chalkboard is given in Table 10.1.

The chalkboard plan

This is essential for all structured lessons and consists of a replica of exactly what the board will look like when the lesson has been completed. More than one may be required if the lesson involves a great deal of material, but if the key points only are written, then one plan should suffice. It is important to leave a margin at the side of the board for impromptu explanations and the plan should indicate the indentations and use of colour. A plan ensures that the chalkboard work is of a high standard and has been carefully thought out for maximum impact.

Table 10.1 Checklist for effective use of chalkboard

A. *Before the lesson*
1. Devise the chalkboard plan.
2. Clean the board.
3. Clean the eraser.
4. Ensure that sufficient chalk is available, in a variety of colours.
5. Check for glare spots by walking around room.
6. Check visibility using a sample heading, and viewing from rear of room.
7. Do pencil outline of complex diagrams.

B. *During the lesson*
8. Adhere to chalkboard plan; use margin for impromptu explanations.
9. Use appropriate lettering.
10. Emphasize by upper case, underlining, colour, encasing.
11. Write slowly enough to be legible.
12. Stop talking when writing.
13. Use template for diagrams, if rapid reproduction required.
14. Allow everyone to see, by using pointer from a distance.
15. Erase only when more space required, or when material will cause interference with subsequent points.
16. Check with learners before erasing.

C. *End of lesson*
17. Use chalkboard material as a summary.
18. Erase completely for next class.

Positioning and illumination

Before the lesson begins, the board should be checked for glare by walking around the room and looking from various angles. If glare spots are identified, then, in the case of a fixed board, the seats should be re-positioned in that section until glare is eliminated. If the board is portable, then it can be re-positioned as required. Illumination serves as a spotlight, focusing the attention of the audience on the message, so it is worth taking trouble to provide adequate lighting.

Chalk and erasers

Chalk can be obtained in two forms, standard and dust-free. The latter is preferable, as it does not deposit dust on the teacher's clothing nor, more importantly, on other audio-visual media present in the classroom. However, it can leave a waxy deposit on some board surfaces, making writing difficult and necessitating cleaning with spirit or repainting. Chalk is made in a variety of colours, but some of the darker ones are not clearly visible from the rear of a classroom. Erasers are invariably used dry, but a board may be wiped clean with a damp cloth, depending on the manufacturer's instructions. Erasers should be kept free of chalk dust by regular cleaning.

Lettering

The art of writing on a chalkboard is to forget the normal style of handwriting, concentrating on making lines and loops from the shoulder. This involves considerable practice, but will pay dividends in clarity and legibility. The size of lettering is often quoted as between one and a half to three inches high, but this will depend mainly on the size of the teaching room. It is useful to write a specimen heading on the board before the class begins and then to check from the rear of the room for visibility.

Lettering is classified into two main types in chalkboard work, upper and lower case. The former are capital letters, and the latter small and the terms are derived from the printing trade, where the cases of letters were placed one above the other, with the capitals in the upper case. Upper-case letters should be used for main headings and also to emphasize key words. All other writing should employ lower case, since the shape of the word is easier to read in this format. When writing on the board the teacher should stop talking, as the voice will not project when the teacher is not facing the audience. Teachers who feel uncomfortable with silences tend to write as quickly as possible, with a resulting loss of legibility. The period spent writing on the board can be used as a mini-break for the students, so that their arousal will increase when the teacher faces them again. Remember, 'if it's worth writing down, it's worth writing legibly'.

Emphasis (or high-lighting) can be achieved by the following devices:

- upper-case lettering,
- underlining,

- encasing the word, and/or
- colouring the words.

Diagrams

These must be large enough to allow the audience to see the details with the labelling written at the periphery and arrows used to pinpoint the component.

Labels should not be written on the diagram itself, since they obscure the detail. If the diagram is complex, then it is useful to do a pencil outline before the lesson begins. Using a soft pencil, the outline is drawn directly on to the board, so that when the time comes to draw it in the class, the outline is simply completed using chalk. Incidentally, the pencil outline is not visible from the class and the dramatic appearance of a complex diagram may earn the teacher an artistic reputation!

Diagrams that have to be reproduced regularly are best done using a template. This is then simply drawn around during the class, and provides a quick way of producing an accurate diagram. Examples of this are shapes of organs, such as the stomach, brain, etc., cut out of cardboard. It is sometimes claimed that students can learn how to draw diagrams by observing the teacher drawing on the chalkboard, but I consider this to be fallacious, since drawing is a psychomotor skill and should be taught using the principles of teaching a skill, for example task analysis, demonstration, practice and feedback. Since these elements are not present in the situation described above, it is more sound to teach drawing skills in a lesson devoted to that end.

Erasing

If a chalkboard plan is used, erasing should not be necessary, as the board builds up during the lesson and serves as a summary at the end. Should it become necessary to erase material, then the teacher must ensure that the students have finished recording it.

Chalkboard variants

Inkboards, commonly termed whiteboards, employ coloured pens instead of chalk. They are cleaned either by using a damp cloth or a dry one, according to the type of board. It is important that the correct type of pen is used for inkboards; it is frustrating on entering a classroom to find that permanent markers have been used to write on boards intended for dry-markers, as such writing is difficult to remove. The use of inkboards is identical to that of chalkboards.

Another similar concept is the magnetic board. This should really be called a magnet-accepting board, since it is only metal, the magnetic part being the tape used to mount the display. This magnetic tape is simply stuck on the back of whatever is to be displayed. The article will then adhere magnetically to the board, in any position. Magnetic boards can present labels, diagrams, pictures and even light objects such as wound drains or ostomy bags. I find this medium particularly useful for demonstrating concepts that involve movement, such as oxygen transport. Small cardboard 'molecules' are used to illustrate the diffusion from blood to tissues, etc.

Feltboards are really a more primitive form of magnetic board, utilizing a felt-covered board to which felt silhouettes will adhere. Special flockpaper is obtainable, which can be used to draw or write material on.

Flipcharts are simply large notepads which can be mounted on a stand or over a chalkboard, and marker pens are used to write or draw. When a sheet is completed, it is simply folded over, revealing a clean one. Material can be prepared in advance and revealed at the appropriate time.

THE OVERHEAD PROJECTOR (OHP)

This is one of the most useful and versatile visual aids. Table 10.2 gives a checklist for the effective use of OHPs.

The principle of the OHP is that light from a halogen lamp passes through a Fresnel lens beneath the window on which the transparency is placed and from there it passes through a mirror and lens in the projection head, which projects the transparency image onto the screen. A fan is employed to cool the lamp and this is usually thermostatically controlled.

Table 10.2 Checklist for effective use of overhead projector

A. Before the lesson
1. Position screen so that everyone can see it, with lower border level with heads of audience.
2. If available, use tilting screen to avoid keystone effect.
3. Obtain correct image size by moving machine backwards or forwards in relation to screen.
4. Focus image sharply.
5. Place masking sheet to hand.
6. Place transparencies in correct order.
7. Check table and head for dust, and wipe if necessary.
8. Ensure that a spare lamp is available in case of blow-out.

B. During the lesson
9. Switch off when:
    (a) placing transparency on table;
    (b) removing transparencies;
    (c) point has been explained.
10. Use pointer to indicate, preferably on the transparency rather than screen. Avoid use of fingers.
11. Use mask to reveal points in a step-by-step fashion when required.

C. After the lesson
12. Do not move the machine while lamp is hot, and never disconnect from mains supply whilst fan is operating.

The OHP is used in daylight, which saves the inconvenience of blackout and the teacher faces the audience whilst using it. It can save time by using transparencies that have been prepared before the lesson and a step-by-step presentation can be done using revelation technique, or overlays. However, there may be some glare from the bright light and some fans tend to be noisy.

Setting up the OHP

The room in which it is used will put constraints on the setting up of the OHP. The screen may be permanently fixed and a dais may limit the distance at which the projector can be placed. However, bearing these factors in mind, the first decision to be made is whether the teacher wishes to stand or sit during the lesson, since this will influence positioning. I prefer to have the overhead projector on my right-hand side, whether I am standing or sitting, but the main criterion is that each member of the audience has an uninterrupted view of the screen image. The bottom edge of the screen should be no lower than head level of the audience and it should be tilted forwards to prevent the 'keystone' effect, indicated by the image being wider at the top than the bottom.

The size of the image should be suitable for those students in the foreground as well as the background and this can be quickly estimated by taking the distance between the screen and the furthest student and dividing by six to give the image width (Ede, 1975).

Although the projector is designed for use in daylight, strong sunlight or artificial light shining directly on the screen may bleach out the image, so, if possible, the lights nearest the screen may be switched off, or blinds drawn. It is often useful, if the screen is portable, to place it across the corner of the room, as this will also permit full use of the chalkboard without obstruction from the screen. Needless to say, all positioning and focusing of the machine should be done prior to the commencement of the session, so that everything is ready for a professional performance.

Preparing transparencies for overhead projection

The use of computer desktop publishing (DTP) packages is by far the best way to design sophisticated, professional transparencies. If this facility is not available, they can be made by writing or drawing directly onto the acetate sheets. Pens specially designed for overhead projection are available in either water-soluble or permanent forms, the latter being much more durable if the acetate is to be used a number of times. Permanent ink can be erased by using spirit-based products, whereas soluble ink needs only a wipe with a damp cloth. When designing acetates, the lettering should be no less than 6 mm in size and it is useful to use lined paper beneath the acetate so that the lettering is kept even.

One of the golden rules of making transparencies is to keep them simple, preferably expressing a single concept only on any one acetate. It is tempting to be economical with acetates by overcrowding them with masses of writing, but this is very bad for the students, who have to cope with trying to write down all the information before it is removed. It is also important to leave a margin at each end of the acetate, or it may be too big for the image area and suffer loss of letters or words at the periphery. When drawing lines of different colours that are very close to each other, it is a good idea to draw one line on one side of the acetate and then turn it over to draw the other; this prevents smudging or blurring of colours. Colour can be added at the end of preparation by the use of coloured adhesive film, producing excellent results on such things as pie diagrams and bar charts. Transparencies can be mounted on cardboard mounts specially designed for the purpose and these provide a safe system for storage as well.

Uses of the OHP

There are three main uses of this medium: projection of transparencies, of silhouettes, and of X-rays and scans.

Projection of transparencies

Presentation of ideas can be extended by the use of revelation and overlay techniques. In the former, the transparency is covered with a sheet of paper, which is then progressively removed to reveal each point. I find it useful to use two sizes of paper as a mask; an A4 size sheet for the initial coverage of the transparency and a small one for the last two or three points. The small mask will conceal the final points effectively, but unlike the larger sheet, will not fall off the projector if the teacher removes his or her hand. Overlays consist of two or more transparencies which build up a concept or diagram. They are constructed by taping a base transparency to a cardboard mount and then taping the overlay transparencies to this, ensuring that the alignment is accurate and that only one side of each overlay is taped. Presentation commences with the base, and then each overlay is hinged into place to build up the transparency. If the order of overlays is fixed, then they should all be taped on the same side of the mount. If the order can be varied, then each can be taped to one of the four sides of the mount and this allows the student's contributions to be added as they arise. If points need to be added to a transparency but the teacher wishes to keep it for further use, then an acetate roll can be attached to the machine and the original transparency slipped beneath it. The teacher then adds the points on the acetate roll, leaving the original unmarked.

Projection of silhouettes

The overhead projector will project a silhouette of any solid object on to the screen, such as the shape of an organ, or of instruments and drains. I have drawn an outline of a leg onto acetate and then added cardboard silhouettes of the two fragments of a fractured femoral shaft to indicate the displacement and the effects of reduction.

Projection of X-rays and scans

Provided that the lamp is bright enough, any good-contrast X-ray should project on the screen. In addition, the silhouette of an object can be added, such as a femoral head prosthesis or intercostal drain, to indicate the position in relation to structure. During the session, it is important to make full use of the 'off' switch, and this should be done whenever a transparency is changed and also if the teacher needs to give a detailed explanation regarding one of the points on the transparency. Switching off the machine will focus the students' attention back to the teacher.

THE SLIDE PROJECTOR

Slide projection is used for showing still pictures to an audience and this is achieved by a powerful light source passing through a lens system and focusing on the screen. The slide itself is inserted into the light beam in the projector and the picture then appears on the screen. There is a variety of projectors available, from simple, manual-loading models to sophisticated automatic ones with remote control and all models take 35 mm slides. In order to obtain a clear image it is necessary to operate slide projectors in darkness, unless back-projection screens are utilized.

A checklist for the effective use of slide projectors is given in Table 10.3.

Table 10.3 Checklist for effective use of slide projector

A. *Before the lesson*
 1. Position screen for maximum visibility.
 2. Align projector so that required size of image is obtained.
 3. Focus sharply using a slide.
 4. Attach the remote lead if required, and position control near teacher's position.
 5. Check blackout. If curtains are used, close them at beginning of lesson and put on lights.
 6. Insert slides if automatic projector, standing behind the projector and turning each slide upside down before inserting into magazine.
 7. If more than one sequence of slides is required during the lesson, insert an exposed black slide between each sequence to prevent continually switching projector on and off.

B. *During the lesson*
 8. Switch off lights when showing slides.
 9. Use a point on the screen.
10. Use remote control lead to re-focus and change slides.

C. *After the lesson*
11. Remove all slides, including the last one in the 'well'.
12. Don't move projector until lamp is cool.

Setting up and using slide projectors

As with all equipment, the slide projector should be set up before the lesson and carefully positioned so that every member of the audience can see the screen. Image size is dictated by the distance of the projector from the screen – the further away it is, the larger the image. The size of the group should determine how large an image is required, and the slides should be inserted with the teacher standing at the rear of the projector and facing the screen. Each slide should be held up to the light so that it is seen and read in the normal manner and then it should be turned upside down before being inserted into the projector. If the projector has an automatic feed the magazine should be filled using the same technique. The projector should then be switched on and the picture focused sharply. If a remote control lead is being used, then it should be tested and then positioned at the teacher's station. Blackout facilities should be operated before the class begins and the lights switched on, as this causes less disruption than doing it during the lesson. If the slide sequence is spread over different parts of the lesson with verbal exposition in between, it is convenient to place an exposed black slide between each of the sequences. This saves the teacher having to keep switching the projector on and off, particularly when teaching in a lecture theatre with a separate projection room.

Slides

Slides can be obtained commercially, or made by the teacher. The former can be useful, as many are produced specifically for nurses in a wide range of topics. Other outside sources that might be useful are the medical photography departments in the hospitals, who may be able to make slides for the use of the college. Teachers can make their own slides using any modern 35 mm camera with a close-up facility. When purchasing film for slides it is important to obtain film for transparencies and not the ordinary film for colour prints. Table 8.3 shows a check list for slide projection.

AUDIO-CASSETTES

Audio-cassettes have a useful contribution to make in both the lecture and the individual situation. The principle of audio-cassette recording is that plastic tape, covered in ferrous oxide or chromium dioxide, is pulled at a constant speed past two electromagnetic heads. This tape is capable of being magnetized and as it passes over the 'erase' head any previous signal is wiped off. It then passes over the 'record' head, where magnetic impulses from the sound source are recorded on it. When the tape is played back, the record head picks up these magnetic impulses and converts them back to the recorded sound via the loudspeaker. The erase head is non-operational during playback, to avoid wiping off the recording. Audio-cassette recordings can be used alone or in combination with slide sequences and can be bought commercially or produced by the teacher. The use of audio-cassettes for long periods during lectures or small-group sessions can become very boring, but it is useful to use 'trigger-tapes' to stimulate discussion. Audio-cassettes are also useful for capturing the feelings and experiences of patients, which makes it a good medium for adding interest to sessions on nursing care. Such recordings are relatively simple to make and the principles are outlined below.

Making audio-cassette recordings

Audio-cassette recordings can be taken 'off-air' from radio and television programmes, or used with the integral microphone. The purpose of making an audio-cassette recording is to capture specific content and make it available to an audience. This does not imply, however, that the quality of the recording is irrelevant, for, indeed, it is very important to ensure that it is of the highest technical quality if people are going to listen to it without distraction. A little attention to the technical points can make all the difference between a good recording and a poor one.

Audio-cassette recorders have built-in microphones that obviate the need for the complicated setting up of external ones. However, in certain circumstances, it may be preferable to use an external microphone, especially if there is a lot of background noise as in a busy ward. There is a wide variety of microphones available, the main ones being moving-coil, condenser, ribbon, crystal and carbon. The last two are not used for high-quality work and of the former ones, the moving-coil (dynamic) microphone provides good quality whilst being relatively inexpensive. Microphones have various directional properties according to the design, and this means that the direction of the sound detected follows a particular pattern. For example, some microphones have an omnidirectional response, which means that they respond to sound coming from all directions. Others have unidirectional responses and receive sounds from one direction only, an important quality when recording interviews, or when a single individual is speaking.

When recording in the wards, a unidirectional microphone may limit some of the background noise and the simplest technique is to position the microphone so that the patient's voice is picked up from the right direction, rather than having the teacher hold the microphone in front of him.

If the recording is being made in the college, a room is required that is free of background noise, including ventilator humming, typewriting and telephones. A totally dead acoustic environment can be a strain to work in and is not as pleasant to listen to. The teacher reading a script for a recording session should be sitting comfortably at a table, with the microphone high enough to avoid having to speak down to it. The head should be held well up and the script must not intervene between the face and the microphone. To prevent the rustling of paper being detected, it is useful to enclose each sheet in a polythene sleeve so that it glides noiselessly to one side.

Recording requires an assistant to switch the machine on and to monitor sound levels. It is important to position the cassette recorder at some distance from the microphone so that amplifier hum is not picked up. If the cassette recorder does not have automatic recording level, the sound level must be monitored by watching the 'VU' indicator on the recorder, ensuring that this does not exceed 0 VU during the recording. On the other hand, it is important to record the signal at a high level, so the level should approach 0 VU but not exceed it. Teachers who are new to recording often feel nervous or embarrassed and this makes their delivery stilted. It is a good tip to have someone sitting opposite the speaker, behind the microphone, to whom the speaker addresses his words. This often makes the tone more natural and conversational.

It is worth mentioning that poor quality recordings may result not only from bad technique, but from badly maintained equipment. The heads on the recorder should be cleaned weekly with head-cleaning fluid and demagnetization should be carried out at monthly intervals using a tape-head demagnetizer.

REPROGRAPHIC HANDOUTS

Handouts are a common strategy in nurse education and consist of a sheet or sheets of paper given to each student for permanent use. The purposes of handouts can be summarized, as follows:

1. *To provide information*   Handouts can be given to provide information to the students, such as lesson objectives, facts or statistics and diagrams and charts.
2. *As a lecture guide*   If the lecture structure is particularly complex, it may be given to the students in the form of a handout that they can follow, adding their own notes.
3. *References and further reading*   If a lecture contains many references, it is useful to record them on a handout so that the exact details are correct. Further reading can also be suggested.
4. *Assessment and questioning*   Handouts in incomplete form are commonly used to assess learning during the course of a lesson. In addition, handouts may be given containing written questions for evaluation at the end of a session.
5. *Worksheets and assignments*   The student is required to complete the instructions on the sheet, which may require information to be sought or problems to be solved. It is commonly assumed that worksheets should be handed in to the teacher for assessment on completion, but the real role of a worksheet is to put the students in the position of having to gain certain knowledge or skills. These can then be assessed using the conventional methods of assessment, rather than trying to mark the wide variety of responses made to a worksheet.

Design of handouts

The principles of design apply to all kinds of media, not just handouts. The following suggestions are made by Brown, Lewis and Harcleroad (1977).

Balance

This can be achieved formally or informally. Formal balance consists of shapes of equal size, formally arranged, while informal balance is fairly casual, but more interesting.

Shape

There are three basic shapes used in layout design: I, T and Z. This means that the material is arranged in the shape of one of these letters across the sheet. For example, in the 'I'-shape the material is arranged vertically down the centre, whereas in the 'T'-shape it also has material in the cross-piece of the 'T'.

Emphasis, contrast and harmony

The use of different styles of lettering and colour will add emphasis to display. Contrasting areas of light and dark will capture the attention of the viewer and the whole layout should be harmonious and well planned.

Methods of reproducing material

Photocopying is almost the only method of reproducing material used in nurse education and is a general term for a variety of copying processes, all of which give exact reproduction of original material. Their simplicity of use is the main advantage, the original is simply placed on the flat table, with the lid closed and at the touch of a button the copy appears. However, copies are relatively expensive and expenditure on photocopying needs careful monitoring. Nurse teachers may still encounter other forms of reprographics and details of these are given below.

Ink-duplicating (Roneo, Gestetner)   Masters can be typed onto stencils, and drawings made freehand. The copies are then run off, preferably at one time. However, the stencil can be stored and used again.

Spirit-duplicating (Banda, etc.)   Material can be typed onto masters, or drawn freehand. In addition, they can be made using heat copiers. It is important to use the correct paper for masters and for running off the copies, if best results are to be obtained. Masters can be stored for re-use.

Heat (thermographic) copiers   These versatile machines can be used to produce spirit masters for spirit-duplicating, overhead projection transparencies, lamination, etc. Original material must first be copied by photocopying and this is then used as the original for the heat copy, since all material must be fed into the machine.

Copyright

Copyright laws are designed to protect authors from the wholesale copying of their works, a very real need in view of the ease with which modern copying machines can reproduce materials. However, copying is an important aspect of good teaching, and there is now a licensing scheme operated by the Copyright Licensing Agency Ltd, that allows copying without permission within clearly defined limits. In higher education institutions the licence enables teaching, administrative and technician staff, librarians and all students to copy for any one course of study in one academic year as follows:

1. up to 5%, or one complete chapter of a book published in the countries listed on the current user guidelines as long as not excluded on those guidelines;
2. the whole or part of a single article from a journal or periodical issue published in the countries referred to in the current user guidelines;
3. from a copy of a chapter or an article which has been made under the terms of the licence and which is kept in a library or reserve collection.

It is a condition of the licence that the number of multiple copies of any one item of copyright material shall not exceed the number needed to ensure that the tutor and each member of a class has one reproduction only. A copy of the User Guidelines must be kept beside the copying machine (Copyright Licencing Agency, 1992).

FILM PROJECTION

Video-recordings have largely replaced films in nurse education, but they may be still in use in some centres.

There are many models of film projector, some being manually threaded and some automatic, but the principle is similar. The film travels clockwise during showing, so the feed-in spool is always at the front. The film is mounted so that the free end hangs down, looking like the shape of a figure 9. Projectors have a threading diagram in a prominent position, which must be carefully followed, paying particular attention to the size of the loops. Automatic threading machines require that the end of the film is cleanly cut, and not uneven. There are three positions on the switch, 'motor', 'lamp' and 'reverse' and in addition, there is usually a fast rewind switch.

Setting up and use

The projector should be set up in advance of the session and the screen checked for visibility. The film should be threaded and run forward a little way, checking the focusing and the volume and tone settings. The loudspeaker is positioned to face the audience. After checking these aspects, the film should be reversed until the point at which the last of the countdown numbers disappears. This ensures that the film starts in the correct place during the session.

Films should be viewed in darkness, and at the end they are rewound according to the supplier's instructions. Some film suppliers do not require their films to be rewound, nor breakages spliced, after showing and the teacher should check the instructions contained in the film carton.

VIDEO

In nurse education, video is a popular learning resource, for both playback of pre-recorded tapes or used with video-cameras. Off-air recordings of television programmes relevant to health care form an important component of library stock, as well as videotapes produced specifically for educational purposes. Video cameras allow teachers and students to make their own video recordings and this has given a new dimension to teaching and learning. The reality of practice-settings can be brought into the classroom to provide authentic material for discussion and analysis. The portability of cameras makes it easy for students to record aspects of the community for analysis back in the college. A less commonly used form of television is closed-circuit television; this does not involve recording, but relays live events to other parts of a building via slave monitors. It is useful for observing events where large numbers of observers would be obtrusive or overcrowded, or for observing interviews without affecting the interaction.

Interactive video and hypermedia

Two very recent developments in information technology are interactive video and hypermedia. Interactive video (IV) utilizes a videodisc player, a computer, and an input device which together offers the student the opportunity to interact with the educational material of the program (Ward, 1992). Hypermedia also utilizes videodisc and advanced programming technologies to allow the student to access information on a multimedia basis. Accessing specific parts of a videotape is notoriously time-consuming, whereas hypermedia technology has random access capability so that virtually instant access can be gained to data in a wide range of media such as video, audio, text, etc. (Merseth and Lacey, 1993).

MEDIA-RESOURCE CENTRES

The term 'media-resources centre' implies a collection of media and resources for learning, with expertise available in the form of a tutor or librarian. These centres are now being called 'flexible-learning workshops' and provide a range of individual facilities for study, including computer-assisted learning, interactive video, tape/slide programmes and many other media.

INFORMATION TECHNOLOGY (IT)

A computer is an instrument for processing information and can be either mainframe, mini-computer or micro-computer. A mainframe computer has a large capacity for processing information and may be shared by a wide network of users via terminals. A mini-computer may offer the same kind of sharing function but on a smaller scale, whilst a micro-computer is a portable device that utilizes micro-electronics and is relatively inexpensive. When referring to computers, it is usual to talk about two major components – hardware and software.

Hardware

Hardware consists of four main components.

1. *Input device*   This is the point at which information is put into the computer and can be a keyboard, mouse, joystick, scanner, etc.
2. *Processing unit*   This contains the micro-processor chips and it is responsible for the information-processing function.
3. *Memory*   Data is stored in the computer's memory, which is internal and external. Internal memory is usually situated within the processing unit and consists of 'random access memory' (RAM) and 'read only memory' (ROM). The RAM is a temporary store holding the data put in by the user or the program, and it is cleared when the computer power is switched off, and the data is completely lost unless it has been saved onto an external memory device. ROM is the memory that contains the data required for the computer to operate and cannot be changed or lost, even by switching off. External memory is stored on floppy disk and hard disk, allowing information to be transfered from machine to machine. Memory capacity (of all forms) is stated in terms of megabytes.
4. *Output device*   This is used to display the data generated by the computer such as visual display unit (VDU) or printer.

Software

Software is the term given to programs, and these are the most important aspect as far as the user is concerned because they carry out the tasks for which the computer is required.

Programs can be written by the user or purchased as software packages from manufacturers. A wide range of software is available for educational purposes and the term courseware is used to describe these.

The term information technology includes the following aspects:

1. information handling, i.e. the storage and retrieval of information;

2. communication technology, i.e. transmission of information; and
3. information transformation, i.e. putting information into a form that is applicable to a particular purpose.

The above aspects encompass the hardware, software, applications and systems appropriate to each. Computer literacy is a closely related term which includes the following (Bostock and Seifert, 1986):

1. psychomotor skills necessary to operate a computer;
2. knowledge of the principles of hardware and software functioning;
3. knowledge of the important applications and social implications of computers; and
4. attitudes to computer use.

There is disagreement amongst experts as to whether computer literacy should encompass the ability to write programs.

It is useful to think of the computer as fulfilling two major roles in the nursing and midwifery curriculum: as subject matter, and as a teaching and learning tool.

Computers as subject matter

'Nursing informatics' is the term given to the use of information technology in nursing practice and nurse education, and can be seen as a combination of computer science and nursing science. Nurses and midwives must be able to manage computer systems so as to gain maximum benefit from the new technology. The younger age-group entrants to nursing will already possess basic computer skills learned in school, but many post-registration or older students will lack these basic computer-literacy skills, so it is important that some time be made available to offer training in basic concepts and skills of computer literacy. A basic computer-literacy course in nursing should introduce students to the fundamentals of computers, i.e. hardware, software, components and keyboard familiarity, as well as some of the main applications such as the use of database systems, spreadsheets, desktop publishing and word-processing. Word-processing is particularly useful for writing coursework assignments. Other applications to practice can be included such as admissions data and bed state, laboratory investigations and care plans. It is also useful to include a visit to the main hospital computer centre to see how the information is processed and accessed via terminals in each of the main clinical areas. However, Lichfield (1992) argues that nursing informatics is developing in isolation from the development of nursing theory, and that its impact on the nature of nursing practice is in danger of being overlooked.

Computers as a teaching and learning tool

There is a wide range of applications of computer technology to learning and teaching and these are given the generic name of 'computer-assisted learning' (CAL) or 'computer-assisted instruction' (CAI).

Computer-assisted learning (CAL)

This is one of the most advanced uses of technology in education and can be defined as 'any of a wide range of educational techniques that rely on a computer to facilitate learning' (Hannah, 1983). The aim of CAL is to teach students the subject matter of nursing or midwifery, and can be carried out using a single computer or in combination with a range of other media as in multimedia CAL. With a single computer approach, the teacher either develops appropriate lesson materials as courseware units, or these can be purchased from manufacturers of educational media. The courseware is selected by the student and loaded into the computer, where it forms the learning experience for the student in whichever mode is appropriate. Computer-assisted learning is only as good as the courseware that goes into it, but computers do have the potential to produce high-quality graphic displays, data storage and retrieval and a host of other effects that would be almost impossible for the individual teacher to emulate in standard teaching situations. Single-computer CAL does have limitations and these can be overcome by the use of multimedia CAL, which consists of a range of media that is used in the same instructional program. It is possible to arrange the computer system to control other types of media such as slides, audio-cassette or video. It is the latter that has opened up exciting prospects for CAL because it is possible to combine the versatility of a computer with the high-quality visual medium of video.

In Chapter 13 (p. 330), the concept of 'open learning' is discussed and it is here that CAL comes into its own; students using a computer can take the material at their own pace, referring back to previous sections as and when they deem necessary. They can answer the questions posed by the program in total privacy, without the embarrassment of having their lack of knowledge exposed in front of a group of peers. CAL can help foster the intuitive kind of thinking that is important for discovery learning, by presenting problem-based information about which the student has to make hypotheses and subsequently checking his or her answers against the computer. CAL can accomplish a number of teaching functions in nurse education, such as presentation of information on new topics, follow-up activities, revision, diagnostic and remedial teaching, in fact most of the activities normally associated with classroom teaching apart from small group work. Even the latter can be catered for by having programs designed for groups rather than individuals and the great advantage of CAL is that it can offer high-quality instruction that eliminates such variables as poor preparation and presentation by the teacher, problems of timing, fatigue, boredom and loss of attention. Of course, the last three can happen in any medium, but at least with CAL the student can switch off and go for a walk to restore concentration.

Gwinnett and Massie (1987) describe the use of 'computer-aided case-studies' (CACS) for teaching care-planning. Students were given basic information on computer, such as the patient's name, age, diagnosis and base-line observations and then were required to interrogate the computer for further information. A maximum of 15 items could be selected and a printout was given of those chosen. Seminars were held afterwards so that students could discuss the case-study and their planning of care.

Evans and Cowley (1985) describe the resources required for writing programs under four headings: expertise, hardware, time and finance. Expertise is required in the form of nurse teachers who are interested and committed, subject specialists who are up to date in clinical nursing, systems analysts who can advise on such aspects as screen lay-out, colour and timing and a programmer who actually writes the program. Awareness of the capabilities and limitations of hardware is important and nurse teachers should not underestimate the demands on finance and teacher time for the proper development of CAL.

Computer-phobia

With the growing proliferation of computers in everyday life as well as the workplace, the concept of computer-phobia becomes increasingly important. Jay (1981) has defined computer-phobia as having:

1. a behavioural component, i.e. a resistance to talking about computers or even thinking about computers;
2. an emotional component, i.e. fear or anxiety towards computers; and
3. an attitudinal component, i.e. hostile or aggressive thoughts about computers.

Studies suggest that computer anxiety is a widespread phenomenon, and is indicated by such behaviours as avoidance of computers and computer areas, excessive caution with computers, negative remarks about computers, and attempts to cut short the necessary use of computers (Maurer and Simonson, 1984). Research suggests that females are likely to have higher levels of computer anxiety than males, although the literature is by no means consistent on this. There appears to be a socialization process that defines computer culture as 'male', and this may account for gender differences in computer anxiety. Brosnan and Davidson (1994) offer the following advice for teaching computing to students with heightened computer-anxiety:

1. initially, anxious students should be separated from other students for teaching purposes;
2. conceptual teaching should be used initially, instead of hands-on computer teaching; and
3. single-sex computer teaching may help reduce computer-anxiety in female students.

REFERENCES

Bostock, S. and Seifert R. (1986) *Microcomputers in Adult Education*, Croom Helm, London.

Brosnan, M. and Davidson, M. (1994) Computerphobia – is it a particularly female phenomenon? *The Psychologist*, **7**(2), 73–8.

Brown, J., Lewis, R. and Harcleroad, E. (1977) *Techology, Media and Methods*. McGraw-Hill, New York.

Copyright Licensing Agency (1992) *Licensed Copying User Guidelines*. CLA, London.

Ede, J. (1975) Primer: overhead transparency projection. *Video and Audiovisual Review*, September.

Evans, P. and Cowley, D. (1985) A software approach. *Nursing Times*, 30 October.

Gwinnett, A. and Massie, S. (1987) Integrating computers into the curriculum 2: transforming a concept into a working tool. *Nurse Education Today*, **7**, 116–19.

Hannah, K. (1983) Computer assisted learning in nursing education: a macroscopic analysis, in *The Impact of Computers on Nursing*, (eds D. Scholes, Y. Bryant and B. Barker), Elsevier Science Publishers, North Holland.

Jay, T. (1981) Computerphobia. What to do about it. *Educational Technology*, **21**, 47–8.

Lichfield, M. (1992) Computers and the form of nursing to come. *International Journal of Health Informatics*, **1**, March.

Maurer, M. and Simonson, M. (1984) Development and validation of a measure of computer anxiety, in *Proceedings of Selected Research Paper Presentations*, (ed. M. Simonson), the 1984 Convention of the Association for Educational Communications and Technology, Dallas, 318–30.

Merseth, K. and Lacey, C. (1993) Weaving stronger fabric: the pedagogical promise of hypermedia and case methods in teacher education. *Teaching and Teacher Education*, **9**(3), 283–97.

Ward, R. (1992) Interactive video: an analysis of its value to nurse education. *Nurse Education Today*, **12**, 464–70.

Assessment 11

Professional practice in nursing and midwifery is under scrutiny as never before, with the professions making major attempts to ensure that practitioners keep their knowledge and skills up-to-date with changing technology and work practices. The UKCC in its final PREP proposals aims to offer a rational, cost-effective framework which matches patient, client and service needs with flexible, responsive educational provision. Teachers of nurses and midwives must be both clinically credible and knowledgeable about contemporary practice. The ENB Framework and Higher Award is also focused on education for professional practice, and in both of these initiatives assessment plays a crucially important role.

Aims of assessment

All types of assessment should conform to the following basic aims:

1. to assess student performance in relation to the aims of the particular programme in question;
2. to be regarded as an integral component of the teaching and learning process, and not simply a means of measuring attainment; and
3. to encourage the student to undertake self-assessment and reflection on their learning.

Assessment can also provide data about the effectiveness of the curriculum and may serve as a source of feedback to the student about progress being made. Some teachers would also claim that assessment acts as a motivator for students, while others would argue that it is a major source of stress within the educational system. What does seem certain is that assessment in some form or other will remain an indispensable part of any educational system for the foreseeable future and this means that nurse educators will need to monitor assessment procedures constantly to ensure their continuing appropriateness to current curricula.

Assessment, then, forms an important component of the nursing curriculum but there is a real danger that it may actually dominate it; in many educational systems it could be argued that the curriculum is geared to the passing of a terminal examination. In other words, the whole system is dominated by the assessment, with consequent restrictions on innovation and creativity. This can be termed 'assessment-led curriculum' and contrasts markedly with its opposite notion of 'curriculum-led assessment'. The latter describes a curriculum that is planned from educational principles, with the assessment component developing logically out of these principles. The terminology relating to the field of assessment may give rise to confusion, as a number of terms tend to be used synonymously. Table 11.1 gives the main distinctions between the most commonly used terms.

In any assessment system, regulations are of vital importance if the system is to run smoothly and students are not to be disadvantaged. Regulations need to be clear, explicit, and easy to understand so that both students and assessors are in no doubt about what is acceptable and what is not. Regulations are discussed later in this chapter.

In nurse education, 'assessment' tends to be the most commonly used term, although it can be seen from Table 11.1 that it is not always appropriate. The key feature of evaluation is that it follows the obtaining of data by measurement or assessment; the nurse teacher first obtains a student's score on an essay test and then makes a value judgement about whether this score is good or poor for the student concerned. In addition to this basic terminology, it is useful to look at the dimensions of the concept of assessment, as shown in Table 11.2.

Formal assessment involves the use of tests to obtain data that is then made available to the institution; the data is often subjected to statistical

Table 11.1 Terminology of assessment

Measurement	A quantitative process involving the assigning of a number to an individual's characteristics
Assessment	A term used instead of measurement when a numerical value is not involved; e.g. checklists of behaviours
Evaluation	The process of judging the value or worth of an individual's characteristics obtained by measurement or assessment
Test	An instrument or tool for obtaining measurements or assessments, e.g. an essay
Examination	A formal situation in which students undertake one or more tests under specific rules

Table 11.2 Dimensions of assessment

Formal	——	Informal
Quantitative	——	Qualitative
Episodic	——	Continuous
Formative	——	Summative
Teacher-centred	——	Student-centred
Norm-referenced	——	Criterion-referenced
Achievement	——	Aptitude/Personality
Paper and pencil	——	Practical/Oral
Local	——	National

analysis and comparisons drawn between other students. Examples of formal assessment in nurse education are modular or unit assessments, unseen written components, and clinical practice assessments. In contrast, informal assessment does not involve comparisons with other students, but is essentially private and subjective to the teacher concerned. Such informal assessment is gleaned from the day-to-day observation of students' behaviour, examination of students' notes, and from informal contact and interviews. Informal assessment, then, is for the private use of a particular teacher and forms an essential part of the total assessment process.

Quantitative assessment refers to the use of numerical data in the assessment of students, whereas qualitative assessment is concerned with the properties or qualities that an individual possesses. Scores obtained on a written test constitute quantitative data; a student's views on what constitutes effective relationships with a patient would be qualitative data. There are two dimensions that are concerned with the timing of assessment, the first being 'episodic' versus 'continuous' assessment. Episodic assessment involves testing the student at specific times or occasions during an educational programme, such as an end of year assessment or a number of specific clinical assessments in particular aspects of nursing. One of the major drawbacks of this system is its reliance on a student's 'one-off' performance on the day of the test and this performance may not reflect the student's typical performance over a longer period. In other words, episodic assessment generates data that is based on a very small and possibly unrepresentative sample of a student's behaviour. A further criticism, which relates particularly to the clinical setting, is that of artificiality, in that episodic clinical assessments are often seen as 'set pieces' which the student may rehearse until 'word perfect' and which bear little resemblance to the student's normal working practices. Continuous assessment attempts to overcome these weaknesses by sampling all of a student's outputs in a course on a continuous basis. In the college setting, this might involve assessing all of a student's coursework, including tests, projects and seminar presentations. In the clinical setting, continuous assessment samples a student's nursing practice on a continuous basis, so that no particular nursing skill can be said to have been 'passed' on a 'once-and-for-all' basis.

The second time-related dimension is that of 'formative' versus 'summative' evaluation and these terms are used in two distinct ways. First, they can be applied to the assessment of a particular student's achievement and second, to the evaluation of a particular aspect of curriculum design, such as teaching media. Formative assessment provides feedback about the progress a student is making whilst the course or unit is being followed, so that modifications can be made to the teaching if necessary. Summative assessment, on the other hand, is done at the end of a course or unit to see if the student has achieved the objectives of the programme and is usually done as a formal test covering the content of the course. Many teachers feel that formative assessment should not be graded for assessment purposes, but used only as feedback or diagnosis of student needs. With regard to the use of these terms for curriculum evaluation, formative evaluation means that instructional material intended for eventual use with students is tested during its formation and modified in the light of these pilot studies. Summative evaluation is the evaluation of such material after it has been used with students in its intended setting.

Another useful dimension to consider is that of 'teacher-centred' versus 'student-centred' assessment. Traditionally, the teacher has been the key figure with regard to the assessment of students in nursing, but with the growth of interest in student-centred learning, there is a move towards much greater involvement of the student in his or her own assessment. Indeed, self-assessment seems to be one of the hallmarks of a professional practitioner in any field, so this is a practice that should be encouraged from the outset.

The next dimension to be considered is that relating to the interpretation of the results of assessment; there are two main ways that these results can be referenced: norm-referencing and criterion-referencing. Norm-referenced assessment means that an individual student's score on a test is compared with scores of other students in a given group, or with published norms for the test in question. Criterion-referenced assessment implies that the score is compared with some criterion or learning task such as achievement of behavioural objectives and is also termed 'content-referenced' or 'domain-referenced' assessment. The main difference between these two forms of referencing is that norm-referenced assessment means that the score obtained by the student is influenced by the performance of the group to which he or she is compared. Criterion-referencing, on the other hand, does not depend an any form of comparison with others, only with achievement in relation to a specific criterion or standard.

Assessment is not only concerned with the measurement of student achievement, but includes such aspects of an individual as attitudes, aptitudes, personality and intelligence. Achievement refers to how well a student has performed in the past; aptitude refers to how well he or she will perform in the future. Assessment of personality and intelligence is usually done using published standardized tests.

A useful distinction can be made between the kinds of tests employed in the assessment of nurses. On the one hand we have the so-called 'paper-and-pencil' tests, which include essays, objective tests and a host of other kinds of written instruments. At the other end of the scale there are the practical, clinical forms of assessment and oral examinations. Practical assessment usually involves observation combined with some form of checklist or rating scale to guide the observer. Oral, or viva voce, tests rely on the spontaneous answering of questions by the student and allow for follow-up and further elaboration on answers given.

The final dimension is that of 'local' versus 'national' assessments. Assessments in nursing are now devolved to the college and devised and administered by the teacher or course-planning team, but there are still examples in general education where assessment is prescribed and formulated by external agencies.

THE CARDINAL CRITERIA

Regardless of the type of test employed or the purpose for which it is used, every effective test must meet the four cardinal criteria: validity, reliability, discriminination and practicality (or usability).

Validity

This is the most important aspect of a test and is the extent to which the test measures what it is designed to measure. In other words, validity is the relevance of a test to its objectives.

Content validity   Assessments should sample adequately the content of the syllabus and if this is the case, then the examination is said to have content validity.

Predictive validity   If a test is designed to predict the future performance of a learner and it fulfils this function, then it is said to have predictive validity.

Concurrent validity   Concurrent validity is the extent to which the results of a test correlate with those of other tests administered at the same time.

Construct validity   A construct is a quality that is devised by psychologists to explain aspects of human behaviour that cannot be directly observed. For example, such things as attitudes, values and intelligence are constructs. Construct validity is the extent to which the results of a test are related to the data gained from observations of individuals' behaviour with regard to the construct in question.

Reliability

Reliability is the term used to indicate the consistency with which a test measures what it is designed to measure. In other words, it should yield similar results when used on two separate occasions, provided that the other variables remain similar.

Test–retest reliability   If a test is administered to a group of students and then re-administered, either immediately or after an interval of time, and the scores are similar on both occasions, then the test is said to have high test–retest reliability.

Parallel-form reliability   If the group is given a different test in the retest phase, but one that measures the same thing, then a positive correlation indicates parallel-form reliability.

Split-half reliability   In this the test items are divided into two halves and the correlation calculated between the two sets of scores.

Discrimination

The purpose of any test is to discriminate between those who answer correctly and those who don't. The term discriminate is used in the sense of 'distinguish between', and not in the equal opportunities sense. If a test makes no discrimination between students, then it has no purpose. The discrimination index will be examined later in this chapter.

Practicality or usability

It is important that a test is practical for its purpose. This implies such factors as the time taken to conduct the test, the cost of using it and the practicality for everyday use.

USING ESSAYS AND RELATED ASSESSMENT METHODS

Essays are very much an 'open' type of assessment in which the student brings a personal response or judgement (CNAA, 1989). They are characterized by requiring the learner to supply an answer that is organized in their own words and presented in their own style and handwriting. There are few, if any, restrictions imposed and there is no single correct answer. The term 'essay-format' covers a number of forms of written assessment; for example, it is used to describe negotiated coursework as well as formal written examinations. There are a number of weaknesses in this form of assessment, which may limit its usefulness.

Weaknesses of essay tests

Low content-validity

Since in essay tests, only a small number of questions are answered, sampling of the syllabus may be inadequate.

Low marker-reliability

Essay tests are notoriously unreliable from the point of view of marking. Every learner knows that some teachers are easy markers and others hard, and the final mark depends to a large extent on the marker. There is often wide variation between markers, and between the same marker at different times.

Often ambiguous or unclear

Essay questions are often difficult for the learner to understand because they are not as clearly stated.

Marking is difficult

Marking essay tests involves a great deal of time and work for the teacher and this in itself makes the reliability open to question.

Student fatigue

This aspect is rarely mentioned in connection with essay tests, but in my opinion it is a very serious disadvantage. In many assessment systems students may have to write for some three hours at a time, which may affect the quality of the answers.

Marks affected by writing ability

The learner's ability to write good prose can influence the mark that is awarded. It is often difficult to separate the content of an essay from the literary style, with the result that a learner may bluff the marker into giving a higher grade than he or she deserves. On the other hand, a learner may be penalized for poor grammar or expression, even though the content is adequately known. Of course, the essay must be legible, but I feel that marks should not be taken off for the grammar or spelling. The teacher may draw attention to this aspect by adding a comment in the margin, without this affecting the mark awarded. It is often argued that written communication is vital to the role of the nurse and I agree entirely with this sentiment. However, we saw earlier that any test must satisfy the criterion of validity, and an essay test that asks for the 'care of a patient following herniorrhaphy' is not designed to test the ability of the learner with regard to written expression and grammar. If this aspect is to be validly assessed, then a test must be designed with this aim in mind, and its reliability evaluated.

Choice is often included

In any essay examination a choice of topics is invariably included, but this practice is open to question on two counts. First, it is difficult to construct problems which have the same degree of difficulty, so that in effect a different test is being offered to each learner. This obviously makes comparison difficult between the achievements of students. Second, the more able students may well be attracted to the more difficult ones and suffer penalties if they fail to do well.

The use of essay tests

Because of the factors indicated above, essays are inefficient for testing recall of knowledge, but are useful for assessing higher levels of cognitive functioning, such as application, analysis and evaluation. These are important areas in nursing, although there may be little correlation between what the learner writes and what he or she does in the real situation (Bendall, 1975). Essay questions can be used as an indirect method of assessing the affective domain of attitudes, values and opinions. The kind of question that asks the learner about caring is an example. Essays require the learners to organize and express their own ideas and this can be a good way of teaching them to organize information efficiently, by providing detailed feedback on her answer.

The problem with formulating essay tests in nursing is that traditionally they have been sub-divided into several parts, as in the following example:

Q: A major part of the nurses' role is the gathering and recording of patient or client information, much of which is confidential.

1. (10%) What is meant by 'confidential'?
2. (30%) Why is confidentiality important?
3. (60%) Critically discuss the methods by which information about patients and clients can be gathered.

If we consider that the time allowance for this question would be somewhere in the region of 45 minutes, which includes reading time, then this format by its very nature will encourage superficial and hurried responses. The student is under pressure of time to move on to the next subsection, and a 10% weighting for the first part trivializes the whole notion of assessment. If nursing and midwifery wishes to encourage students to become critical, analytical thinkers and reflective practitioners, how can the above kind of assessment encourage the development of such characteristics. It would be far better to have a single question worth 100%, so that the students could at least get their teeth into the topic. This would also make marking much easier for the teacher, who could expect a reasonable degree of analysis and thoughtful discussion in a 45-minute essay on a single question.

Essay-type assessments that encourage critical thinking

In the light of my foregoing criticism of essays in nurse education, I feel obliged to offer some alternative types that can measure higher levels of cognitive functioning. The following are examples of essay-type assessment questions that require critical thinking skills on the part of the student.

Interpretive essay

Q: The accompanying table relates accidents at work to the type of industry, i.e. manufacturing, construction, railways, coal mining and agriculture. Comment on the relative risk of accidents for the types of industry represented in the table.

When answering this type of question, the student has to interpret the table in order to come up with the relative risk for each industry, and this requires high-level cognitive functioning.

Hypothesis-formation essay

> Q: You are the chair of a committee charged with making recommendations for the siting of a new hostel for the mentally-handicapped in a quiet suburban area of town. Speculate on the likely planning objections to your proposal.

In this case, the student has to consider all the relevant facts and present a hypothesis about the likely planning objections. This essay cannot be written by a simple reliance on memorized facts, but requires higher-order synthesis.

'Doing-it' assessment

> Q: Read this article from the *Journal of Advanced Nursing* and comment on the author's underlying assumptions about the nature of nursing.

This assessment requires the student to explore the article thoroughly and to search for the writer's assumptions. These assumptions may not be obvious, and the student may have to analyse the text deeply before they become apparent.

Inquiry-based assessments

> Q: Carry out an investigation into the provision for disabled people in terms of access to public buildings within the Newhampton district.

> Q: Design a small-scale survey to ascertain the need for a Community Centre in Oldhampton town.

These two assessments require the student to undertake some form of inquiry in order to answer a question.

Synthetic assessments

> Q: Select a patient or client within either a hospital or community setting in consultation with your mentor. Participate in the care for this patient/client over a period of one week, maintaining a diary of your interactions and interventions. Write a commentary on the care given, within the context of relevant theory from both nursing and social and biological science. Make particular reference to any incongruities between your experiences and your theoretical analyses.

Table 11.3 Checklist for formulating essay tests

Commence planning the test well in advance of the time it is needed.
Check the content validity of the questions proposed.
Write the questions clearly and without ambiguity.
State the action-verb for the learner's performance, for example state, describe.
State the limits of the question, and include them in the statement, for example 'normal ageing', 'first 24 hours'.
Write the instructions clearly, indicating time available, percentage weighting, and policy regarding grammar and spelling.
Do not give choices unless the learner's experience has been different.
Employ questions which test the higher levels of functioning, such as application and problem-solving.
Consider using questions which have short answers, so that the sampling of content can be extended.
Ensure that time allowance is sufficient for the question to be fully answered.
Prepare a marking key and check it with a colleague.

This somewhat long-winded assessment requires the student to synthesize information gained by both experiential learning and study in order to identify any gaps between them. This is high-level cognitive functioning.

Table 11.3 offers a check list for formulating essay tests.

Marking or grading of essay tests

Marks or grades are assigned to students' essays to indicate the degree of achievement they have attained and there are two systems for assigning grades. Absolute grading awards marks depending on how well the student's essay has met the requirements of the model answer and is usually expressed as a percentage. Relative grading rates the student's essay answer in relation to other students doing the same test, by indicating whether or not it was average, above average or below average. Relative grading usually uses a literal scale such as A, B, C, D and F. Some teachers would argue that two grades are the best way of marking, so that students are given either a pass or fail grade. This overcomes the problem of deciding what constitutes an 'A' or 'C' grade but does reduce the information conveyed by a particular grade, since no discrimination is made between students who pass with a very high level of achievement and those who barely pass at all.

When using absolute grading to a specific criterion, it is useful to use the analytic method of marking and with relative grading, the global method is best. In the former, the marking key is prepared in advance and marks are allocated to the specific points of content in the model answer. However, it is often difficult to decide how many marks should be given to a particular aspect, but the relative importance of each should be reflected in the allocation.

Table 11.4 illustrates the analytical method of marking for an essay question. This method has the advantage that it can be more reliable provided the marker is conscientious, and it will bring to light any errors in the writing of the question before the test is administered.

Table 11.4 Example of analytical method of marking essays

Essay question
A male patient aged 30 is admitted to the ward accompanied by his wife. He is unconscious, and a diagnosis of meningitis has been made.

   (a) *List* the micro-organisms which can cause meningitis   10%
   (b) *Describe* his total nursing care and management during the first
        48 hours in the ward.   90%

Analytical marking scheme
   (a) Virus 2; *Neisseria meningitidis 2, Streptococcus pneumoniae 2;*
        Haemophilus influenzae 2
        Others, e.g. *M. tuberculosis 2.*
   (b) Care of the unconscious patient

Maintenance of airway	4	Hygiene	4
Position in bed	4	Mouth care	4
Pressure areas	4	Eye care	4
Physiotherapy	4	Nutrition and fluids	4
Catheter care	4	Psychological – talking to him etc.	4

Isolation nursing
   Outline of technique and reasons   10
Treatment and observations
   Investigations, e.g. lumbar puncture   10
   Antibiotics – detail and reasons   10
   Neurological observations – details and reasons   10

Care of the wife
   Support, instructions reisolation, counselling   10

The global method of marking still requires a model answer, but in this case it serves only as a standard of comparison. The grades used are not percentages, but descriptive scales, such as

    excellent
    good
    average
    below average
    unsatisfactory,
    or literal scales, such as A, B, C, D, F.

Scales can be devised according to preference, but it is important to select examples of answers that serve as standards for each of the points on the scale. The teacher then reads each answer through very quickly and places it in the appropriate pile, depending whether it gives the impression of excellent, good, etc. The process is then repeated and it is much more effective if a colleague is asked to do the second reading. This method is much faster than the analytical one and can be quite effective for large numbers of questions.

    When marking essay answers it is important to eliminate the 'halo' effect, which is the term used to describe the influence that the preceding answer has on the marker. If all the answers from one learner were marked together, then the chances are that this would create an impression, favourable or otherwise, that would influence the marking of the remainder of the answers for that learner. It is thus important to mark all the answers for one question before proceeding to the next. It has been suggested that answers should be shuffled randomly after each question has been marked, so that the position of any paper will not consistently be affected by the quality of the preceding ones. Anonymous marking helps to eliminate bias, but is rather tedious to organize. It is good policy to have answers monitored by colleagues and this can be easily arranged by having each teacher circulate one or two papers to the rest of their colleagues.

So far, no mention has been made of feedback to the learner. Some examinations are designed to assess the students' achievement, so feedback comments are not done and the papers are not returned to the students. Some colleges do return these papers, but, without comments they are of little use. The question of how much feedback to give is a difficult one, since for some answers the teacher would have to write out the entire essay again to indicate the improvements required. In addition, feedback is time-consuming, whereas it is fairly easy simply to assign a mark without comments. However, feedback is very important for students' learning, provided they review such feedback rather than just filing their essay away. It is often better to return marked essays to the student during a tutorial so that the main feedback points can be discussed.

Variants of the essay test

Some essay examinations allow the candidate to see the paper some weeks prior to the examination and may even allow them to bring notes into the examination up to 100 words. The 'seen-paper' test is used to evaluate the candidate's ability to select sources and to organize the information in a meaningful way. Another variation of the essay is the 'open-book' examination in which the candidate is allowed to look up information in a book during the examination. It removes over-reliance on memorizing facts and is closer to the reality of professional behaviour, where information has to be looked up most of the time. Gray (1993) suggests that there are several benefits of open-book examinations, such as deeper study of course notes, development of important professional skills, easier marking of exam scripts, and a reduction in students' exam anxiety.

USING OBJECTIVE TESTS FOR ASSESSMENT

The limitations of the essay test led to the development of the objective test, the word 'objective' referring to the marking of the test, which is not influenced by the subjective opinion of the marker. However, the actual writing of the test may be as subjective as an essay, depending on the expertise of the writer. In current terminology, an objective-test question is termed an item and this seems quite logical, since many items are written in the form of statements. In comparison with essay tests, objective tests have perfect marker reliability, because the answer is predetermined. Content validity is also very high in this form of test, as the large number of items ensure that the syllabus is adequately sampled. Furthermore, the marking is economical of teacher time, since it can be done by clerical staff and the items can be kept in a bank and used time after time. The question of marker fatigue does not arise, as objective tests take much less time to answer. However, they are very time consuming to write, and tests of the higher levels of intellectual functioning are difficult to formulate.

Objective tests are commonly classified into those that require the answer to be selected from amongst alternatives and those that require the answer to be supplied by the learner.

Multiple-choice item

This consists of three parts: the 'stem' containing the problem or statement, the 'key', which is the correct response, and 'distracters', or incorrect responses. There should be at least three options given, to reduce the chances of guessing. For example:

(*Stem*)	The epithelium lining the colon is called:
(*Distracters*)	*a* squamous
	b cuboidal
	c transitional
(*key*)	*d* columnar

The multiple-choice item is a very versatile test that can measure a variety of levels of functioning. It is less susceptible to guessing and is popular with students.

Matching item

This consists of two lists in columns; the learner is required to match items from column A with responses in B, e.g.

A	B
1 Yellow discoloration of skin	*a* Bile salts
2 Severe itching of skin	*b* Unconjugated bilirubin
3 Clay-coloured stools	*c* Bilirubinaemia
4 Dark urine with yellow foam	*d* Jaundice
	e Haemolysis
	f Obstruction

Matching items are useful for testing both knowledge of terminology and specific relationships between facts.

True–false item

True–false items are statements which may be true or false and the learner has to decide which. There is a large risk of guessing with this type of item.

Also, it is often difficult to select items that are categorically true or false, e.g.

The commonest form of mental illness in Great Britain is schizophrenia. True/False

Assertion–reason item

This test presents two statements, an assertion and a reason. The learner is required to decide whether each statement is true and then whether the reason is a correct explanation of the assertion, e.g.

| *Assertion* | *Reason* |
| Pressure in the glomerular capillaries is 70 mm Hg | The efferent arteriole has a smaller calibre than the afferent. |

Short-answer items

In this item, there is a statement or question that has a missing word that the learner must supply, e.g.

The part of the brain which contains the visual cortex is called the . . . lobe.

This type is used to test knowledge of terms, but is not very useful for higher levels of functioning. There is often more than one answer which will fit the blank and this item may encourage rote learning.

Multiple completion items

This involves the selection of more than one correct response, from a choice of combinations. The learner is looking for the incorrect option, so this item is often termed reverse multiple-choice. For example:

Which of the following would indicate occurrence of cardiac arrest?

  a Apnoea
  b Dilated pupils
  c Chest pain
  d Absence of pulse

Interpretive items

This form of objective test uses a common problem or source of data and the student is required to select the correct answers from a series of related items. An example is given in Table 11.5.

Table 11.5   An example of an interpretative item

Accidents at work in Great Britain in 1980

Type of industry

	Manufac- turing	Con- struction	Railways	Coal- mining	Agri- culture
All accidents					
Number	133,164	29,492	4391	36,758	4248
Rate per 100,000 at risk	2900	3000	2400	15,200	1400
Fatal accidents					
Number	125	128	30	42	24
Rate per 100,000 at risk	3	13	14	17	8

Directions: The following statements refer to the table above. Please read each one and then mark your answer as follows:
Circle: T if the statement is true; F if the statement is false

1. The occupation with the highest risk of death through accidents is construction.

    T   F
2. The likelihood of having an accident at work is greatest in the coal-mining industry.

    T   F
3. Agriculture is the safest industry out of the five to work in.

    T   F
4. Railway workers are at greater risk from fatal accidents than manufacturing workers.

    T   F

Source of data: Donaldson and Donaldson (1983).

Interpretive items are useful for assessing the higher levels of the cognitive domain, including the ability to recognize relevant information, or warranted or unwarranted generalizations, to apply principles and to recognize assumptions and inferences (Gronlund, 1985).

Guidelines for writing objective tests

Multiple-choice items

The stem should include:

- the clearly stated problem;
- only material which is essential for clarity; and
- novel material to test higher levels.

Examples 1–3 illustrate this point. In example 1, the stem does not contain the problem. The learner has to examine each option to decide what is required. In example 2, the stem contains the problem, but also contains non-essential material, namely, 'one of the water-soluble B group of vitamins'. In example 3, the stem contains a novel problem which requires application and synthesis of knowledge to solve.

Example 1
Vitamin B_{12}
    a. contains iron
    b. is absorbed by mouth
    c. is stored in liver
    d. is given for haemolytic anaemia

Example 2
Vitamin B_{12}, one of the water-soluble B group of vitamins, is necessary for
    a. prevention of haemolytic anaemia
    b. formation of haemoglobin
    c. formation of thrombocytes
    d. maturation of red corpuscles

Example 3
A female patient aged 60 is admitted with a history of fatigue, dyspnoea on exertion, and fainting attacks. Her Hb is 7 g and tests reveal achlorhydria.
The likely diagnosis is
    a. iron deficiency anaemia
    b. haemolytic anaemia
    c. pernicious anaemia
    d. folic acid deficiency anaemia

The options should:

- be three or more, to limit guessing,
- be in logical or quantitative order,
- be as short as possible, but clear,
- avoid repetition,
- be homogeneous,
- make limited use of negative forms, and
- avoid 'all of these' and 'none of these'.

Examples 4–9 illustrate these points. In example 4, the options should be in rank order i.e. 7, 10, 14, 18. In example 5, the options are repetitious, as each one contains the '2 black dots joined by'. This can be included in the stem. The options in example 6 are not homogeneous, in that peritoneum is not part of the thoracic cavity. A better choice is ribs. In Example 7, the negative should be clearly indicated by capitals or underlining. This example would be better stated in a positive form, i.e.: Which of the following is an abnormal constituent of urine . . . . Examples 8 and 9 illustrate poor use of all/none. In example 8 if the learner recognizes one wrong option, or two correct ones, option (d) can be discarded in the former, and accepted in the latter. 'None of these' should only be used when the answer is clearly right or wrong. It should be the key every so often if used.

Example 4
The normal Hb level in men, in grams is
   a. 14
   b. 7
   c. 18
   d. 10

Example 5
A patient's blood pressure when lying down is charted using
   a. 2 black dots joined by an interrupted horizontal line
   b. 2 black dots joined by a continuous vertical line
   c. 2 black dots joined by a continuous horizontal line
   d. 2 black dots joined by an interrupted vertical line

Example 6
The inferior boundary of the thoracic cavity is
   a. sternum
   b. thoracic vertebrae
   c. diaphragm
   d. peritoneum

Example 7
Which of the following does normal urine not contain
   a. urea
   b. albumin
   c. phosphate
   d. chloride

Example 8
Which of the following occurs in dehydration
   a. inelastic skin
   b. oliguria
   c. constipation
   d. all of these

Example 9
Amount of energy released by one gram of fat, in kilojoules is
   a. 7
   b. 17
   c. 37
   d. none of these

The distractors should be plausible. In example 10 sweat and cerumen are plausible distractors, but it is unlikely that any learner would consider option c.

Example 10
The secretion of the sebaceous glands is called
   a. cerumen
   b. sebum
   c. semen
   d. sweat

The key should be:

- the single best or most likely answer, and
- free of specific determiners.

In example 11, the item writer made b the key, but it is debatable if any one option is clearly right or best.

Example 11
A patient in the ward develops diarrhoea. The nurse's first priority is
   a. increase his fluids
   b. isolate him
   c. send stool to laboratory
   d. commence fluid balance recordings

Specific determiners are clues contained in the item, but not linked to knowledge of content. There are several types to be aware of:

- constant position of key in options,
- length of key in relation to distractors,
- opposite options,
- grammatical inconsistency, and
- use of words like 'never' and 'always'.

Example 12
Hypertension is a state of
   a. high blood sugar
   b. high blood pressure
   c. low blood sugar
   d. low blood pressure

Example 13
Diaphragmatic breathing is usually seen when a patient is
   a. running
   b. standing
   c. bending
   d. asleep

Learners will often see the key as being one of the opposites, as item writers commonly choose statements which are opposite to the one they have selected. It can be remedied by including another pair of opposites, as in example 12. In example 13, there is grammatical inconsistency in option d, which gives a clue to the key.

The guidelines for multiple-choice items also apply largely to the other types of objective item. However, there are some specific ones for other types of item and these will be outlined.

Matching items

When writing matching items, there are two specific points to watch out for. The number of choices should always exceed the number of statements, so that guessing is reduced. Also, the longer statements should be used as the premisses, so that the learner has the shorter responses to scan when searching for the answers.

True-false items

The specific points when writing these are to:

- have an equal number of true and false statements;
- ensure that items are clearly true or false; and
- avoid trick questions.

Short-answer items

The specific points when writing these are:

- Leave only important words blank.
- Avoid excessive blanks in a statement.
- Ensure that it is factually correct.

Analysis of objective-test items

One of the more useful characteristics of objective-test items is that they can be stored and used again, but this can only be the case if the item has been validated. Validation is performed after the test has been marked, and there are two aspects that are considered, facility and discrimination. The facility index is the percentage of students who answer the item correctly, and the discrimination index indicates the extent to which an item discriminated between the more knowledgeable and the less know-ledgeable students.

Facility index   This is calculated by the following formula:

$$\frac{\text{Number of students who answered correctly}}{\text{Total number of students tested}} \times 100$$

For example, if 40 students take the test, and 20 answer the item correctly, then the facility index is

$$\frac{20}{40} \times 100 = 50\%$$

Discrimination index   This is normally calculated by arranging the test papers in order from the highest to lowest mark, and then putting them into high and low groups. The top 27% from the high group and the bottom 27% of the low group are then examined to see how many students answered item correctly. If N is the total number of students tested, and N_b (N_t) the number of students who answered item correctly in bottom (top) 27%, respectively, then

$$\text{Discrimination} = \frac{N_t - N_b}{0.27N}$$

The figure of 27% is not rigidly fixed, and if $N < 40$ it is better to use the top and bottom halves of the group. The index range is from $+1.00$ to -1.00.

Example If a batch of 200 test papers is used and the number of correct answers for the top 27% is 40, and for the bottom 27% is 20, then the calculation will be as follows:

$$\frac{40 - 20}{54} = 0.37$$

Interpretation of indexes The facility index is generally considered ideal when it is 50%, but the acceptable range is from about 25–75%. It is often desirable to include some easy items at the beginning of the test and then for it to became progressively more difficult. The index of discrimination ranges from $+1.00$ to -1.00 and zero indicates no discrimination. Positive discrimination is accepted at 0.3 and above. If the index shows a negative figure, this implies that the less knowledgeable students are getting more correct answers for an item than the more knowledgeable ones and may indicate that the item is ambiguous or the wrong key has been chosen.

The writing of objective-test items is made easier if the college has regular 'shredding' sessions, consisting of three of four teachers who look at new test items to decide whether or not they are suitable for inclusion in pre-testing.

THE ASSESSMENT OF NURSING COMPETENCE

The primary aim of nurse education is to provide education that will equip nurses and midwives to maintain and develop their competence as practitioner of nursing. However, competence is a very difficult concept to pin down, and the literature abounds with varied definitions. Benett (1989) suggests that the term has several dimensions such as task competence, job competence, functional competence, occupational competence, and vocational competence. The Further Education Curriculum Unit (FEU) offer the following definition: 'competence is the possession and development of sufficient skills, knowledge, appropriate attitudes and experience for successful performance in life roles' (FEU, 1984). Benner (1984), on the other hand, places competence only midway in her stages of nursing skill development; novice, advanced beginner, competent, proficient, and expert. The competent stage, according to Benner, is characterized by conscious, deliberate planning based upon analysis and careful deliberation of situations. The competent nurse is able to identify priorities and manage her work, and Benner suggests that she can benefit at this stage from learning activities that centre on decision-making and planning. It is interesting to note that she makes a distinction between competence and proficiency; unlike the competent nurse, the proficient nurse has the ability to home in directly on the most relevant aspects of a problem because she is able to perceive situations holistically. It is clear from this description that Benner views competence as a fairly basic level of performance, and this accords with the lay concept of competence as equating to mediocrity. Competence is commonly perceived as synonymous with safety, in that safety is the main criterion for competence. However, it is quite possible for a nurse to perform her role without putting the patient at risk, but she may lack the necessary interpersonal skills that would make for competent practice. Hence, safety is a necessary but not sufficient condition for competence; one cannot be a competent practitioner without safety, but safety alone does not make a competent practitioner.

Approaches to the assessment of practice performance

The main method of assessing competence is by observing the student's performance. This observation is usually combined with some form of checklist or rating scale that serves as a guide for the assessor.

Checklists

A checklist is simply a list of student behaviours associated with a particular nursing intervention, with a space for the assessor to check or tick off whether or not that particular behaviour occurred. There is no means of indicating how well a behaviour was carried out, and this limits the usefulness of checklists. A checklist may contain only the desired behaviours, or may also include the behaviours that constitute poor performance. Table 11.6 shows a behavioural checklist that contains descriptions of both effective and ineffective behaviours and it should be noted that the respective columns are not pairs of opposites. The right-hand list of behaviours consists of common faults that reduce the effectiveness of nursing.

Rating scales

Rating scales provide an indication of the degree or amount of a particular characteristic and use either numbers or descriptions.

Table 11.7 shows a numerical rating scale and Table 11.8 gives three examples of descriptive rating-scales.

Behaviourally anchored rating scales (BARS) is a type of rating scale that involves identifying the qualities that the organization values, such as communication skills, reliability, etc. These attributes are then put before a panel of appraisers who are asked to give definitions in their own words of the kinds of behaviours that would constitute excellent, adequate and poor levels of each attribute. Only those definitions that are measurable can be included and these form the anchors for the rating scale.

Table 11.6 Checklist for assessment of clinical competence

Place a tick against any behaviours you observe during the assessment. Aspect of assessment: *Admission of patient from waiting-list*			
The effective nurse:	Tick	The ineffective nurse:	Tick
Prepares bed and locker area in advance.		Conveys an impression of unreadiness to patient.	
Greets patient (and companion) by introducing herself.		Excludes companion from process of admission.	
Conducts patient to bed area.		Emphasizes procedural aspects of admission rather than welcome and reassurance.	
Ensures privacy whilst patient is unpacking and changing.		Omits provision of amenities, e.g. jug of water.	
Introduces patient to fellow patients adjacent to him/her.		Overloads patient with detailed explanations.	
Shows patient the ward layout.		Leaves patient to provide his or her own orientation.	
Allows ample opportunity for questions.			
Gives only essential explanations initially.			
Makes appointments for further explanation and discussion.			
Employs appropriate procedures with regard to patient's property.			

Another type of scale is the 'self assessment, identification of needs and teaching of work skills' (SAINT) system (Dunn, 1991) which involves self-assessment in six important work areas: social skills, management skills, communication skills, practical skills, teamwork skills and teaching skills.

Categories or descriptions of nursing behaviours are notoriously difficult to write with any precision, as many interventions involve value judgements about quality and will vary between assessors. There are many ways that a nurse can establish rapport with a patient and it may be that the only sure way of telling whether or not it has occurred is to ask the patient whether he felt that a rapport existed. Even then, the patient may

Table 11.7 Numerical rating scale

Aspect of assessment: *Performance of a surgical dressing*

Please circle the number that describes the nurse's performance; 1 means poor performance and 6 means excellent performance.

1.	Establishng rapport	1	2	3	4	5	6
2.	Explaining procedure	1	2	3	4	5	6
3.	Preparation of equipment	1	2	3	4	5	6
4.	Preparation of patient	1	2	3	4	5	6
5.	Hand-washing	1	2	3	4	5	6
6.	Removal of dressing	1	2	3	4	5	6
7.	Observation of area	1	2	3	4	5	6
8.	Use of equipment	1	2	3	4	5	6
9.	Application of dressing	1	2	3	4	5	6
10.	Removal of equipment	1	2	3	4	5	6
11.	Attending to patient	1	2	3	4	5	6
12.	Disposal of equipment	1	2	3	4	5	6
13.	Recording of intervention	1	2	3	4	5	6

Table 11.8 Examples of descriptive rating scales

A. *Bipolar description*

X	X applies	Marked tendency to X	Some tendency to X Y	Y applies	Y
Work shows a consistently high standard of attention to detail and finish					Work does not always show sufficient attention to detail and finish

B. *Single-word category*

Gives a full explanation to patient prior to commencing a procedure	Always	Usually	Occasionally	Never

C. *Phrase description*

Working in partnership with another nurse	Takes a leading role	Shares equal responsibility with partner	Allows partner to lead most of the time

be reluctant to say that rapport did not exist; the patient might feel this would be letting the nurse down, or that such a comment might influence the quality of care required for the rest of their stay.

One way of generating behavioural descriptions of nursing practice is CIT (critical-incident-technique) (Flanagan, 1954). This involves the observation of qualified nurses as they practise nursing, noting down any particular desirable or undesirable incidents. These particularly critical incidents are written down as descriptions of behaviours rather than as evaluative comments and then large numbers of these incidents are classified by nursing experts to see if there is agreement about whether or not they represent particularly good or bad practice. The incidents that are agreed by the experts are then used to provide descriptions of effective or ineffective job performance and can then be used as check lists for observational assessment. CIT is also a useful tool for teaching students, and is discussed in Chapter 8 (p. 192).

Factors influencing validity and reliability of practice assessments

There are three major factors influencing observational assessment: the assessor, the student and the methodology.

The assessor

Accurate assessment requires care and effort if it is to be objective and there may be a lack of time and interest for this. An assessor may be biased in their perception of the performance and this can take a number of forms. The 'halo' effect occurs when the assessor is influenced by the general characteristics of the student: if given a good impression of the student, then the student is likely to be rated highly on the performance – and if the impression is unfavourable, then the reverse will occur. Another common factor is the central-tendency error, in which the rater gives everybody an average mark. The generosity error occurs when the rater gives a higher score than is warranted and the explanation for this is the tendency to feel that our nursing role is to care for students, so this the assessor does unconsciously. In addition to the above factors, assessors will be subject to the same influences on their interpersonal perception as everyone else, namely past experience, motivation and personality.

The student

The main factors that influence assessment from the student's point of view are: state of preparation, level of anxiety and the presence of others. The first point is self-evident, in that the student must have adequate preparation in the aspects that are being assessed. Anxiety has the effect of degrading decision-making, which could make a difference to an assessment in which decisions are required. The presence of others, i.e. the assessor, may have the effect termed diffusion of responsibility (Latane and Darley, 1968), which might account for a student's indecision

Table 11.9 Examples of performance criteria for drug-round assessment

Example of criterion	Comments
1. Understands the reason for giving the drugs	No indication of the level of understanding required
2. Shows knowledge of scheduled drugs and controlled drugs	No indication of amount and level of knowledge required
3. Works well with assisting nurse	No indication of what 'working well' means
4. Practises safe, intelligent administration of medicines	No indication of what 'intelligent' administration is

in the assessment. The work of Latane and Darley is discussed in Chapter 2 (p. 28).

The methodology

The criteria chosen for the observation schedule will have implications for reliability and validity and it is exceedingly difficult to formulate objective criteria for checklists or rating scales. The problem is that most criteria are fairly general and this may be of necessity because it is impractical to state them in a more precise way. Table 11.9 gives examples of performance criteria for assessing a drug round, with comments on their formulation.

These examples illustrate the dilemma referred to earlier about trying to make accurate descriptions of nursing behaviours. Some teachers have resorted to identifying a list of behaviours similar to the behavioural objectives approach, which gives more detailed criteria; for example, the following criterion might apply to the drug round: 'Describes the action, dosage, route of administration, unwanted side-effects and contraindications of a given drug, to the level indicated in the current edition of the British National Formulary.' This criterion is certainly more specific and does give the student an idea as to the kind of level of questioning to expect. However, it is rather lengthy and one can imagine a checklist of skills required for a drug round being stated in several pages of text. Another problem is that such objectives are reasonably meaningful when applied to knowledge or motor skills, but how do we go about writing criteria for the interactional elements of a drug round? We could try: 'Displays warmth and friendliness towards patients during the drug round.' This is certainly an important aspect of nursing care, but the difficulty lies in the assessor's interpretation of the behaviours that are considered to be warm and friendly. At first glance it may seem fairly straightforward, until we begin to wonder what the borderline is between friendliness and familiarity and between humour and offence.

One way round the problem would be to adopt a stance advocated by Stenhouse (1975) who suggests that the teacher, as an expert in the field of nursing, can judge the quality of what is observed without having to define what that quality might consist of in advance. In other words, a competent teacher-practitioner can tell whether a student has done a satisfactory drug round or not without having to go through any kind of checklist. The problem arises when different assessors hold different views on competence, but perhaps it is naïve to expect any real consensus in nursing, or in any other social-science endeavour, since there are so many variables to be considered. In the world of the arts, an art critic makes judgements about the merits of a work of art without having to specify in advance what the work of art should look like. I am often asked by students: 'How should I approach this topic in order to get an 'A' grade for my assignment?' All I can say in reply is 'I can't tell you in advance what an 'A' assignment will look like, but I will recognize one when I see it.'

SELF-ASSESSMENT AND PEER-ASSESSMENT

One of the dimensions of assessment outlined earlier was that of 'teacher-centred' versus 'student-centred' assessment and it was suggested that increasing importance was being given to the latter. If one of the goals of nurse education is the development of an autonomous professional, then self-assessment is an important means towards this goal. Students could, in theory, use any of the assessment methods already outlined in this chapter to assess their own learning, such as marking their own essays. Indeed, this can be a very useful way of encouraging self evaluation; the student is given the opportunity to mark his own essay according to the criteria that the teacher has devised and then they both discuss their respective marking with each other. Interviews are another useful way of getting students to undertake self-assessment; the teacher can facilitate this by careful use of probing questions that focus attention upon aspects of the student's performance. Questionnaires provide an alternative method for this and are less time-consuming, but both methods are open to distorted reporting by the student. It is best not to grade these self-assessments to ensure honest and unbiased reporting, although the teacher may wish to negotiate with the student about the final grade of work, taking into account these self-assessments. Another method is to keep a self-assessment diary or commentary about progress on a course and this involves writing down the reflections of the student's experiences and feelings.

Self-assessment is not the only way in which student-centred assessment can be used; peer-assessment is the assessment of a student by his or her peer group, and there are a number of ways in which this can be done. The presentation of course material by a single student can be assessed by the peer group to whom it is presented, or essays can be exchanged between students and then marked by them prior to returning to the writer. Of course, the teacher needs to beware of fixing of marks, especially if these are to be taken into account towards a final grade. Students might soon realize that if each of them gives a high mark to the other, then the overall marks will be very high for everyone. It is therefore best if these peer-assessments are used as feedback rather than as final grading, to ensure honesty of feedback. Many peer-assessment techniques are used in the context of small-group evaluations, so this issue will be examined below.

ASSESSMENT/EVALUATION OF SMALL-GROUP PROCESSES

Assessment of achievement in small groups utilizes all the techniques discussed so far, but the evaluation of the processes involved in small-group learning needs a range of additional methods. Many of these methods have been discussed elsewhere in this book, so the reader should refer to the relevant chapters.

Individual-response evaluation

Reflective diary

Group members are invited to keep a diary of the events and feelings they have, about the group meetings over a period of time. These comments may be disclosed to the group or the tutor, and can give much insight into the group process. However, the fact that the diary may be seen by other people may inhibit the students revealing some aspects of their experiences.

Individual impressions

Students are asked to jot down two aspects of the group they did not like and two aspects they did like, for feedback to the tutor, the group or both.

Face-to-face interview

Here, the tutor spends time with a group member discussing her perceptions of the group and the usefulness of the process. It can be time-consuming, but worthwhile, provided both parties are trusting enough to be honest and open.

Sociometry

This technique involves individual group members privately writing down which other group members they would choose to spend time with on a particular activity. Sociometry is described in Chapter 2 (p. 31).

Group-response evaluation

Do-it-yourself evaluation

This involves each group member in writing three statements about the group and then forming 'snowball' groups of two, four and eight people to modify and hone the statements. A plenary is called and the group must edit the list, after which the finished statements are put up on a notice board. Each group member then has to rate each statement on a six-point scale ranging from 'strongly agree' to 'strongly disagree' and record their rating in the form of large blobs that can be easily seen. The whole exercise provides a forum for discussion and exchange of feelings.

Group consensus

Group members form 'buzz' groups to ascertain whether they have common likes or dislikes about the group and are required to reach a consensus of opinion.

Group interview

Similar to the face-to-face interview with one group member, this involves the total group in interview with the teacher. Again this requires skilful handling if it is to be effective and not just tokenism.

'Sculpting'

This is a technique for evaluation that uses physical position to indicate group processes. One member is asked to volunteer to be the 'sculptor' and the rest of the group is asked to remain in any position the chosen member would like to put them in. He or she is asked to 'sculpt' the way they see relationships within the group; the leader is often put on a chair to show their elevation above the rest of the group. Trust is essential among members if this is to work well, particularly as some may find themselves in the role of outsider or isolate. Following the sculpting, there is group discussion and debriefing about the exercise.

Third-party evaluation

Observation

This can take place during normal group interaction, where a non-group member observes the process of group interaction. The main problem is the Hawthorne effect, i.e. the presence of an observer may alter the natural behaviour of the group.

Video-recording

This can provide a good alternative to a live observer, since it will not interpret the events, only record them. During the analysis playback, group members comment on the process.

Group-interaction analysis

This is a formal system of observing group interaction using a variety of measures including video, flow diagrams and categorization. The most familiar system is Bales' Interaction Process Analysis, which is described in Chapters 7 (p. 149) and 18 (p. 427).

ASSESSMENT OF ATTITUDES

Although attitudes are of fundamental importance in professional practice, the assessment of them presents major problems for the teacher. Attitudes are much less easy to pin down than practical or intellectual skills, but they are just as important for quality nursing and midwifery care. Traditionally, attitudes have been assessed almost intuitively by teachers and supervisors, and students' placement reports might contain reference to their attitude to patients or other staff. However, as the requirements for assessment have become focused on specific behaviours, supervisors are more cautious in their comments about students attitudes because of the difficulty in stating exactly what the problem is. For example, a skilled practitioner can often 'feel' that a student has the 'wrong attitude' to patients, but trying to pin it down to specific incidents is not easy.

Attitudes are commonly described as having three components: a cognitive component or belief, an effective component or feeling, and a motor component or tendency to action. Attitudes predispose an individual to act in a certain way towards stimuli and are thus powerful influences on learning and behaviour. Some people may adopt an anti-smoking attitude and this would consist of a set of beliefs about smoking plus a set of related feelings of disgust, bafflement or aggression towards smokers. The third component is the action tendency, which would make the individual react to smokers in a typical way, probably avoidance or confrontation. Student nurses, nurse teachers, patients and other staff will have their own particular attitudes towards most things in their environment, but the nurse teacher may want to find out specifically about his students' attitudes towards nursing and education.

However, a note of caution is required here; the methods of assessing attitudes outlined below include a wide range of techniques, most of which require a qualified psychologist to administer and interpret.

Measurement of attitudes

Self-report

In this approach, the students are asked to write down their attitudes towards something, either anonymously or otherwise, depending on the degree of trust and the honesty of the respondent.

Table 11.10 A Likert scale for attitude measurement

	Strongly agree	Agree	Uncertain	Disagree	Strongly disagree
	5	4	3	2	1
1. Nursing gives me a great deal of job satisfaction.					
2. Academic nurses don't make good practical nurses at the bedside					
3. Enrolled nurses are the best bedside nurses.					

Published inventories

These are standardized scales for measuring attitudes to various things, such as attitudes towards college. They are more useful than home-made tests because they claim to have high validity and reliability, but they may not meet individual teachers' exact requirements.

Likert scaling

In this technique, a pool of items is devised to cover the attitude in question, and then a scale is drawn up that rates each item under five points, ranging from 'strongly agree' to 'strongly disagree'. These five points are scored from one to five, and the teacher can choose whether the high score of five is to mean a favourable or unfavourable attitude towards the statement in question. Once this has been decided, the inventory is given to subjects, who are asked to tick the appropriate response for each item and then the total score is calculated. This score gives an indication of the subject's attitude towards the thing in question, either favourable, unfavourable or neutral. Table 11.10 shows an example of a Likert scale for attitude measurement.

The semantic differential

This kind of rating scale consists of a number of bi-polar rating scales, each with seven points between them. (Table 11.11 gives an example of this scale applied to attitudes towards the College of Nursing.) At either end of the scales there are adjectives that are the opposite of each other, such as black/white and each respondent is required to select a point on the scale that they feel represents their feelings about the item in question.

Table 11.11 Semantic-differential technique for attitudes to College of Nursing

Hot	.	.	.	.	.	.	.	Cold
Slow	.	.	.	.	.	.	.	Fast
False	.	.	.	.	.	.	.	True
Colourful	.	.	.	.	.	.	.	Colourless
Strong	.	.	.	.	.	.	.	Weak
Passive	.	.	.	.	.	.	.	Active
Wise	.	.	.	.	.	.	.	Foolish
Child	.	.	.	.	.	.	.	Adult
Soft	.	.	.	.	.	.	.	Hard

The 'semantic differential' can assess not only physical properties of things, but also aesthetic and value based ones as well.

Projective techniques

The most famous of these is the 'ink-blot' test, but others include the 'word-association' test and the 'thematic apperception' test (TAT). Projective techniques aim to reach behind the mask that people put up consciously or otherwise to prevent access to awareness. In the ink-blot test the subject is required to study patterns to see what things they represent. In the word-association test the subject has to respond very rapidly to the experimenter's prompt words by saying a word that comes into his or her mind that is associated with the first word. In TAT the subject is shown a picture and asked to make up a story about what they think is going on.

THE MANAGEMENT OF THE ASSESSMENT SYSTEM

There are probably few areas of nursing and midwifery education that have more potential for problems and errors than that of assessment. The assessment system requires meticulous attention to detail, and sound management if problems are to be avoided. One of the most important aspects of assessment are the assessment regulations; these act as an absolute guide to the whole assessment system for a given course or pathway, and should be followed meticulously by the course or pathway Director.

Assessment regulations

Although assessment regulations will be specific to a given course or pathway, there are some generic aspects that apply to most:

Student referral

The first time a student is unsuccessful in an assessment is termed referral. There would normally be one opportunity for retrieval for each unit assessment, and there is usually a maximum grade that can be obtained, which is less than the highest grade possible.

Compensation

This refers to a situation where a good grade in one assessment can compensate for a weaker grade in another. Some courses allow this, others do not.

Submission date for assessments

There should be a published date for submission of assessments, after which the student will be deemed to have been referred. In exceptional circumstances the student may be granted an extension by the unit leader. A request for such an extension must be made in writing before the original due date.

Failure on re-submission of assessment

In the event of students being referred and then failing upon being re-assessed, they would normally be counselled to reconsider their programme of study. The failed unit may then be retaken only at the discretion of the course director.

Planning for assessment

Assessments in nursing and midwifery education can be classified into course-work, examinations, and assessment of competence in practice. Regardless of the nature of the assessment, careful planning is required to get the best out of the system. Assessment regulations normally state that the requirements for assessment of each component will be notified to every student in writing at the start of the component.

Planning coursework assignments

Coursework assignments are by far the commonest form of written assessment in nursing and midwifery education and often allow a degree of negotiation between teacher and student. In CAT schemes, course-work is linked to individual units or modules that comprise the pathway, each unit having its own assessment. This can make for a large number of assessments, but it may be possible in some institutions to combine assessments from more than one unit.

Planning a written examination paper

Planning a written examination paper requires careful formulation to ensure that it has high content validity for the course or unit in question and the best way to do this is by use of a specification grid or blueprint.

Table 11.12 Test specification grid or blueprint: 'Nursing the burned patient'

Subject matter	Cognitive domain categories						Total %
	1	*2*	*3*	*4*	*5*	*6*	
Admission of patient	2	4	8	1	1	4	20
Structure of skin	0.5	1	2	0.25	0.25	1	5
Pathophysiology of burns	1	2	4	0.5	0.5	2	10
Observations	1.5	3	6	0.75	0.75	3	15
Infection control	0.5	1	2	0.25	0.25	1	5
Pre- and post-operative care	2	4	8	1	1	4	20
Fluids/drugs	1.5	3	6	0.75	0.75	3	15
Rehabilitation	1	2	4	0.5	0.5	2	10
Total %	10	20	40	5	5	20	100

The best time to formulate the blueprint is during the planning phase for the particular unit, when the learning outcomes have been formulated. Table 11.12 shows a blueprint for planning an examination paper for a unit on 'Nursing the burned patient'.

It is a two-way matrix, with content areas derived from the objectives down one side and the categories of Bloom's cognitive domain across the top. The right-hand side shows the amount of weight given to each aspect of content in terms of a percentage of the total content of the unit. For example, the item 'admission of a burned patient' is weighted at 20%, whereas structure of the skin is only given 5%. At the foot of each of the cognitive-domain categories, there is another total percentage that applies to the percentage weighting given to each category of intellectual functioning. For example, this unit emphasizes the application of knowledge, rather than the mere recall of specific facts, so category 3 (application) receives a weighting of 40%. The two columns of percentages should both add up to 100 and the percentage of test items for each aspect of the unit can now be calculated. For example, taking the component called 'admission of the patient' we see that it has a total weighting of 20% of the unit; this figure is now multiplied by each of the figures at the foot of the cognitive-domain categories to give the percentage for each cell in the matrix. Thus, under the category of knowledge, admission of a burned patient receives 20% of 10%, i.e. 2%. This means that 2% of the total test must comprise questions about terminology relating to the admission of a burned patient. If we wish to know the percentage of the test that should be devoted to pre-operative/post-operative care of a burned patient, at the level of application (category 3), we calculate 20% of 40%, i.e. 8%. The use of a test blueprint ensures that the test reflects the weighting given to both the subject matter and the level of objectives during the particular unit.

Conduct of written examinations

The room should be prepared the evening before, with desks spaced evenly, and the appropriate materials distributed. Clocks must be clearly visible and synchronized, and a room plan with seat numbers should be displayed outside the room. Before the commencement of the examination the teacher should provide water to drink and a sufficient number of glasses. The lighting and ventilation will need careful monitoring during the examination. The name of each candidate should be checked before entry to the room or hall and personal property should be stored separately in a cupboard, or at the rear of the hall. Candidates should bring no books or paper unless specifically requested to do so. If there are a large number of candidates, a microphone and public-address system may be required. At the commencement of the examination, the invigilator should read out any instructions (such as beginning each answer on a fresh page) and point out the procedure for leaving the room for purposes of visiting the toilet.

The examination papers can then be distributed, face down on each desk and the candidates requested not to turn them over until instructed. The teacher asks them to turn the paper over and to check that they have the correct one. The instructions at the top of the paper are read out and the candidates are told when time checks will be given. The word is given to commence the examination and the invigilators are responsible for observing the candidates throughout the examination.

Time is called at the end, and candidates requested to put their pens down. They check each question to see if they have numbered it correctly and are then dismissed. The invigilators collect and arrange the papers in order, checking them against the attendance register.

MODERATION OF MARKED ASSESSMENT WORK

Before marked work is handed back to the students, it undergoes two kinds of moderation, internal and external. The purpose of moderation is to ensure consistency and fairness of marking amongst the unit markers. Inter-marker reliability, i.e. consistency, is notoriously low, and internal moderation seeks to expose marked papers to a second scrutiny so as to determine the consistency of marking standards between different unit markers. External moderation is carried out by the external examiner appointed to the pathway, and the aim here is also to monitor consistency and standard of marking to ensure that students are being assessed fairly. In addition, the external examiner can compare the standard of work with that on similar courses nationally.

Internal moderation

Internal moderation can be carried out in a number of ways, but the principles remain the same, i.e. to ensure fairness and consistency of marking across the pathway. Internal moderation normally consists of the scrutiny of a sample of students' work across the range of marks. It is important to distinguish internal moderation from double marking; in the latter, two teachers independently mark a student's work, and come to an agreement about the final mark awarded. Whilst this is an added safeguard for individual students' marks, it is not a substitute for proper internal moderation. Effective moderation requires scrutiny of a sample of the entire student work, whereas double marking focuses on a limited number of student assessments. Internal moderation is a resource-intensive activity and as such requires careful planning. Whatever system is used, it will have to be agreed by the pathway committee and the board of examiners. One effective way to carry out internal moderation is to select from each marking teacher a sample of marks they have awarded at each grade or percentage band. Hence, the scrutineers will have a sample of each grade or percentage band for every marking teacher, and are then in a position to ascertain the degree of consistency between markers for each grade or percentage band. If only one unit is being assessed, then the internal moderation will sample only in relation to that unit. For example, each teacher is asked to provide a 10% sample from each of the grade or percentage bandings they have used in their marking. For a typical pathway using a literal grading system, this might involve three or four papers marked at Grade A, and a similar number from each of Grade B to D, including all borderline and referred papers. One point that often causes confusion is whether or not internal moderators should alter individual student marks. Generally speaking, moderators should only adjust student marks if all the assessments within a category have been moderated, e.g. all borderline or referred papers. Since moderation involves only a sample of students' assessments, there will be considerable numbers of students whose work is not moderated. If the moderators were to alter individual students' marks, this could give an unfair advantage or disadvantage to those students whose work was sampled.

In CAT schemes it is more likely that a number of units are being assessed at the same point, such as at the end of a semester, and in this case it is possible to moderate across different units. The principle is the same, but the scrutineers task is more difficult, in that they have to judge the consistency of marking at each grade or percentage band across a number of different units.

External moderation

External moderation is undertaken by the external examiner, who will inform the pathway director of the procedures to be adopted. Normally, the external examiner would receive all referred papers and all papers awarded the highest grade, as well as a sample of papers from each grade or percentage band.

Once the internal moderation system has been completed, assessment work can be returned to students. Assessments are made available for collection at the department office. Students should note that any mark awarded is provisional at this stage; the final mark is determined at the Board of Examiners' meeting. A unit pass list is sent to each successful student as soon as possible after the Board of Examiners' meeting. Students who were unsuccessful are informed individually by letter.

External examiners

The external examiner plays a crucial role in the assessment process, and must be present at any Board of Examiners' meeting where conferment of awards are recommended. A decision of the external examiner is normally taken as final, except in extreme cases such as disagreement between external examiners, when the matter would be referred to the academic board of the institution. External examiners should be experts in the relevant subject area and be experienced in the assessment of students at the level of the pathway in question. Their judgements must be impartial and not influenced by previous association with either students or staff of the institution. The typical responsibilities of an external examiner are to:

1. approve proposed examination papers and other assessments;
2. consider, and if appropriate, agree proposed changes to assessment regulations;
3. undertake moderation of students assessment work, including scrutiny of all students work proposed for the highest and referred grades;
4. compare students assessment performance with that of students on comparable courses elsewhere;
5. report on the consistency and standard of internal marking;
6. attend meetings of the Board of Examiners at which recommendations are made for conferment of academic awards; and
7. provide reports to the institution on the assessment process.

Board of Examiners

The Board of Examiners carries out vitally important functions in relation to assessment; typical terms of reference are:

1. oversight of assessment procedures;
2. ensuring students are assessed fairly;
3. maintenance of the standard of awards;
4. ensuring compliance with assessment requirements;
5. making decisions about student progression and reassessment; and recommending students for academic awards.

The *typical composition of a Board of Examiners* is:

- Appropriate senior manager (Chair)
- Other senior managers with involvement in the pathway
- Pathway director
- Representative of staff teaching on the pathway as internal examiners
- External examiner
- A representative from the Academic Registry will normally attend meetings to record the proceedings and to offer advice regarding regulations

It is one of the responsibilities of the pathway director to make arrangements for meetings of the board of examiners, in consultation with the chair and the external examiner. He must arrange the production of all papers, including draft results lists and pass lists, for each meeting, and be prepared to comment on individual students' performance, and where necessary, on any mitigating circumstances, as required by the board. Following the meeting of the Board of Examiners, the pathway director must arrange for the mailing of pass lists and referral/fail letters to students, and also the entering of the results on the registry database for the pathway.

Appeals against a decision of the Board of Examiners

All institutions have procedures for appeals by students, and the grounds of appeal are carefully defined. Students may not appeal against the academic judgement of the markers as ratified by the Board of Examiners, and there are normally only three grounds upon which an appeal may be based:

1. illness or other factors which the student claims affected their performance, but which he or she was unable or unwilling, for legitimate reasons, to make known to the Board of Examiners before it made its decision;
2. the occurrence of an administrative error or other irregularity affecting the assessment; and
3. the assessment not being carried out in accordance with the regulations for the pathway.

Appeals are conducted by an Appeals Committee whose typical composition includes a deputy vice-chancellor, the dean of faculty, a head of department from a different faculty, a member of the academic board of the institution, and a student nominee of the students union. No member of the committee should have had previous involvement with the student in matters regarding the appeal.

STUDENT PROFILES

Once the nurse teacher has gathered in all the data from the various assessments we have discussed, it must be recorded in some permanent form in the student's records. One recent development in this area has been the concept of student profiling, which arose out of dissatisfaction with a system of record keeping that only gave grades for areas of study. Profiling aims to give a balanced picture of the strengths and competencies of the student so that potential employers get a much better picture of the candidate. Student profiling is discussed in Chapter 9.

REFERENCES

Bendall, E. (1975) *So You Passed, Nurse*. RCN, London.
Benner, P. (1984) *From Novice to Expert: Excellence and Power in Clinical Nursing Practice*, Addison-Wesley, London.

Benett, Y. (1989) The assessment of supervised work experience (SWE): a theoretical perspective. *The Vocational Aspect of Education*, XLI, **109**, 53–64.

Council for National Academic Awards (1989) *How Shall We Assess Them?*, CNAA, London.

Donaldson, R. and Donaldson, L. (1983) *Essential Community Medicine*, MTP, Lancaster.

Dunn, D. (1991) *SAINT*, Assessment Dunn, Sidcup.

Further Education Curriculum Unit (1984) *Towards a Competency-Based System*, FEU, London.

Flanagan, J. (1954) The critical incident technique. *Psychological Bulletin*, **51**, 327–58.

Gray, T. (1993) Open book examination. *The New Academic*, **3**(1), 6–9.

Gronlund, N. (1985) *Measurement and Evaluation in Teaching*, 5th edn, Macmillan, London.

Latane, B. and Darley, J. (1968) Group inhibition of bystander intervention in emergencies. *Journal of Personality and Social Psychology*, **10**, 215–21.

Stenhouse, L. (1975) *Introduction to Curriculum Research and Development*, Heinemann, London.

The curriculum: 12
principles and
application

The business of Colleges and Departments of Nursing and Midwifery is the provision of professional education and training that meets the needs of service. This provision takes a variety of forms, from short in-house courses through to long formal courses leading to academic awards, and is made available as taught courses or open learning. The two main categories of provision are pre-registration and post-registration education. The former consists of courses or pathways leading to both an academic award, such as a Diploma of Higher Education, and entry to the register of nurses. Post-registration provision, on the other hand, is much more diverse and includes study days for qualified staff, longer modules or units for specific staff development, e.g. Supervision and Mentorship Skills, and pathways leading to named academic awards such as first degrees or higher degrees. With the advent of Credit Accumulation and Transfer (CAT) schemes, the tendency is for colleges and departments to offer all their post-registration provision in the form of modules or units which carry a credit rating. These credit points can then be accumulated towards an academic award.

Whatever the nature or mode of educational delivery, the term curriculum is used to describe the plan or design upon which this provision is based. For example, nurse teachers might refer to the curriculum for a Project 2000 DipHE course, or the curriculum for a post-registration BSc in Professional Practice. It is less common to find the term used to describe smaller educational provision such as a study day, although its use would still be appropriate here.

This chapter explores the concept of curriculum, discusses the principles of curriculum design and implementation, and examines curriculum innovation, all within the context of nurse education.

THE NATURE OF CURRICULUM

Curriculum theory is an established field of study within education, but examination of the literature reveals that the concept is by no means straightforward. There is wide variation between definitions and a number of writers – Lewis and Miel, (1972) Tanner and Tanner (1980) Saylor, Alexander and Lewis (1981) – have attempted to categorize these. Four main interpretations of the concept emerge.

1. Curriculum as objectives

   'Any statement of the objectives of the school should be a statement of changes to take place in students'. (Tyler, 1949).

2. Curriculum as subject-matter

   'A curriculum is the offering of socially valued knowledge, skills and attitudes made available to students through a variety of arrangements during the time they are at school, college or university' (Bell, 1973).

3. Curriculum as student experiences

   'Curriculum is all the learning which is planned and guided by the school whether it is carried on in groups or individually, inside or outside the school' (Kerr, 1968).

4. Curriculum as opportunities for students

   'A curriculum is all the educational opportunities encountered by students as a direct result of their involvement with an educational institution' (Quinn, 1988).

Skilbeck's (1984) categorization has considerable overlap with the above, but additionally the aspect of culture is introduced:

1. Curriculum as a structure of forms and fields of knowledge
2. Curriculum as a chart or map of the culture
3. Curriculum as a pattern of learning activities
4. Curriculum as a learning technology

This categorization has been adapted by Beattie (1987) in his Fourfold Model of Curriculum, described later in this chapter. Other writers – Stenhouse (1975) Saylor, Alexander and Lewis (1981) – take a more generic view of the concept, seeing it as an overall plan or design for learning:

'Curriculum is an attempt to communicate the essential principles and features of an educational proposal in such a form that it is open to critical scrutiny and capable of effective translation into practice' (Stenhouse, 1975).

'Curriculum is a plan for providing sets of learning opportunities for persons to be educated' (Saylor, Alexander and Lewis, 1981).

'Curriculum refers to the learning experiences of students, in so far as they are expressed or anticipated in educational goals and objectives, plans and designs for learning and the implementation of these plans and designs in school environments' (Skilbeck, 1984).

The concept of curriculum has been further subdivided by some commentators and the more common ones are as follows.

- Official Curriculum: the curriculum laid down in the policy of the institution.
- Actual Curriculum: the curriculum as implemented by teachers.
- Hidden Curriculum: the attitudes and values transmitted by the teachers

How are nurse teachers to make sense of these widely differing approaches to curriculum in their everyday work as a teacher? My own approach is to go straight to the heart of the concept; my definition of curriculum is a plan or design for education/training that addresses the following questions:

- *Who* is to be taught? Who will learn? This is the *consumer* of the curriculum, i.e. the student, course member, colleague, etc. who will experience the curriculum.
- *What* is to be taught and/or learned? This is about both the *intentions* and the *content* of the curriculum. Intentions may or may not be stated overtly, according to the education ideology underpinning the curriculum. Where outcomes, goals, or objectives are overtly expressed, these statements also indicate to some extent the nature of the curriculum content.

    If the intentions are covert, then content is usually indicated by a list of topics in a syllabus.
- *Why* is it to be taught and/or learned? This is the *ideology* of the curriculum, i.e. the beliefs and values that underpin the curriculum approach.
- *How* is it to be taught and/or learned? This is the *process* of education, i.e. the teaching, learning and assessment approaches or opportunities available to the consumer.
- *Where* is it to be taught/learned? This is the *context* of the curriculum, i.e. the faculty, department, school, college, campus, rooms, etc. It also refers to the place of a given curriculum within the range of awards of the education provider institution.
- *When* is it to be taught and/or learned? This is the *programming/ timetabling* of the curriculum, i.e. the length, pattern of attendance etc.

Curriculum terminology

Understanding of curriculum theory is not made any easier by the plethora of terminology used within the literature. Three key concepts in common use are outlined below.

Curriculum theory

The purpose of theory is to try to understand and explain phenomena, and curriculum theory attempts to relate educational scholarship to pragmatic everyday aspects of educational practice. Theories provide a rationale for making decisions about the curriculum and can be thought of as having a basic structure. The basic building blocks are 'concepts' and these can be defined as classes of objects, events or situations that possess common properties. Concepts are not specific entities, rather they are mental constructs with which we make sense of the environment. We are able to classify most things we encounter instantaneously, because we compare the specific stimulus with our concepts to see where it fits most easily. If the specific stimulus fits into a concept category, it can be confidently classified as a member of the concept and this process means that the individual can very quickly make sense of the myriad of stimuli impinging upon his or her senses every day.

Concepts are thus the basic building blocks of theory, but they need to be combined together in the form of statements if they are to constitute a theory. Statements in a theory can be either non-relational or relational (Walker and Avant, 1983). Non-relational statements may simply state that something exists, or they may go further and actually define the concept. Theories can be developed either deductively or inductively; deduction is the making of inferences from something already known, such as the development of a theory from an existing theory in another discipline. Induction is the making of inferences from data that has been gathered. In curriculum studies, theories are often expressed as models of curriculum, the terms being used interchangeably.

Curriculum model

A model is a physical or conceptual representation of something; physical models are replicas of objects, and may be actual size or built to scale. Curriculum models are conceptual models, i.e. simplified representations of reality in graphic, mathematical or symbolic form. Models of curriculum help to clarify thinking about the nature of curriculum and a number of models have become well established within the literature. These are discussed in detail later in this chapter.

Curriculum ideology

A nurse teacher's concept of the curriculum is shaped by the system of beliefs and values held about education; in other words, the educational ideology to which he or she subscribes.

Curriculum ideologies

A number of such educational ideologies have been identified (e.g. Davies, 1969; Scrimshaw, 1983), each with its own adherents who share common values and beliefs about the educational enterprise, and whose views may conflict with those of adherents to other ideologies. The essential features of the prevailing curriculum ideologies are outlined below.

Conservative/classical humanism

These ideologies focus on the nation, and view education as the transmission of the cultural heritage of a nation, and key values are stability and a sense of continuity with the past. Curricula are differentiated for the elite and the non-elite and the curriculum is subject-centred and teacher-dominated. Motivation is extrinsic, with an emphasis on discipline.

Democratic/liberal humanism

The emphasis here in on the role of education in the creation of a common democratic culture, with educational opportunity for all. Key values are quality, relevance and lifelong education. Curricula are common core and teacher–pupil negotiation features as a teaching strategy.

Romantic/progressivism

These ideologies see education as meeting the needs, aspirations and personal growth of the individual. They emphasize the process of learning by experience, group discovery, and mutual dialogue between teacher and pupil.

Revisionist/instrumentalism

In these utilitarian ideologies, education must be relevant to the economic and social needs of society by producing a skilled workforce. Vocational relevance is a key principle of curricula and the teaching of science and technology is emphasized. Scrimshaw (1983) further subdivides instrumentalism into traditional and adaptive: the former concerned with the learning of specific vocational skills, while the latter aims to equip the learner to be adaptable to the changing needs of society.

Reconstructionism

This ideology sees education as means of bringing about social change through analysis, discussion and reconstruction of social issues. The key teaching approach is small-group methods. The above review of ideologies portrays them as mutually incompatible, but in practice elements are often combined to meet the needs of a given curriculum design. For example, curricula for health care professionals are by their very nature instrumental in ideology, in that their purpose is to produce a skilled professional workforce. However, they also reflect a progressive ideology in their emphasis on the personal and professional growth of the individual and by the adoption of such strategies as student/teacher negotiation and learning by experience.

CURRICULUM MODELS

The behavioural objectives (product) model

Although having its origins in certain writings at the turn of the century, this model is usually ascribed to Ralph Tyler. In his book *Basic Principles of Curriculum and Instruction*, Tyler (1949) articulated a rationale for effective curriculum, viewing education as 'a process of changing the behaviour patterns of people, using behaviour in the broad sense to include thinking and feeling as well as overt action' (Tyler, 1949, p.5). He identifies four fundamental questions to be answered in developing a curriculum (1949, p.1):

1. What educational purposes should the school seek to attain?
2. How can learning experiences be selected that are likely to be useful in attaining these objectives?
3. How can learning experiences be organized for effective instruction?
4. How can the effectiveness of learning experiences be evaluated?

This notion of rational curriculum planning was taken up by a number of writers and led to the generic model of curriculum as consisting of four main components; objectives, content, method and evaluation. Hence, the emphasis on this model is on the achievement of objectives by the student. In other words, it is an output model. Tyler stressed the importance of stating objectives in terms of student behaviours: 'any statement of the objectives of the school should be a statement of changes to take place in students' (Tyler, 1949, p.44). This emphasis on student behaviours was taken up by other proponents of the model and led to a move to limit behavioural objectives to observable, measurable changes in behaviour, leaving no room for such things as 'understanding' or 'appreciation'. The behavioural objectives model has influenced education throughout the world; indeed, in 1977 the then General Nursing Council for England and Wales (1977) issued a circular which espoused the behavioural objectives model for nursing curricula and by the early 1980s, such objectives were almost universally applied in both classroom and clinical settings.

Implementing a behavioural objectives model

There is no universally accepted terminology with regard to the formulation of educational goals, but the following guide may serve to clarify the concepts involved

Educational outcome

This is the end result of an educational experience and is the most general of all terms associated with goals.

Educational aim

This is the term used mainly in Britain, which equates with the American term 'general goal'. An aim is a broad, general statement of goal direction, which contains reference to the worthwhileness of achieving it. The educational aim is the most important part of the goal system, since all the other objectives are derived from it. The following is an example of an educational aim in nursing: 'Understands the nature of malignant disease, so that she may perform skilled nursing care of the patient with such disease.' This statement gives a very general indication of the goal to be achieved, namely the understanding of malignant disease. It does not give details as to what this understanding should consist of, but it does stress the value of achieving this goal, which is the skilled care of the patient. Some authorities subdivide these general goals into immediate and long-term goals and in nursing, it is likely that teachers will need to state goals for the learner that apply to practice after qualification and so are long-term goals.

Secondary-level goals

These are subdivisions of the general goal that specify particular areas within its framework. For example, the general goal outlined above can be subdivided into a number of secondary-level goals, such as: 'Understands the factors that contribute to the development of malignant disease.'

Specific behavioural objectives

Also termed instructional objectives or terminal objectives, these are highly specific statements that describe the changes in behaviour that constitute learning. They must always contain a verb that indicates exactly what the learner must do in order to achieve the objective and this verb should describe an observable action so that achievement can be measured. Behavioural objectives are derived from the secondary goals, for example: 'List five factors which predispose an individual to malignant disease.' The word 'list' describes an observable action on the learner's part, which can be measured simply by asking them to write down the list on paper.

If the curriculum uses a behavioural objectives approach to the formulation of goals, then the following guidelines may be helpful:

1. Formulate the educational aims, ensuring that there is some indication of the worthwhileness of achieving them.
2. Formulate the secondary-level goals, which will break down the material into manageable sections for study.
3. Formulate specific behavioural objectives from the secondary-level goals.
4. Formulate any experiential objectives from the secondary-level goals.

Behavioural objectives present the most difficulty in formulation, so it is important to examine them in some detail. Most authorities agree with Mager's (1962) suggestion that there are three parts to any objective, namely a verb indicating the learner's observable behaviour, an indication of the conditions under which the achievement will be demonstrated and a standard or criterion by which the performance is evaluated. Let us take each of these and examine them in relation to nursing.

Learner's observable behaviour

Unless the learner's behaviour is observable it is impossible to assess whether or not an objective has been achieved. Take the objective which states: 'The learner will understand the structure of bone.' How will the nurse teacher know that the learner has achieved this objective? It is not possible to measure understanding as such, but it can be inferred from certain behaviours. For instance, if the learner can write a description of the structure of bone in their own words and without referring to notes or textbooks, then one might safely assume that they have comprehended or understood the material. Thus, it would be much more accurate to state the objective as follows: 'Describe in writing the structure of bone.' The word 'describe' is the action verb, which indicates the learner's observable behaviour. It is important to select verbs that are as unambiguous as possible and which do not rely on the interpretation of the individual who is reading them.

Conditions under which achievement will be demonstrated

Although not always strictly necessary, this can be an aid to clarity in an objective. Conditions are usually such things as time constraints, use of materials or special situations. For example, an objective may state that the condition under which achievement is demonstrated is 'on a patient in bed'. In the example quoted above, the condition is 'in own words, without notes or textbooks'.

Standard or criterion of performance

In the following objective the criterion of performance is 'without danger or discomfort to the patient': 'Remove a drain from the wound of a patient using aseptic technique and without danger or discomfort to him.' Note that the objective cannot be achieved simply by removing the drain; it must be done according to the criteria.

This objective contains all three components, the action verb 'remove', the condition 'using aseptic technique' and the criterion of 'without danger or discomfort to the patient'. Criteria and standards are useful whenever there is doubt as to the level of performance required in an objective.

Levels of objective

In order to perform their role adequately, nurses need a variety of behaviours. They must be able to remember and understand the theoretical aspects of nursing, such as pathophysiology, therapeutics and behavioural sciences. In addition, nurses must possess a wide variety of skills that demand physical ability and co-ordination, such as assisting patients who have difficulty performing activities of living. But the behaviour that is most closely associated with the role of the nurse is the caring aspect, which involves feelings, emotions, attitudes and values, and which puts the nurse in a unique position with regard to helping patients. Of course, most aspects of nursing involve a combination of all three types of behaviour. In order to perform a blanket bath, the nurse must utilize certain theoretical behaviours such as remembering the patient's condition and relating it to the procedure to be adopted. An assessment of the patient will be needed before commencing. Is the patient in pain? Does he or she require specific help, etc.? Knowledge of the normal and abnormal responses is integrated with information gained from the assessment, to give an overall picture. The nurse must perform many nursing skills, such as stripping the bed, removing the patient's clothing, altering their position and so on. There is an accepted way of washing and drying a patient that takes a little time to learn. In addition to these 'theoretical behaviours' and 'practical skills', there are the elements of caring, namely interpersonal skills, feelings of empathy, consideration and such. A simple blanket bath is far from simple when analysed, although it is often argued that anyone with common sense can perform it, as we each take care of our personal hygiene when in normal health. This procedure is often delegated to health care assistants because of this viewpoint, but I maintain that there is a world of difference between a blanket bath that merely leaves patients clean and one which leaves them clean, undistressed and with many of their queries or anxieties relieved.

If the role of the nurse requires this wide range of behaviours, then objectives will need to be stated for each of these categories of activity. In addition, it is important that they do not simply require factual recall of information, since nursing involves the ability to apply theoretical knowledge to a practical situation and also to analyse, synthesize and evaluate information. In order to assist the teacher in formulating objectives at different levels and for different kinds of behaviours, Bloom (1956) developed a system of classification called the taxonomy of educational objectives. A taxonomy is a classification, and the best known one is that of Linnaeus, which classifies all living things according to general and then subsequently more detailed, similarities of structure and function. The taxonomy of educational objectives classifies objectives into three main spheres or domains and each of these is further categorized according to level of behaviour, progressing from the most simple to the highly complex. The levels are arranged in the form of a hierarchy, so that the behaviours at any given level will incorporate those of the levels below.

The three domains are cognitive, which is concerned with knowledge and intellectual abilities, affective, which is concerned with attitudes, values, interests and appreciations and psychomotor, concerned with motor skills. The taxonomy for the affective domain was published by Krathwohl, Bloom and Masia (1964) and taxonomies for the psychomotor domain have been developed by Simpson (1972) and Harrow (1972).

The cognitive domain

Table 12.1 gives the classification of the cognitive domain. There are six levels of objective, each of which is divided into subcategories. Table 12.2

Table 12.1 Taxonomy of educational objectives: cognitive domain (Bloom, 1956)

Level		Category		Sub-category	
1.00	Knowledge	1.10	of specifics	1.11	of terminology
				1.12	of specific facts
		1.20	of ways and means of dealing with specifics	1.21	of conventions
				1.22	of trends and sequences
				1.23	of classifications and categories
				1.24	of criteria
				1.25	of methodology
		1.30	of the universals and abstractions in a field	1.31	of principles and generalizations
				1.32	of theories and structures
2.00	Comprehension	2.10	Translation		
		2.20	Interpretation		
		2.30	Extrapolation		
3.00	Application				
4.00	Analysis	4.10	of elements		
		4.20	of relationships		
		4.30	of organizational principles		
5.00	Synthesis	5.10	Production of a unique communication		
		5.20	Production of a plan, or proposed set of operations		
		5.30	Derivation of a set of abstract relations		
6.00	Evaluation	6.10	Judgements in terms of internal evidence		
		6.20	Judgements in terms of external criteria		

Table 12.2 The hierarchical nature of the cognitive domain

Knowledge	= Knowledge
Comprehension	= Knowledge + Comprehension
Application	= Knowledge + Comprehension + Application
Analysis	= Knowledge + Comprehension + Application + Analysis
Synthesis	= Knowledge + Comprehension + Application + Analysis + Synthesis
Evaluation	= Knowledge + Comprehension + Application + Analysis + Synthesis + Evaluation

shows the hierarchical nature of the levels and the requirement for each, and Table 12.5 (p. 282) gives examples of behavioural objectives for each of the six levels.

Level 1.00 Knowledge At this, the most basic level, all that is required is the bringing to mind of such things as specific facts or terminology, as stated in the subcategories. Typical verbs used to indicate this level are: defines, describes, identifies, labels, names, states, lists, etc. However, it is important to remember that it is the context of the verb rather than the verb itself that will decide the level, as some verbs can be used at more than one level.

Level 2.00 Comprehension This refers to understanding, which is usually demonstrated by the learner making limited use of the information. Such activities as paraphrasing a communication whilst maintaining the intent of the original would constitute translation. Interpretation can be observed by the learner summarizing or explaining information in their own words and extrapolation is involved when information is projected beyond the given data. Typical verbs used at this level are: paraphrase, translate, convert, explain, give examples, etc.

Level 3.00 Application The learner is required to apply rules, principles, concepts, etc., to real situations. These should be sufficiently unfamiliar to avoid the mere recall of previous behaviours. Typical verbs used at this level are demonstrates, discovers, prepares, produces, relates, uses, solves, shows, etc.

Level 4.00 Analysis This involves the ability to break down information into its component parts, which may be elements of information, relationships between elements, or organization and structure of information. Its purpose is to separate the important aspects of information from the less important, thus clarifying the meaning. Typical verbs are: differentiates, discriminates, distinguishes, etc.

Level 5.00 Synthesis At this level the learner is required to combine various parts into a new kind of whole. Creativity is present because the learner produces something unique, such as a plan or design. Typical verbs used are: compiles, composes, creates, devises, plans, etc.

Level 6.00 Evaluation This implies the ability to make judgements regarding the value of material and involves the use of criteria. Typical verbs are: compares, contrasts, criticizes, justifies, appraises, judges, etc.

Table 12.3 Taxonomy of educational objectives: affective domain (Bloom, 1956)

Level	Category
1.00 Receiving (Attending)	1.1 Awareness 1.2 Willingness to receive 1.3 Controlled or selected attention
2.00 Responding	2.1 Acquiescence in responding 2.2 Willingness to respond 2.3 Satisfaction in response
3.00 Valuing	3.1 Acceptance of a value 3.2 Preference for a value 3.3 Commitment
4.00 Organization	4.1 Conceptualization of a value 4.2 Organization of a value system
5.00 Characterization by a value or value complex	5.1 Generalized set 5.2 Characterization

The affective domain

This domain has particular significance for nursing because it deals with the realm of feelings and attitudes, which constitute the caring functions. While many schools of nursing have stated comprehensive behavioural objectives for the cognitive and psychomotor domains, it is unusual to find the same coverage of the affective domain. It is perhaps useful at this point to clarify what is meant by the terms attitude and value. Both of these are constructs, that is terms invented by psychologists to explain things which cannot be observed directly, but which must be inferred from the person's own account or their behaviour. 'Values' refer to the person's concept of what he or she considers desirable, and so has a large emotional component. A person's values may include sincerity, compassion, respect, etc. 'Attitudes', on the other hand, are positive or negative feelings about certain things and consist of both cognitive and affective aspects. People who feel that smoking is antisocial and that it endangers health, are demonstrating a negative attitude towards smoking.

The affective domain consists of five levels, each of which is subdivided into categories, as shown in Table 12.3; examples of nursing objectives at all six levels are shown in Table 12.6 (p. 283).

When writing objectives for this domain, it is essential to include within the written statement both the attitude or value in question, and the behaviour that will indicate the particular value or attitude.

Level 1.00 Receiving (attending) At this level the learner is sensitive to the existence of something and progresses from awareness to controlled or selected attention. It is difficult to tell when a learner is receiving or attending to something, so the best indicator is verbal behaviour. Typical verbs are: asks, chooses, selects, replies, etc.

Table 12.4 Words associated with the affective process of caring

Appreciative	Empathic	Obliging
Attentive	Feeling	Patient
Charitable	Friendly	Respectful
Comforting	Gentle	Sincere
Compassionate	Helpful	Sympathetic
Condolent	Honest	Thoughtful
Considerate	Humane	Understanding
Consoling	Integrity	Valuing
Courteous	Kind	Warm

Level 2.00 Responding This is concerned with active response by the learner, although commitment is not yet demonstrated. The range is from reacting to a suggestion through to experiencing a feeling of satisfaction in responding. Typical verbs are: answers, assists, complies, conforms, helps, etc.

Level 3.00 Valuing Objectives at this level indicate acceptance and internalization of the values or attitudes in question. The learner acts out these in everyday life in a consistent way. Typical verbs are: initiates, invites, joins, justifies, etc.

Level 4.00 Organization Having internalized the value, the learner will encounter situations in which more than one value is relevant. This level is concerned with the ability to organize values and to arrange them in appropriate order. Typical verbs are: alters, arranges, combines, modifies, etc.

Level 5.00 Characterization This is the highest level, and having attained this level the learner has an internalized value system which has become their philosophy of life. These are the values that characterize an individual. Typical verbs are: acts, discriminates, listens, etc. Nurse students, unlike schoolchildren, will have acquired mature attitudes and values systems, because they enter nursing mature. However, this domain is still most applicable to nurse education, as the learner may have to acquire new attitudes and values, or modify existing ones. Table 12.4 shows a list of words that come under the heading of 'caring', and which might form the basis of affective objectives for nursing.

The psychomotor domain

Taxonomies is this domain have been developed by Harrow (1972) and Simpson (1972), the latter having more application to the type of skilled performance involved in nursing.

Level 1 Perception This basic level is concerned with the perception of sensory cues that guide actions and ranges from awareness of stimuli to translation into action. Typical verbs are: chooses, differentiates, distinguishes, identifies, detects, etc.

Level 2 Set This is concerned with cognitive, affective and psychomotor readiness to act. Typical verbs are: begins, moves, reacts, shows, starts, etc.

Level 3 Guided response These objectives refer to the early stages in skills acquisition where skills are performed following demonstration by the teacher. Typical verbs are: carries out, makes, performs, calculates, etc.

Level 4 Mechanism At this level, the performance has become habitual, but the movements are not so complex as the next higher level. Typical verbs are similar to the previous level.

Level 5 Complex overt response This level typifies the skilled performance, and involves economy of effort, smoothness of action, accuracy and efficiency, etc. Again, verbs are similar to level 3.

Level 6 Adaptation Here, the skills are internalized to such an extent that the nurse can adapt them to cater for special circumstances. Typical verbs are: adapts, alters, modifies, reorganizes, etc.

Level 7 Origination This is the highest level, and concerns the origination of new movement patterns to suit particular circumstances. Typical verbs are: composes, creates, designs, originates, etc.

Tables 12.5, 12.6 and 12.7 give examples of behavioural objectives for each of the levels in the three domains.

Gronlund (1978) has suggested an alternative approach to the detailed documentation of single objectives. A general instructional objective is first stated, such as:

Understands the structure and function of the human body.

Then a representative sample of the types of behaviour that constitute understanding of the subject in question are given. For example:

Identifies the organs of the body. Describes the structure of a given organ. Describes the function of a given organ.

This approach has the distinct advantage that the objectives can be used for more than one module or unit. It is based on the premise that it is impossible to list all the behaviours that constitute understanding of something, so only a representative sample of behaviours is included. It also emphasizes that the main goal is understanding of the structure and function of the human body, the objectives are only means to this end, and not ends in themselves. Gronlund's system can be effectively applied to the formulation of objectives for the clinical field, where difficulties might be experienced with objectives for different wards. Rather than having exhaustive lists for each ward, general instructional objectives can be stated for the main areas, with a representative sample of behavioural objectives. For example, the following might apply to every ward in the hospital:

> General instructional objective: 'carries out admission procedure for a waiting-list patient'. Specific behavioural objectives: 'prepares bed and bedside area; assembles charts and equipment; conducts patient to bedside, employing appropriate interpersonal skills to allay anxiety.

A critique of the behavioural objectives model

Although remaining influential in the design of curricula, the behavioural objectives model has been the subject of considerable criticism in the literature. Table 12.8 summarizes the viewpoints of both proponents and opponents of the model.

Perhaps a real-life example may help to show how much of the richness of the learning experience is lost by adhering strictly to a behavioural objectives model. I sat in on a lecture entitled 'The Care of a Child with Leukaemia' and the teacher's stated objectives for the students were:

1. recall the normal leucocyte blood picture;
2. state how the blood picture is altered in leukaemia;
3. deduce some resulting signs and symptoms of leukaemia;
4. suggest appropriate nursing care for an eight-year-old child undergoing chemotherapy and radiotherapy in hospital; and
5. demonstrate an interest in the bone-marrow transplant form of treatment.

These objectives seem perfectly acceptable outcomes for the lecture, but such was the skill of the teacher that by the end of the lecture I was feeling a range of emotions that I subsequently wrote down to try to capture their essence:

1. feelings of empathy and caring for those children with leukaemia;
2. admiration for medical science and its new technology, which can offer treatment for children who would have been considered incurable a few years ago;
3. real appreciation of the frightening nature of treatment for leukaemia, especially the necessary isolation of the child during treatment for bone-marrow transplant;
4. feelings of pride for the courage of my fellow man;
5. understanding of the principle of bone-marrow transplantation, and
6. motivation and a desire to help patients suffering from leukaemia and their relatives.

It does seem from the list that there were many outcomes that could not have been anticipated by the teacher, yet they were very important results for me. One might argue that in the longer term they are much more important than the behavioural list that the teacher gave to the students,

Table 12.5 Examples of nursing objectives for the cognitive domain

Level 1.00 Knowledge
States the four stages of the nursing process.
Defines the term psychoneurosis.
Identifies the functions of the health education officer.
Outlines the three stages of normal labour.
Defines the term anaesthesia.
Names the stages in child development as described by Piaget. It should be noted that all of these objectives are normally to be achieved without reference to notes or textbooks, so it is not necessary to include this in each statement.

Level 2.00 Comprehension
Translates the term haematemesis into its English equivalent.
Summarizes section 26 of the Mental Health Act 1959.
Gives three examples of the facilities available for the elderly in the community.
Explains in own words the methods available for contraception.
Gives one example of a potential threat to patient safety in the operating department.
Distinguishes between the clean and dirty dressing rooms in the Accident and Emergency Department.

Level 3.00 Application
Given the characteristics of ageing, *relates* these to the needs of the elderly in hospital.
Given the principles of care for a patient with pneumonia, *relates* these to the care of a particular patient with this condition.
Given the guidelines for handling violence in hospital, *applies* these to the care of a patient with a psychopathic disorder.
Using the rules for calculation of an infant feed, *calculates* correctly the feed requirements of an infant of given weight and age.
Given a list of community facilities for the handicapped, *formulates* a plan for discharge of a handicapped child to the community.
Given the principles of aseptic technique, *applies* these when preparing trolleys for surgical operations in the operating department.

Level 4.00 Analysis
Given a list of twelve statements about the aetiology of diabetes mellitus, *differentiates* between those which are factual and those which are assumptions.
From a videotape depicting the performance of a surgical dressing, *points out* two instances of unsafe technique.
Given a series of 12 assertion–reason statements on psychiatric disorders, *identifies* at least four in which the reason is inaccurate.
Given a simulated case history of a community patient, *distinguishes* two inappropriate interventions.
Given a list of surgical instruments for laparotomy, *identifies* three omissions.
Given a list of nursing interventions in the Accident and Emergency department, *discriminates* between those which are important and those which are unimportant, in relation to cardiac arrest.

Table 12.5 *continued*

Level 5.00 Synthesis
Writes an original essay on 'The role of the nurse in care of the in-patient with
   multiple sclerosis'.
Devises a nursing care plan which meets the needs of a patient who has
   undergone cholecystectomy.
Produces an outline design for an Accident and Emergency department, which
   allows for the following:
   (1) one-way flow through the department;
   (2) prevention of cross-infection;
   (3) separate resuscitation area.
Given a list of personnel, *designs* an off-duty rota for a labour ward, which
   gives adequate coverage on all shifts.
Writes an original essay on 'The role of behaviourism in psychiatry'.
Devises a plan to meet the needs of a newly discharged lower-limb amputee in
   the community.

Level 6.00 Evaluation
Evaluates the arguments for and against the use of pertussis vaccine in infants.
Given three methods of contraception, *judges* which one is best, stating how
   this decision was reached, and what criteria were used.
Justifies the continued use of bottle feeding as opposed to breast feeding of
   infants.
Compares and evaluates two approaches to the treatment of depression, stating
   the criteria used.

Table 12.6 Examples of nursing objectives for the affective domain

---

Level 1.00 Receiving (Attending)
Indicates an awareness of the value 'consideration for others' by *contributing* to
a discussion on the subject.

Level 2.00 Responding
Demonstrates interest in the value 'consideration for others' by *reading* the
assigned literature for the topic.

Level 3.00 Valuing
Shows a high degree of commitment to the value 'consideration for others' by
actively *encouraging* colleagues to display consideration for others.

Level 4.00 Organization
Demonstrates organization of the values 'consideration for others' and
'personal autonomy' by *writing* an essay which requires interaction of these two
values.

Level 5.00 Characterization
Indicates characterization of the value 'consideration for others' by consistently
approaching others in a considerate way.

Table 12.7 Examples of nursing objectives for the psychomotor domain

Level 1. Perception
Detects the need for pharyngeal suction in a patient, by listening to the sound of his breathing.

Level 2. Set
Demonstrates the correct bodily position for lifting a patient.

Level 3. Guided response
Performs urine testing as demonstrated by the instructor.

Level 4. Mechanism
Sets a tray for an intramuscular injection.

Level 5. Complex overt response
Applies with skill a stump bandage to a lower-limb amputee.

Level 6. Adaptation
Modifies surgical dressing technique to suit a particular patient's circumstances.

Level 7. Origination
Devises an original way of securing a dressing which has tended to come loose soon after application.

Table 12.8 Viewpoints of proponents and opponents of behavioural objectives model

Proponents
They provide the student with clear direction as to what must be learnt.
Their use encourages the teacher to examine his or her goals more carefully.
It is relatively easy to assess students' achievement, as behaviours are observable.
They can aid self-instruction.
They are accessible to public scrutiny.
They offer a rational system for curriculum planning.
Students on the whole tend to welcome the clarity that behavioural objectives bring to learning.
They provide a basis for comparison between similar courses in different institutions.
They offer a system for evaluating the performance of the teacher.

Opponents
They act as a set of blinkers that narrow the learning field.
They are difficult to formulate for higher-level outcomes and hence encourage trivialization of learning by focusing on lower-level outcomes.
They are almost impossible to formulate in the affective domain.
They ignore unanticipated outcomes of instruction.
It is impossible to state objectives for every learning outcome, even if this was desirable.
They are unsuitable for arts subjects such as music, poetry and drama.
They are unsuitable for science subjects, as they emphasize the learning of factual information rather than scientific enquiry.
Their use reflects a training approach rather than an educational one.
They encourage conformity rather than diversity.
It is wrong for one individual, i.e. the teacher, to dictate how another individual i.e. the student should behave.
They are extremely time-consuming to formulate and require continuous updating.

since I am more likely to remember and understand the principles of the lecture because of these feelings.

Stenhouse's process model of curriculum

One of the major critics of the behavioural objectives model was the late Lawrence Stenhouse, who formulated an alternative approach known as the 'process' model. He saw the use of behavioural objectives acting as a filter that distorted knowledge in schools (Stenhouse, 1975, p. 86):

> The filtering of knowledge through an analysis of objectives gives the school an authority and power over its students by setting arbitrary limits to speculation and by defining arbitrary solutions to unresolved problems of knowledge. This translates the teacher from the role of the student of a complex field of knowledge to the role of the master of the school's agreed version of that field.

Stenhouse's (1975) minimum requirements for a curriculum are that a curriculum should offer:

1. *in planning*
   (a) principles for the selection of content – what is to be learned and taught;
   (b) principles for the development of a teaching strategy – how it is to be learned and taught;
   (c) principles for the making of decisions about sequence;
   (d) principles on which to diagnose the strengths and weaknesses of individual students and differentiate the general principles (a) (b) and (c) above to meet individual cases;
2. *in empirical study*
   (a) principles on which to study and evaluate the progress of students;
   (b) principles on which to study and evaluate the progress of teachers;
   (c) guidance as to the feasibility of implementing the curriculum in varying school contexts, pupil contexts, environments and peer-group situations;
   (d) information about the variability of effects in differing contexts and on different pupils and an understanding of the causes of the variation; and
3. *in relation to justification*
   (a) a formulation of the intention or aim of the curriculum which is accessible to critical scrutiny.

Stenhouse believed that it was possible to organize the curriculum without having to specify in advance the behavioural changes that should occur in students; indeed, he argued that the purpose of education was to make student outcomes unpredictable. Knowledge does not consist of 'known facts' to be remembered, rather, it provides a basis for speculation and conjecture about a discipline. The content of a curriculum can be selected on the basis that it is worthwhile in itself and not merely as the means to achievement of a behavioural objective. Hence, we could argue that the content in a nursing curriculum can be chosen for its worthwhileness in providing examples of the key concepts, procedures and criteria of nursing science. Similarly, teaching methods and learning experiences can be specified in terms of their worthwhileness as learning activities. Stenhouse refers to these statements of worthwhileness as 'principles of procedure' and it is important to note that the principles of procedure for teaching are couched in terms of what the teacher will do rather than what the students will be able to do. For example, 'to encourage students to reflect on their experiences'.

The role of assessment in a process curriculum is very different from that in a product model, being that of critic rather than marker. The teacher is cast in the role of critical appraiser of the student's work, with the emphasis on developing self-appraisal in the student. According to Stenhouse (1975, p.95):

> The worthwhile activity in which teacher and student are engaged has standards and criteria immanent in it and the task of appraisal is that of improving students' capacity to work to such criteria by critical reaction to work done. In this sense, assessment is about the teaching of self-assessment.

A critique of Stenhouse's process model

The most common reservation expressed in nurse education with regard to the process model centres on the issue of evaluation. If no terminal behaviours are prescribed, how can the teacher assess whether a student is competent or not? It seems that nurse teachers have forgotten that there was life before behavioural objectives! Indeed, it is only a decade and a half since the movement towards the product model was endorsed by the General Nursing Council for England and Wales (1977). How did nurse teachers evaluate student progress prior to 1977? Interestingly enough, it was by reference of a specification of course content, namely, the 'syllabus for training'. This gave an outline of the main topic headings, e.g. 'The effects of the environment on health', but no fine detail was included, this being left to the individual teacher to decide. A 'schedule of practical skills' was also available to identify clinical skills required for nursing practice and such skills were assessed by both clinical nurses and nurse teachers. The criteria for these skills must have been internalized by each assessor, in the light of what was considered to be good nursing practice by the institution and the profession. It is also worth reminding ourselves that large sections of education have never espoused the behavioural objectives model at all, particularly the university sector of higher education.

The greatest weakness of the process model is identified by Stenhouse as its dependence upon the quality of the teacher. In this model, the teacher's commitment to professional development is vital; teachers need to see themselves as learners rather than as experts, and to be continually striving to improve their performance and judgement. Table 12.9 shows

Table 12.9 Comparison between key concepts of product and process models of curriculum.

Product model	Process model
An *output* model, i.e. emphasis is on the achievement of behavioural objectives; the *product* of education.	An *input* model, i.e. emphasis is on learning experiences; the *process* of education.
Curriculum activities are seen as *means* to an *end*, i.e. achievement of terminal objectives.	Curriculum activities are seen as being *worthwhile* in themselves.
Learning is seen as a change in *observable* behaviour.	Acknowledges that much learning is *not observable*.
Teaching is geared to producing *predictable* outcomes.	Teaching is geared to encourage *unpredictable* outcomes.
Teacher specifies *content* in terms of the student's achievement of behavioural objectives.	Teacher specifies *content* but cannot know in advance what the student will *do* with that content.
Evaluation is done by assessing the student's achievement of behavioural objectives.	*Evaluation* is done by critical appraisal of the student's work, using the criteria intrinsic to the discipline concerned; .includes self-assessment by the student.

the main differences in approach between the two models, as a basis for comparison.

Lawton's cultural analysis model

Lawton's model was a reaction against what he saw as the dangers of the behavioural objectives model. As the name implies, this model proposes a curriculum planned on the technique of cultural analysis. Culture is defined as the whole way of life of a society and the purpose of education is 'to make available to the next generation what we regard as the most important aspects of culture' (Lawton, 1983). Cultural analysis is the process by which a selection is made from the culture and in terms of curriculum-planning, Lawton suggests cultural analysis will ask the following questions:

1. What kind of society already exists?
2. In what ways is it developing?
3. How do its members appear to want it to develop?
4. What kinds of values and principles will be involved in deciding on question 3, and on the educational means of achieving it?

Lawton (1983) offers a five-stage model for this analysis:

1. *Cultural invariants* This stage examines all the aspects that human societies have in common, such as economic and moral aspects, beliefs and other systems.

2. *Cultural variables* This stage involves analysing the differences between cultures in each of the systems.
3. *Selection from the culture* This stage consists of comparing the cultural analysis of the systems with the existing school curriculum.
4. *Psychological questions and theories* This stage is not in direct continuity with the previous stages, but is seen as an important consideration for any curriculum development.
5. *Curriculum organization* In this final stage the curriculum can now be planned on the basis of the cultural analysis carried out in the previous stages, bearing in mind the important psychological questions and theories that influence learning and instruction.

Critique of Lawton's cultural analysis model

Lawton's model of curriculum attempts to apply a rational system of analysis to the problem of curriculum content; it is designed for the school curriculum for children and approaches the task of curriculum planning in a broader way. As Lawton points out in his preface 'the problems of young people growing up in a complex urban, industrialized society have been seriously underestimated; schools have generally failed to take seriously the moral, social and political aspects of culture in relation to curriculum planning' (Lawton, 1983).

Beattie's fourfold model

Beattie's (1987) fourfold model of the curriculum draws upon his experience with nursing curricula. He suggests that there are four fundamental approaches to the task of planning a curriculum for nursing, each with its own particular strengths and weaknesses:

1. The curriculum as a map of key subjects As the name implies, this approach consists of mapping out the key subjects in the nursing curriculum, preferably integrating them by means of themes such as 'the human lifespan' to avoid the danger of an isolated collection of topics.

2. The curriculum as a schedule of basic skills This approach emphasizes the explicit specification of basic skills of nursing, these skills being culled from recent empirical research into nursing practice. A behavioural objectives approach can be appropriate here, provided that it is not used dogmatically for all aspects of teaching, particularly in relation to the knowledge base for clinical practice.

3. The curriculum as a portfolio of meaningful personal experiences This approach puts the student at the centre of things by organizing the curriculum around their interests and experiences. This is done by using a variety of experiential techniques such as action-research, critical incidents, role-play and the like. There will always be a degree of tension between the unpredictability consequent upon student autonomy and the need to ensure sufficient opportunity to cover key areas.

4. The curriculum as an agenda of important cultural issues This approach avoids giving detailed subject-matter, focusing instead on controversial issues and political dilemmas in nursing and health care. These issues are chosen because they are open to debate and have no single correct answer, thereby stimulating discussion and enquiry, e.g. 'nurse power or patient power'.

How can nurse teachers use these ideas in practical curriculum planning? Beattie suggests that there are three ways of combining the fourfold framework. The first one he calls the 'eclectic curriculum', in which the four approaches are mixed together in some sort of combination. The main problem with this is that the more traditional approaches tend to dominate, leaving only the marginal inclusion of student-centred ideas. Another way is to negotiate each of the key areas with the consumers, the 'negotiated curriculum'. The third way Beattie calls the 'dialectical curriculum', in which the curriculum designer 'goes out to do battle', as it were, to engage in a deliberate, principled and committed struggle to combat, challenge and contest the dominant codes of curriculum (Beattie, 1987, p.31). In his 'fourfold model of curriculum' Beattie argues that 'curriculum planners in nursing can and must move beyond simple-minded, "single-model" approaches and towards complex, multifaceted strategies' (Beattie, 1987, p.32).

THE SHORTCOMINGS OF CURRICULUM MODELS IN NURSE EDUCATION

The classic models outlined above were, with the exception of Beattie's model, developed with the education of children in mind. The various educational ideologies underpinning the models are beliefs about childhood education, as evidenced by references to 'transmission of the cultural heritage of the nation', 'creation of a common democratic culture', 'meeting the needs, aspirations and personal growth of the individual' and 'education relevant to the social and economic needs of society'. The classic models are usually adapted in some way to meet the needs of curriculum developers in nursing and midwifery, but these tend to be relatively superficial adaptations which leave the essential principles of the model unchanged. It is highly significant that none of the curriculum models, including that of Beattie, take into account the views and needs of service managers/employers about the outputs they require from education and training to fulfil their own service contracts. Until the advent of the Government White Paper, *Working for Patients: Education and Training Working Paper 10* (HMSO, 1989) employers had to take whatever education and training was on offer from the College of Nursing. Contracting for education has made dramatic changes in the respective power base of education and service. Colleges of Nursing now have corporate status, many within HE, and a competitive training environment has been introduced. Colleges are no longer automatically funded to provide pre- and post-registration courses, but are required to bid through Regional Health Authorities for educational contracts with NHS Trusts/District Health Authorities. These service providers have become clients of the Colleges of Nursing, and as such will require them to provide education and training that meets identified staff development needs. This has necessitated a shift in orientation from a teacher-led to a client-centred approach to education, and if colleges cannot meet the requirements of the service providers, contracts will go elsewhere. Contracting for education is a means of ensuring that service providers obtain the education and training that best suits their staff development needs. As an alternative to sending staff on existing college courses, the service providers will be able to state precisely their specific education and training requirements.

They will also be able to monitor the quality of the educational provision and give feedback to the college. In turn, the colleges will have to adopt a client-centred approach to curriculum design and delivery, and teaching staff may have difficulty initially in accepting the shift of control from themselves to the service providers. They may also be anxious about the competitive contracting process, and what might happen if they fail to win contracts.

Hence, educational contracting has major implications for curriculum development in nursing and midwifery; Humphreys and Quinn (1994) offer a detailed analysis of the impact of the market on health care education.

CURRICULUM DEVELOPMENT AND IMPLEMENTATION

The basic principles of curriculum development apply to both pre-registration and post-registration provision, although there are some differences in approach between these. Pre-registration courses or pathways in nursing and midwifery tend to be offered in both full-time and part-time modes, whereas post-registration continuing education programmes are largely part-time.

Since pre-registration pathways form the entry gate to the nursing or midwifery professions they must meet the criteria laid down by the UKCC and the appropriate National Board for Nursing, Midwifery and Health Visiting. Post-registration pathways and units are, on the whole, less constrained by such requirements and provide scope for curriculum designers to be much more flexible and imaginative.

Curriculum development needs to be distinguished from curriculum design at this point. Curriculum design is a focused activity concerned with questions of structure, content and process. For example the curriculum philosophy and model, content-mapping, organization and sequencing of content, etc. Indeed, curriculum design may be mistakenly perceived as the sole activity involved in curriculum development, but there are other aspects of the process that have equal importance. Curriculum development is a much broader concept that encompasses all the processes involved in the production and implementation of a curriculum, from the initial idea through to monitoring and review.

Stages of curriculum development

There are four stages in the curriculum development process: exploratory, design, implementation, and monitoring and review.

Exploratory stage

Within the market environment, it is important that college staff liaise closely with service providers to identify gaps in the provision of nursing and midwifery education so that new courses or pathways can be developed to meet those needs. Ideas for new provision need to be carefully explored before either adopting or rejecting them, and a core team should be set up to this effect. Market research is vitally important to ascertain the views of employers and other interested parties such as statutory bodies. The availability of resources and expertise within the college needs to be explored, and the estimated costs of development will have to calculated for eventual inclusion in any contract. It is useful to undertake an initial critical path analysis for the development so that a realistic idea of the timescale is gained.

Design stage

If a decision is made to go ahead with the development, a curriculum planning team should be set up to prepare the course or pathway for validation and subsequent implementation. The actual process of design and validation is discussed in the next section of this chapter.

Implementation stage

In this stage students have been recruited, all systems are in place, and the curriculum is fully operational. In the early days of implementation a few teething troubles can be expected until the systems have been fine tuned. For example, in CATS pathways the offering of a choice of option units to students may result in some units being under-subscribed and others over-subscribed. During the implementation stage, curriculum evaluation is ongoing by means of unit evaluation. This does not refer to the assessment of students achievement of unit outcomes, but to the systematic collection of their opinions about the quality and usefulness of the units.

Monitoring and review stage

Although the evaluation of pathway units is an ongoing process, the monitoring and review stage can be usefully seen as a distinct phase in the curriculum. In HE, pathway directors – in consultation with pathway committees – are required to produce an annual pathway monitoring report. This report is retrospective for the previous academic year, and requires the pathway director to reflect upon the quality of the pathway using data gathered from a variety of sources such as students' evaluations of units, external examiners' reports, and the views of employers. This report is scrutinized at a series of meetings before being discussed at a Faculty Board or Academic Board. Annual pathway monitoring is therefore an important mechanism for ensuring quality on the pathway. Pathway monitoring is further discussed in Chapters 14 and 15 (p. 367).

When a pathway receives approval following validation, a timescale for pathway review will be proposed. The length of approval ranges from as little as one year through to indefinite approval, but regardless of length, continuation of the pathway is dependent upon a satisfactory pathway review. A review is very similar to a validation event, but the pathway team are required to produce a detailed review of the operation of the pathway over the prescribed timescale. Proposals for changes must be accompanied by a well-argued rationale and supporting evidence. Hogg (1990) describes a curriculum evaluation and development model that utilizes a problem-solving approach. There are four stages in the model as follows:

1. *antecedent stage* – formative evaluation prior to a major course innovation;
2. *interactive stage* – concerned with curriculum development and involves evaluation by students, teachers and clinical facilitators;
3. *implementation stage* – formative evaluation during the trial period of the new development; and
4. *consequential stage* – involves formative evaluation of the established development and also summative evaluation at the completion of the programme.

Within the model, evaluation data collection from students, teachers and clinical facilitators is both quantitative and qualitative, and the author comments positively on the simplicity, flexibility and user-friendliness of the model in practice.

Design of curricula

This constitutes the second stage of the curriculum planning process as outlined above. The small core team, formed during the exploratory stage to consider the feasibility of the development, now needs to be augmented by a small number of other individuals possessing the required knowledge and experience with reference to the curriculum in question. In curriculum development groups for nursing and midwifery, particularly for pre-registration programmes, the range of representation commonly includes teaching staff, students, and hospital and community service managers. The latter represent the various specialisms of nursing such as learning difficulties, community nursing, and children's nursing, and are usually chosen to reflect representation from each health district or trust to which the college or department relates.

Whilst this wide representation seems like a good idea in principle, in practice there are a number of shortcomings. Curriculum development groups tend to meet very frequently, putting severe demands on the service representatives' time, who then respond with frequent apologies for absence. Another problem is the terminology and concepts of curriculum and education; teaching staff are thoroughly familiar with curriculum models, conceptual mapping and the like, but to service colleagues and students they may seem as obscure as a foreign language. While the teachers argue about the merits of one particular model over another, or the application of Gagne's conditions of learning (p. 74) to the curriculum, the service and student representatives have to sit in mystified silence, as they are not privy to these concepts. It seems to me there is little point in trying to induct service colleagues and students into the complexities of education and curriculum, since it has taken teachers years of education and training to become familiar with them. Also, the timescale for curriculum development is always relatively short and time is simply not available for explanations of complex curriculum concepts to non-educationalists. A much more sensible alternative is to solicit the opinions of these specialists, either by interview or co-option, as the need for their expertise and experience becomes evident. In my opinion it is quite sufficient for the views and experience of appropriate specialists to be used to inform the development process, and I consider it wasteful of resources for service colleagues to participate as full members of the development team. Indeed, in a market environment for education the service managers might well question why they are paying the college or department for curriculum development when so many of their own staff are heavily involved in it.

The curriculum development group should have a chairperson, and it is sufficient to have notes of the decisions made at meetings rather than formal minutes.

Critical path analysis

One of the first issues to be addressed by the group should be a critical path analysis which identifies deadlines for each aspect of the development. It is useful to work backwards from the proposed date of the validation event, allowing a minimum of three weeks before the event for the documentation to be available to validation panel members. Other deadlines that need to be included are the first draft of the validation document, the internal validation event, and the printing of the document. A specimen critical path analysis for curriculum development is shown in Figure 12.1. Another issue that needs to be addressed early in the development is the question of curriculum 'givens'. These are regulations and requirements from the university or college, and from the statutory bodies where appropriate. For example, curriculum development groups would have no choice but to use a CATS structure if the

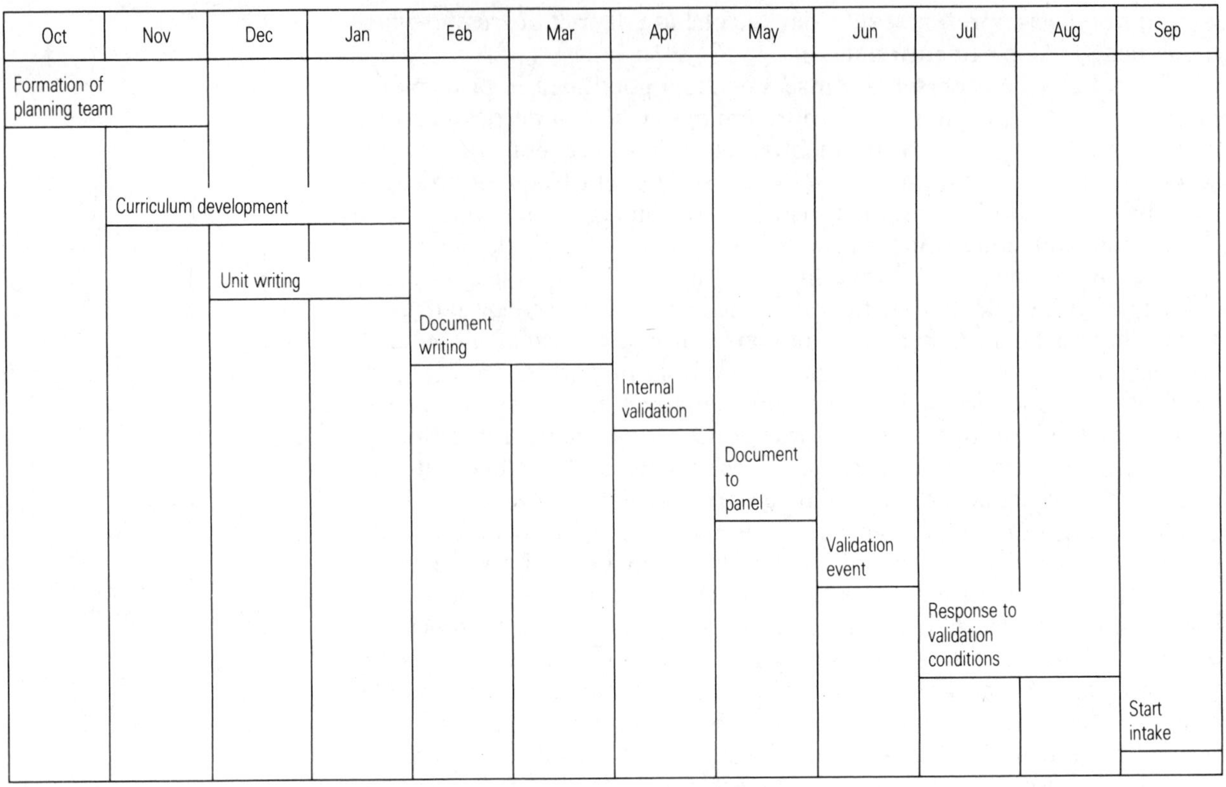

Fig. 12.1 Specimen critical path analysis for curriculum development.

institution operates on the basis of a CATS framework. Similarly, the institutions' regulations on admissions and assessment would have to be followed, and if a statutory body is involved in validation or accreditation of the curriculum, the respective regulations must be followed.

Approval in principal

Institutions of higher education and statutory bodies have mechanisms for granting approval in principle, which is normally required before the team can proceed with curriculum development. In HE, this is typically a brief outline of the proposal, including resource implications, presented to a committee for approval to proceed in principle. Application for approval in principle to the English National Board for Nursing, Midwifery and Health Visiting requires the following details (ENB, 1993):

- rationale and outline of the proposed programme,
- teaching staff details,
- details of other courses in the department,
- administrative support,
- dates and intake numbers,

- results of consultation about availability of practical experience, and
- funding arrangements.

Approval in principle for the ENB Higher Award requires evidence that the institution has a CATS system, quality assurance mechanisms, ability to teach and assess to a minimum of first degree level with honours, and a commitment to staff development.

Writing the validation document

Another key component of curriculum development is the validation document and the writing of this should be the responsibility of one person, although informed by the team. The document should be written in parallel with the development so that key aspects are captured as they happen. HE institutions differ in their requirements for validation documents, but there is a general structure common to all. The format for pathway documentation used in the University of Greenwich Credit Accumulation Framework (University of Greenwich, 1992) is:

1. Award(s) to which pathway leads
2. Pathway title
3. Modes of study
4. Faculty
5. School
6. Introduction and rationale
7. Aims
8. Learning outcomes
9. Access
10. Structure and levels
11. Assessment strategy: summary of requirements and regulations
12. Pathway management
13. Staffing and staff development
Appendices
    Unit information and Outlines
    Staff details

This format does not include teaching and learning activities, since these are included within the unit information and outlines in the appendices.

The requirements of the ENB for Course Submission Documents are more detailed:

1. Course details, including teaching staff details
2. Financial arrangements
3. Course management team
4. Course curriculum, including philosophy of care, and rationale
5. Course content, structure and organization
6. Practical experience
7. Assessment of competence
8. Methods for internal evaluation of the course

Curriculum rationale and model

Two of the key sections of the validation document are sections 6 and 7, the rationale and aims of the pathway. The purpose of the rationale is to outline the philosophy and model upon which the curriculum is based, and all other components of the pathway must be congruent with this rationale. For example, the rationale for a nursing curriculum may define the student as an autonomous, reflective individual who is responsible for his or her own learning. Hence, the timetable should provide adequate time for private study and reflection, but if the day is fully programmed with lectures and teaching contact, then there is clearly a mismatch between the rationale and the teaching and learning process. Such incongruence would be seriously questioned at a validation event. The development team may decide to use any one of the curriculum models outlined earlier in this chapter, in their curriculum. On the other hand, they may wish to adapt an existing model to fit their ideas, or devise an entirely new one. Curriculum development teams may be tempted to include a model in their validation document simply because it is expected, but unless the model helps to conceptualize the curriculum it will quickly be detected as irrelevant by the panel.

Devising a curriculum model is not difficult, and an example is shown in Figure 12.2.

The example I have devised is a generic model of curriculum for nursing and midwifery, consisting of three main components, imputs, process, and outputs.

1. Curriculum inputs These are the elements influencing the curriculum design, and consist of educational perspectives, employer requirements,

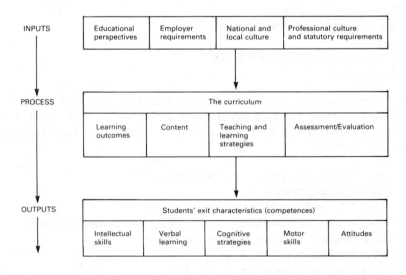

Fig. 12.2 A generic model of curriculum for nursing and midwifery.

national and local culture, and professional culture including requirements of statutory bodies.

2. Curriculum process This is the curriculum as experienced by the
student, and consists of learning outcomes, content, teaching and learning
strategies, and assessment/evaluation.

3. Curriculum outputs These can be subsumed under the general
heading of professional competence, but in the model I have used Gagne's
five learning capabilities which together constitute the students' characteristics on exit from the curriculum.

   This model can therefore be used to conceptualize curricula for nursing
and midwifery, and being a generic model could apply to a wide range of
curricula at different levels. For example, it could be equally appropriate
for a pre-registration midwifery course or a post-registration ENB course
in intensive-care nursing. The nature of the curriculum inputs, process
and outcomes would differ markedly between these two examples, but the
basic structure of the model would remain the same.

Organizing and sequencing of curriculum content

The curriculum rationale guides the selection of content, but not the
sequence and organization of that content into some form of logical order.
The latter is important if students are to be able to make sense of the
programme of study and is achieved by means of a conceptual framework
or model. Bernstein (1971) identifies two approaches to content organization in curricula: collection and integration. In a 'collection' curriculum,
subjects are taught as separate, isolated entities with clear-cut boundaries,
the emphasis being on depth of treatment. In contrast, 'integrated'
curricula focus on common themes that unite various subjects and the
emphasis is on breadth of coverage. Collection curricula are typified by
timetables containing 'slots' with separate subjects such as 'anatomy and
physiology' and 'psychology'. Integrated curricula, on the other hand,
themes consist of broad themes such as 'the individual in pain'. Simmons
and Bahl (1992) describe an integrated approach to curriculum development at post-registration level. In nurse education, they see integration
having two main meanings. Integration of content can be achieved by
linking academic disciplines, and also theory and practice. Integration
also applies to student groups, where students from different branches of
nursing, or from other professions, learn together. They describe their
PEP curriculum model for post-registration education as developing
individual practitioners in three areas: professional development, educational development, and personal development.

Academic validation of curricula

Academic validation is the pathway or course approval process used in
HE. It consists of a carefully selected panel of academics that engages the
pathway team in discussion about the pathway curriculum, and decides

whether or not the pathway is approved to run. Validation needs to be distinguished from an allied concept, accreditation. Many pathways and courses in HE involve professional education and training, and as such are subject not only to university regulations, but also to the requirements for professional recognition by the appropriate professional body. These requirements are safeguarded by the process of professional accreditation, which may consist of scrutiny of the pathway documentation alone, or by an accreditation event. The latter is usually combined with a validation event, so that both academic validation and professional accreditation are undertaken at the same time. In nursing and midwifery, however, there is an additional category called conjoint validation, in which HE and a National Board for Nursing, Midwifery and Health Visiting are equal partners in the validation process.

Once the curriculum development work has been completed the pathway can be advertised provided that it states 'subject to validation'.

The validation event is seen as the culmination of the work of the curriculum development team, and if carried out in the right spirit can be a stimulating academic debate between peers. There are a three types of validation: internal, mock and full validation. In cases where nurse education is part of HE, internal validation is carried out by the institution. Where Colleges of Nursing remain separate, internal validation is conducted in partnership with a HE institution, but the process is the same in both circumstances. Internal validation is a formal component of the quality assurance mechanism of the institution, and consists of a meeting between the curriculum development team and selected members of the institution. The curriculum submission is scrutinized in a similar way to a final validation, using a small panel of internal members of the institution who have no direct involvement with the curriculum in question. Feedback from internal validation is incorporated into the draft validation document, after which it is sent for printing. Mock validation is the name given to a practice validation event which is conducted exactly like a real event, the aim of which is to test the team's cohesiveness and ability to defend their curriculum design. Full validation is a major academic event in which a panel of academic staff is assembled to engage and challenge the pathway team on their curriculum design.

Membership of validation panels

HE has strict guidelines for the choice of panel members, and typical membership is as follows:

- chair: a member drawn from the committee responsible for academic standards in the university, who is not from the faculty submitting the pathway;
- at least one other member from the above committee, who is not from the faculty submitting the pathway;
- at least one member of the university teaching staff drawn from the faculty submitting the pathway; and

- at least two members external to the university who are nominated by the faculty submitting the pathway – of these, at least one member should have subject-matter expertise relevant to the pathway, at least one member should have experience of validation and review, and at least one member should be a practising professional in an appropriate field.

The validation event

Pathway development teams usually experience some anxiety when approaching a validation event, since it is important for them to achieve a successful outcome. However, a validation event is one of the few opportunities that educators have to engage in real academic debate about philosophical and practical educational issues. The pathway development team will have received in advance the key agenda issues that the panel wish to cover, but should be prepared also for other issues to be raised during the event.

The most important aspect of a pathway is the quality of the staff who will be teaching on it, so the pathway team must project a confident, informed and cohesive impression. This means that contributions should be distributed amongst the entire team, and not dominated by any one individual. Having said this, it is equally important that the pathway director designate should maintain a high profile during the event, and this can be done by taking the lead in some areas of questioning, and by inviting other members of the team to answer particular questions. It is useful to have decided in advance of the event which team member will answer questions on a particular area, such as assessment or admissions. This ensures that no team member should be caught out by not having a satisfactory answer ready. Self-confidence and conviction are the keys to successful validation; the panel are fellow educationalists and peers, so the pathway team need not feel intimidated by them. The chair of the event has an important role in keeping the dialogue constructive rather than confrontational, although it is important to encourage an atmosphere of rigorous challenge and debate.

There are a number of possible outcomes of a validation event:

1. approval for an indefinite length of time, with review at a given time, e.g. every five years;
2. approval for a fixed length of time, e.g. five years, after which the pathway is then subject to review;
3. approval that is conditional upon fulfilment of certain requirements within a specified time scale; and
4. approval withheld.

Conditional approval is a very common outcome of validation events, and conditions can be imposed for any aspect of the curriculum. For example, the assessment strategy may need to be amended, certain regulations modified, an evaluation carried out by the end of the first year, or a students' handbook produced. Conditional approval will always carry a date by which the conditions must be met, and this can vary from a few weeks to a whole year. The pathway development team must make a satisfactory response to the conditions, and this is sent to all panel members by the academic validation unit of the institution. Once the panel has agreed that the conditions have been met, the amendments are incorporated into the validation document, and this then becomes the definitive pathway or course document. This is housed in the library for general access by students and anyone else who is interested in the pathway.

Staff development for key players

Whilst the curriculum group is developing its work, there needs to be a parallel development with the in-service training department to plan for the anticipated training needs of qualified staff who will be involved in the new curriculum. Opportunities must be made available for such staff to spend time in workshops and study days that relate to specific aspects of the new curriculum. For example, if experiential learning is to be a major strategy, then staff will need to be given training and information about this. Other innovations will also need to be explored with qualified staff, as it is likely that new curricula will contain ideas with which most staff will be unfamiliar.

CURRICULUM CHANGE AND INNOVATION

Innovation is literally the bringing in of something new, even if it is an established procedure nationally yet new to a particular institution. It has been defined as 'acceptance over time of some specific item, idea or practice by individuals, groups or other adopting units, linked by specific channels of communication to a social structure, and to a given system of values or culture' (Katz, Levin and Hamilton, 1963). Curriculum innovation may be classified on a number of dimensions of change (Hoyle, 1972) as shown in Table 12.10.

It is unlikely that the rate of change will ever slow down to give the stable periods that were common in the past, so the implication is that we must adapt to living with rapid change and adjust accordingly.

Table 12.10 Dimensions of change (Hoyle, 1972)

Dimension	Range
Rate	Rapid . . . . slow
Scale	Large . . . . small
Degree	Fundamental . . . . superficial
Continuity	Revolutionary . . . . evolutionary
Direction	Linear . . . . cyclical

The scale of change is difficult to trace, except for the policy decisions that affect colleges or departments of nurse education. Other changes may affect only one or two institutions. Degree of change implies that fundamental changes may be implemented in name only. Under the dimension of continuity, nursing has, in the past, tended to change in an evolutionary way over a long period, but the last decade has been little short of revolutionary. The direction dimension goes from a linear form to a cyclical one, the former implying permanent change and the latter a change that is later superseded by another, which returns the situation to its original state.

Innovation implies a new idea or practice, but it is also a process by which these are adopted. Hoyle (1972, p. 15) sees innovation as a continuum, from invention through to adoption. Invention is the creation of something new, whereas adoption involves accepting an innovation that was devised by an outside agency. In nursing, as in general education, there is rarely any innovation that can be described as completely new. Most innovations are modifications of existing ideas, although the development of interactive video would count as invention. Similarly, adoption of other people's ideas is rare without some form of adaptation to suit the local requirements. There is a crucial difference between the acceptance of an innovation and its subsequent institutionalization, the latter implying that the innovation has been incorporated into the total function of the institution. Innovation can be introduced in any component of the curriculum, and in more than one at any given time.

The climate for innovation and change

There are many constraints on innovation in nurse education, the most obvious being that of resource limitations. Innovation requires time, finance and energy if it is to be done well and nurse teachers may already be overstretched with existing commitments. Another major influence is that of the 'health of the organization' which is profoundly influenced by the leadership and management style of the head of the college or department. Colleges and departments of nursing vary enormously in their climate; some are alive with enthusiasm and ideas, while others maintain a more traditional status quo. Innovation is much more likely to occur in a setting where there is little hierarchical authority evident, where autonomy is emphasized and where morale is high. The latter results from an awareness of common goals and a sense of purpose and value in the job that is being done.

Miles (1975) coined the phrase 'organizational health' and this is related to the climate of the institution. He lists a number of dimensions of organizational health:

1. *Goal focus*   Goals are clear to members and relatively well accepted by them.
2. *Communication adequacy*   Information is well-distributed.
3. *Optimal power utilization*   Influence is fairly equally distributed, so that the influence of subordinates can be felt at high levels.

4. *Resource utilization* These are used effectively, particularly personnel resources.
5. *Cohesiveness* There is a sense of identity between members.
6. *Morale* There is a feeling of well-being among members rather than dissatisfaction.
7. *Innovative-ness* Moves are made towards new goals, and new procedures are invented.
8. *Autonomy* The organization is relatively autonomous and independent of outside influences.
9. *Adaptation* Structure is constantly adapting to meet new demands.
10. *Problem-solving adequacy* The effective system copes well with problems.

Role of the Principal or Head of Department

The Principal, or Head of Department or Dean, occupies a central position with regard to innovation, as he or she carries traditional authority and also has an overall perspective of the organization. This role involves one of leadership rather than administration, the former being concerned with the innovation of new ideas and policies, while the latter is mainly concerned with the efficient running of the existing system. This pivotal role cannot be over-emphasized, since the style of leadership will profoundly affect the climate of the whole department of institution.

The style of decision-making is also important and four styles of decision can be identified (Loubser, Spiers and Moody, 1975):

1. *Tell* – the Head makes the decision, either because it is so important or so trivial.
2. *Sell* – the Head knows that there is only one course of action, and so tries to persuade others so that it will have a chance of success.
3. *Consult* – the Head obtains opinions from all staff concerned, but takes the final responsibility for making the decision.
4. *Share* – the Head allows other staff to share the decision-making process and accepts the joint decision.

The first two styles may lead to the appearance of mutual consent among staff, but this may be superficial if they feel the decision has been imposed unilaterally. The third style is one of the most common, since it has clear lines of responsibility. It follows the 'management are there to manage' philosophy and also maintains the notion of effective leadership and management as being largely due to personality variables. The fourth style is often thought of as being democratic, with most issues and decisions being put to a vote. However, this is open to abuse if factions develop outside of the meetings in order to block or prevent innovation. Another problem is that consensus often implies some kind of neutral, middle ground or compromise and this may not foster creative innovation.

Clearly then, the role of the Principal or Head of Department has great influence and the combination of this with staff behaviour can be a guide to the climate. Halpin (1966) identifies a continuum of climates from open to closed as follows:

Open The Head is hard-working, flexible and prepared to make rules and criticize when necessary; monitoring is not too close and staff needs are seen as important. Staff morale is high and relationships are good.

Autonomous The Head is less obvious than in the open style, allowing staff more autonomy but providing less positive leadership. Staff social needs are less well catered for, but teachers feel a sense of accomplishment of tasks.

Controlled The Head makes the staff work hard and is authoritarian, with little scope for staff satisfaction socially. Staff respond to this and gain task achievement satisfaction.

Familiar The Head gives very little leadership, but creates a happy atmosphere for staff. Morale is low because they lack direction.

Paternal The Head has little influence over the staff, and is seen as interfering rather than leading. There is not much achievement even though staff 'get on with the job' and the Head's approach to social needs is seen as insincere.

Closed The Head is distant and aloof, giving no leadership and taking no personal interest in the staff as people. There is little job satisfaction.

Guidelines for innovation and change

We have so far considered the factors that influence innovation and in this section, some guidelines are offered for implementing innovation.

Hoyle (1976), for example, has identified three types of innovation strategy:

- The innovation is made by powerful bodies such as the UKCC or ENB and the innovation is aimed mainly at the structure of education. Communication is one-way, from authority to professional practitioner.
- The target here is the attitudes, values and opinions of a group of teachers. The communication is two-way, between the 'expert' and the practitioners, and it is non-directive. This might be such things as the Principal or Head attempting to alter the teachers' attitudes to open learning.
- This strategy aims to change the curriculum rather than the individual, and is backed by expertise. Communication is one-way, and usually consists of films, lectures or books on innovation.

It is quite possible for the leader to introduce innovation by using his or her authority, but this has fundamental weaknesses. The co-operation of teachers is essential, since it is they who will have to implement the changes.

Innovation is more likely to be accepted if the changes are generated from within the organization, rather than by outsiders. Innovation is also likely to be acceptable if it involves a reduction in workload, or an emphasis towards something that the teacher desires. For example, if a curriculum innovation is planned that provides more time for clinical involvement by the teacher, then it is likely that most teachers would accept this willingly.

Group discussion is vital if the innovation is to be accepted, and sufficient time must be allowed for this. Opportunity for teachers to put their points of view, and for questions to be asked are essential steps in the innovative process. It is useful to attempt to meet in a hotel for 'away-days' to discuss such issues, since this removes people from their traditional roles and associations and allows them to be more themselves. Resistance to change can arise out of peer-group norms; it is interesting to see that new nurse teachers, when they leave the teacher-training institution, are keen to make innovations but within a year or so of being in the 'real world' most of this has evaporated! Georgiades and Phillimore (1975) talk about the myth of the 'hero-innovator':

> The idea that you can produce, by training, a knight in shining armour who, loins girded with new technology and beliefs, will assault his organizational fortress and institute changes both in himself and others at a stroke. Such a view is ingenuous. The fact of the matter is that organizations such as schools or hospitals will, like dragons, eat hero-innovators for breakfast.

They offer six guidelines for change:

1. try to work with those supportive forces within the organization, rather than against those who are resistant to change;
2. aim to produce a self-motivated team of workers who are powered from within themselves;
3. work with the 'healthy' parts of the system, i.e. those who have the motivation and resource to be improved, rather than on lost causes;
4. ensure that the people you are working with for change have the freedom and authority to implement the proposed changes;
5. try to obtain involvement of key personnel in the change programme, but make this realistic and appropriate; and
6. protect team members from undue stress and pressure.

It would seem from the foregoing discussion that the successful manager of change and innovation requires a combination of personal qualities and expertise. He or she needs to have good interpersonal skills in order to manage the staff and minimize anxiety, yet should be prepared to be unpopular if this is necessary to implement decisions. The manager needs to feel secure enough to allow staff to be involved in some of the decisions about change and be prepared to question assumptions when difficulties arise. Management of change requires vision and belief in oneself, but at the same time the manager's feet must be kept on the ground if their ideas are to be put into practice. It is extremely important that the manager of change should avoid getting enmeshed in the finer details of the system; his or her role is to be able to have a 'bird's-eye' view of the whole thing to ensure a holistic outcome.

Gibbs (1990) offers useful guidelines for curriculum innovation and the management of change in relation to a curriculum leading to registration in mental health.

CURRICULUM INNOVATION IN NURSING AND MIDWIFERY EDUCATION

One of the most significant curriculum innovations in recent years is the ENB Framework and Higher Award for Continuing Professional Education for Nurses, Midwives and Health Visitors, which aims to meet the needs of the majority of practitioners who work in practice settings. Another significant innovation that spans all sectors of post-compulsory education is Credit Accumulation and Transfer Schemes (CATS), and in particular the Accreditation of Prior Experiential Learning (APEL). The ENB Framework and Higher Award utilizes a CATS system for the delivery of modules. Open Units are another innovation within CAT schemes which demonstrate an extension to the notion of contract learning. This section on innovation concludes with a discussion of nursing theories and models, and the multicultural curriculum.

The ENB Framework and Higher Award for continuing professional education for nurses, midwives and health visitors

The ENB Framework and Higher Award began operating in April 1992 and emphasizes the pivotal importance of continuing education in helping practitioners to keep up-to-date with changing technology and work practices (ENB, 1991). The Board was concerned about the haphazard nature of continuing professional education, particularly the varying availability of provision and the repetitive nature of courses. Continuing education needs to be related to quality of care, and this means that the traditional definition of clinical skills must be broadened to embrace an integrated approach to management of information, innovation, decision-making, setting and maintaining standards, and health promotion. The Framework and Higher Award are open to all practitioners on the live professional register, but is particularly relevant to those in day-to-day practice. Practitioners may choose to undertake the Higher Award or simply use the framework to plan their professional development.

The framework is a partnership between the practitioners, managers, and educationalists, and there are five stages to be considered when a practitioner commences the framework:

1. *Review* The practitioner reviews their expertise and achievements with their current client group in relation to the key characteristics, and index for the Higher Award if desired.
2. *Contract* With the collaboration of the manager, a contract is entered into with the educational institution to identify learning outcomes for the award.
3. *Delivery* The practitioner then participates in the educational activities to achieve the learning outcomes, including maintaining an individual professional portfolio.
4. *Assessment* Achievement of learning outcomes is demonstrated by assessment, and recorded in the portfolio.
5. *Quality assurance* Practitioners, educationalists and managers will review the relevance and effectiveness of the learning experiences undertaken.

Ten key characteristics

Ten key characteristics are identified as representing the knowledge, skills and expertise necessary for the provision of quality care to meet changing health needs, and the integration of all these can be recognized by the Higher Award. This is at a minimum of first-degree level and requires demonstration of mastery of the ten key characteristics into a field of professional practice. The ten key characteristics are (ENB, 1991):

1. Professional accountability and responsibility
2. Clinical expertise with a specific client group
3. Using research to plan, implement and evaluate strategies to improve care
4. Team working and building, multidisciplinary team leadership
5. Flexible and innovative approaches to care
6. Use of health promotion strategies
7. Facilitating and assessing development in others
8. Handling information and making informed clinical decisions
9. Setting standards and evaluating quality of care
10. Instigating, managing and evaluating clinical change

The outcomes for the Higher Award can be achieved through a range of activities such as in-service courses, open learning, self-instruction, and taught courses. Practitioners working towards the Higher Award are required to maintain a personal Professional Portfolio.

ENB professional portfolio

This is provided as part of the indexing process for the Higher Award, and is a means of recording the practitioner's professional and personal development, qualifications, and professional experience so as to provide a complete picture of this. The portfolio constitutes a basis for reflection and critical analysis of experiences and also for negotiating a learning contract with their manager and colleagues in education. The portfolio centres around the ten key characteristics listed above, and should be reviewed periodically, particularly when considering undertaking a course, or seeking a new post.

Accreditation of prior experiential learning

The principles of Credit Accumulation and Transfer (CAT) Schemes are outlined in Chapter 13 (p. 319), including the Accreditation of Prior Experiential Learning. In this section the process of making an APEL claim is explained.

Making an APEL Claim

There are seven steps in making a claim for Accreditation of Prior Experiential Learning (Butterworth, 1993).

1. Focus on the area of learning and summarize it in a learning claim. The first step in putting together an APEL claim is for students to decide upon which part of their past experience they wish to base their claim, and this can be one large experience or more than one, provided that it is reasonably substantial. It is not possible to use many small experiences to build up a claim, as this would lack the necessary coherence.
2. Clearly identify and list the learning outcomes derived from the experience. Learning outcomes need to be stated in a precise form rather than vague, general statements, and must encompass all the knowledge and skills that were learned.
3. Check that the learning is relevant and at the right level for the award which is being sought. The claim must be current, i.e. the experience should have been within the last five years, sufficient, and relevant to the award being sought.
4. Collect sufficient documentary evidence to support the claim, together with at least one suitable testimonial authenticating it. Direct evidence constitutes the student's own work, such as reports, plans, materials that have been designed, etc. that will demonstrate achievement of the learning outcomes. Indirect evidence refers to testimonials and other evidence from external sources.
5. Produce a reflective commentary which describes the experience(s) and analyses them to show how they produced the learning that is being claimed. This is a very important stage, as it demonstrates the student's ability to reflect upon and conceptualize the experiences.
6. Present an outline of APEL portfolio at a formative assessment tutorial. This involves discussion with the APEL counsellor about the appropriateness and sufficiency of the claim, and the quality of the reflective commentary.
7. Collate all this material and organize it in the form of a portfolio that can be presented to an assessor. The portfolio is not assessed by the APEL counsellor, but by a 'gatekeeper' who has not been involved

with the student's preparation. The portfolio should contain a contents page and each chapter should be clearly labelled.

OPEN UNITS IN CATS

Negotiation of learning contracts between student and teacher is an important aspect of the educational process in CAT schemes and is taken to its ultimate in the negotiation of an Open Unit. An Open Unit has the same kind of specification as any other unit, but the major difference is that the student designs it in negotiation with the tutor. This provides the student with an opportunity to study areas of particular interest or relevance, as well as conveying a sense of ownership of his or her own learning. Tables 12.11 and 12.12 give a specification for an open unit, and an example of an open unit negotiated by a health visitor in the community.

THEORIES AND MODELS OF NURSING

The use of terminology in describing theories and models of nursing is not very consistent, and the literature reveals the same author using several terms interchangeably when describing their own work (Meleis, 1985). However, the two most common terms in use are 'nursing theories' and 'nursing models'.

Nursing theories

The purpose of science is to explain things and its hallmarks are objectivity and empirical research. Empiricism means the pursuit of knowledge by observation and experiment and this systematic process of research makes for evidence that is much more valid than that obtained by other methods (Kerlinger, 1979). There are, however, different types of explanation in science. Psychology, for example, offers cognitive, behaviourist, humanist and psychoanalytic explanations for human behaviour, each of which may well suit a particular phenomenon better than others. It is useful to think of science as having two levels of organization of explanations: 'empirical generalization' and 'theory formation'. Empirical generalization involves explanations that state the relationships between observable things, whereas theory formation involves the introduction of unobservables into the explanation (Hyland, 1981). Explanations that are confined to observable phenomena tend to be descriptive rather than explanatory; in psychology, behaviourism explains behaviour by looking at relations between observables, i.e. between stimuli and responses without specifying any unobservables between these two concepts. Cognitive approaches, on the other hand, specify unobservables such as memory to explain phenomena and attempt to say why things occur. These comments apply to all kinds of science, including nursing science,

Table 12.11   Unit specification for an open unit

Title: Open unit

Credit points and level: 15 at either Level 2 or 3

Co-ordinator: The unit will be staffed by the Course Director or a nominated specialist tutor.

Introduction and rationale: In order to further develop their health professional interests or meet the needs of their employing institutions, course members may choose to use this unit to design their own learning in consultation with the unit tutor.

  Students are permitted to undertake a maximum of two open units within the pathway.

Aims: The aim of this unit is to support students in establishing their own personal/professional aims within the broader aims of the course, and to support them in devising an appropriate strategy to achieve these.

Learning outcomes: There are no prescribed outcomes for this unit. Instead, the course member will negotiate a personal set of learning outcomes with the unit tutor, which must be of an appropriate level and focus for 15 credit points at either Level 2 or 3. These outcomes will form the criteria for the unit assessment.

Prerequisites: Nil.

Process of learning and teaching: The activities set out below will normally be carried out in conjunction with the Course Director or a nominated specialist tutor. The unit will consist of a number of stages:

1. Negotiation with the tutor to establish the course member's personal/ professional aims and to establish outcomes which are appropriate for either Level 2 or 3.
2. The planning with the tutor of a sequence of activity that will enable the student to demonstrate that they have met the outcomes as set out in Section 1 above. The tutor will establish that the activity will involve some 40 hours of learning time.
3. The planning with the tutor of an assessment task that the student can carry out which will enable them to demonstrate that they have met the outcomes as set out in Section 1 above.
4. The carrying out of the activity agreed in Section 2 above, and the submission of the agreed assessment work.

Assessment: Evidence as agreed by the tutor that demonstrates achievement of the negotiated learning outcomes.

so it can be seen that the use of theory in nursing is an important way of explaining the nature of nursing science. A distinction can be made between basic and applied research; the former is aimed solely at explanation for its own sake, whereas the latter is concerned with the solution of problems in everyday life. Since nursing is very much a practical pursuit it seems likely that nursing theories will be directed towards the improvement of care by systematic explanations of the concept of nursing.

  Theories in any science can be thought of as having a basic structure as illustrated in Figure 12.3. The basic building blocks of theory are

Table 12.12 Specimen open unit on mentorship and supervision in community practice

---

Title: Mentorship and supervision in community practice

Level: 10 credit points at Level 2

Rationale: Student nurses are regularly allocated to the community to gain understanding of the role of the health visitor. The learning environment is not always conducive to learning, with the students often left to their own devices in making use of the experience. This can lead to demotivated and disillusioned students, which in turn may potentially have a negative effect on the relationship between health visitor and client.

Aims: My aim is to increase my understanding of the nature and skills of supervision, mentorship and preceptorship, and to be able to utilize these to provide a learning environment that facilitates students' learning in the community practice setting.

Learning outcomes:

1. Understand the nature and role of supervisor, mentor and preceptor in the community setting.
2. Describe the interpersonal skills required for effective supervision and mentorship in the community setting.
3. Analyse the relevant literature on supervision and mentorship in the community, and relate teaching strategies to this literature.
4. Discuss the nature of negotiation, including use of learning contracts in a mentoring relationship.

Pattern of learning activities:

1. Analysis of primary and secondary source material from relevant journals and textbooks.
2. Interviews with existing supervisors/mentors/preceptors in the Community Trust to ascertain their approach to their role, the strategies they prefer, and the problems they encounter.
3. Interviews with newly qualified nurses to ascertain their views on the effectiveness of the supervision/mentorship/preceptorship they experienced during their training.
4. Reflective diary of supervision/mentoring/preceptorship encounters with students.

Assessment: Presentation of a reflective diary which contains the following:

1. a descriptive, reflective record of supervision, mentoring and preceptorship encounters with students during the course of the unit;
2. an analysis of these encounters using theory derived from the relevant literature; and
3. a list of recommendations for future practice based upon the analyses of the above encounters and the relevant literature.

'concepts' and these can be defined as classes of objects, events or situations that possess common properties. Concepts are not specific entities, rather they are mental constructs with which we make sense of the environment. We are able to classify most things we encounter instantaneously, because we compare the specific stimulus with our concepts to see where it fits most easily. If the specific stimulus fits into a concept category, I can confidently classify it as a member of the concept

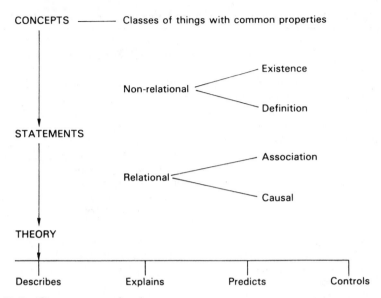

Fig. 12.3 Components of a theory.

and this process means that I can very quickly make sense of the myriad of stimuli impinging upon my senses every day.

Concepts are thus the basic building blocks of theory, but they need to be combined together in the form of statements if they are to constitute a theory. Statements in a theory can be either non-relational or relational (Walker and Avant, 1983). Non-relational statements may simply state that something exists, or they may go further and actually define the concept. Hence, it might be that a theory of nursing states that nursing exists in society without actually defining what nursing is; on the other hand, it may define the term precisely. Relational statements are of two kinds, association and causal statements; an association statement merely says that two or more concepts are related without implying a causal relationship. Causal statements do postulate a causal relationship between concepts; for example, a nursing theory may suggest that the use of nursing process causes (leads to) greater patient satisfaction with nursing care.

These various components of theory are seen by Meleis (1985) as levels of nursing theory. The first-level theory is that which identifies and labels the concepts, e.g. 'restlessness'. Once these concepts have been labelled, it is possible to move on to second-level theories, which make relationships between concepts. Third-level theory involves making predictions based upon causal relationships, such as the influence of pre-operative information on the post-operative uptake of analgesia. Fourth-level theory is the ultimate goal for nursing theory and it is at this level that theoretical notions become reality. At this level, theory influences changes in the clinical situation by prescribing interventions and procedures to bring about desired goals. Theories can be developed either deductively or inductively; deduction is the making of inferences from

Table 12.13 Definitions of theory and model from a variety of sources

Theory	*Model*
Chapman (1985) A statement describing the relationship between phenomena or concepts which have been shown (by research) to exist.	A conceptual framework capable of explaining or illustrating a complex situation.
Hyland (1981) A way of describing how the world works.	A heuristic for constructing theories. When one uses a model one simply borrows the form for a new theory from somewhere else. Hence, a model is an isomorphic theory.
Meleis (1985) An articulated and communicated conceptualization of invented or discovered reality pertaining to nursing for the purpose of describing, explaining, predicting or prescribing nursing care.	Models have to model another entity, while a theory may or may not model other properties, structures or functions.
Walker and Avant (1983) An internally consistent group of relational statements that presents a systematic view about a phenomenon and which is useful for description, explanation, prediction and control.	A graphic representation of theory which is necessary to quantify and clarify the relationships between concepts in any theoretical work.

something already known, such as the development of a nursing theory from an existing theory in another discipline. Induction is the making of inferences from data that has been gathered, such as the use of nursing observations to develop a theory. In practice, it is likely that a combination of these will be used. Table 12.13 gives some definitions of a theory and contrasts these with definitions of a model.

Nursing models

A model is a physical or conceptual representation of something; physical models are replicas of the things they represent and may be actual size or built to scale. Architects and town planners build scale models of civic developments that aim to show, in miniature, a replica of houses and commercial properties that are to be built. In colleges of nursing, students are encouraged to examine models of the organs of the body so as to understand the structure. Other kinds of model do not represent concrete entities, but concepts. Such conceptual models are usually in graphic or mathematical form and attempt to represent abstract concepts such as nursing and health. It can be seen from Table 12.13 that there is no easy distinction between the terms 'theory' and 'model'. However, from our earlier definition of a model as being a representation of something, it is

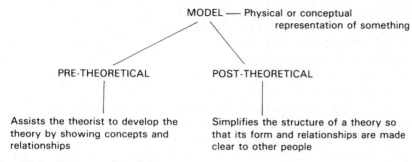

Fig. 12.4   Concept of model.

clear that a model and a theory are not the same. A model may well represent a theory, but it cannot be a theory itself; on the other hand a theory may well serve as a model for another theory, as in the case of isomorphic theory. It is quite possible to use an existing theory as a model for a new theory; for example, one could suggest that the Atomic Theory, with its notions of a central nucleus surrounded by shells of electrons could serve as a model for a theory about the structure of the ward-management team. Sister or staff nurse would be seen as the nucleus and the various grades of trained and untrained staff would occupy the inner and outer shells of responsibility. Both of these theories have identical forms and are thus said to be isomorphic, the new theory being modelled on the old. A useful way of distinguishing between definitions of model is to think of models as being either pre-theoretical or post-theoretical, as shown in Figure 12.4.

A pre-theoretical model is used to help the theorist develop the theory by showing some of the concepts and relationships. The model can then be altered and extended as the theory formation proceeds. A post-theoretical model has quite a different function, in that it is a way of simplifying the structure of a theory so that its form and relationships are made clear to other people.

Meleis argues strongly for the use of the term 'theory' rather than 'model' or 'conceptual framework', suggesting that these alternative terms merely devalue the work that nurses are doing in the realm of theory and minimize the impact of such theorizing. The following checklist for analysing nursing theories and models provides an aid to evaluating their usefulness.

1. Perform an introductory *overview* by reading the theory/model and:
   (a) identify key concepts and definitions;
   (b) establish whether development is inductive or deductive; and
   (c) read any research generated by the theory/model.
2. Consider the *internal consistency* of the theory/model by:
   (a) examining relational statements to see if they are logical;
   (b) ascertaining if any empirical support is available; and
   (c) if empirical support is available, checking whether the methodology and conclusions are sound.

3. Consider how *useful* the theory/model is for:
    (a) giving better insight into phenomena;
    (b) enabling better predictions to be made; and
    (c) influencing nursing practice.
4. Consider how far the theory/model will *generalize* by examining its use in a wide range of settings.
5. Consider how *parsimonious* the theory/model is by comparing it with another theory/model to see if it explains the same data more simply.
6. Consider whether the theory/model is *testable* by:
    (a) examining if it can generate hypotheses which can be tested empirically; and
    (b) examining its predictive power by identifying potential falsifiers.

THE MULTICULTURAL CURRICULUM IN NURSING AND MIDWIFERY

The term 'culture' refers to the civilization and customs of particular people or groups, their whole way of life, in fact. Great Britain is very much a multicultural society by virtue of its rich mix of individuals and groups with ethnic differences. This does not refer solely to differences in skin colour, since cultures can vary considerably within a relatively small area. There are marked differences in customs between the North, the Midlands and the South of England and such cultural differences form part of the richness of society.

Immigration has brought a much wider range of cultures to British society, each with its own particular values, beliefs and customs, and a true multicultural society will give equal status to every culture. In practice, however, it appears that ethnic minorities, particularly black people are exposed to racial discrimination and racism in their daily lives in Britain. Racial discrimination means that an individual or group receives less favourable treatment in comparison to another by virtue of their racial origins. Discrimination is not always obvious, as in the case of regulations regarding nurses' uniforms, which forbid certain forms of dress in violation of cultural requirements. Racism is a broad term that implies the use of power to support racist beliefs, such as the superiority of white people.

Nurse educators need to be aware of the implications of multicultural education in nursing and these can be thought of in terms of two specific aspects, the students' own cultural requirements and their need to understand aspects of the culture of patients with whom they will come into contact. It is common to find that curricula in nursing deal with aspects of diet in relation to other cultures and also the specific beliefs and procedures to be followed when a patient dies. It is much less common to find that other aspects of culture are included. Awareness of cultural values as a topic needs to be seen as crucial if nurses are to practise their profession effectively in a multicultural society.

Nursing draws its recruits from a variety of cultural backgrounds and they will practise very much in a multicultural setting in both hospitals and community. The importance of multicultural education in nursing can be underlined by the development of a multicultural policy by the health district; such a policy can provide a forum for discussion and allow representation of ethnic minorities. It can also provide guidelines for the recruitment of staff and can monitor the effectiveness of its anti-racist measures. The following questions form a useful checklist for multicultural issues in nurse education (FEU, 1985).

1. Culture

   (a) Is the college aware of the range and variety of cultures amongst its members?
   (b) Is adequate provision made for the religious or cultural needs of all students?
   (c) Does the college draw, in appropriate circumstances, on the resources provided by the local (in some cases, multicultural) community?
   (d) Are ethnic minority organizations encouraged to use college premises?
   (e) Is provision made for special dietary needs?

2. Curriculum content and methods of assessment

   (a) What procedures are available in the college to review its own practice in relation to a multicultural society, through the work of an Academic Board, departments, subject/course teams, curriculum development committees?
   (b) In what ways can mainstream subject curricula reflect a multicultural society?
   (c) How can positive strategies reflecting a multicultural society be introduced into different subjects and disciplines?
   (d) Are assessment criteria and methods appropriate for all types of student?

3 Staff development, guidance and counselling

   (a) Does the local authority (health authority) run courses in education/training for a multicultural society?
   (b) What other courses are available to be matched with training needs of this kind?
   (c) Are specialist staff needed to advise students in a multicultural college; if so, what type of staff are these?
   (d) How can the local community be involved in guidance and counselling?

Curricula in nursing and midwifery education should acknowledge the multicultural nature of a trust or health authority by including study of the cultures represented in that particular community. This should not be represented as a minority interest, but as part of a balanced approach to the study of society in general.

Another way in which multicultural aspects can be brought into nurse education is during actual classroom teaching; when presenting materials and information, the teacher should present ideas and examples from a variety of cultures rather than solely from Western European culture. It is important that visual media and books contain members of ethnic minorities as well as the indigenous white population and that case studies and simulations should include names and characters from ethnic minorities.

REFERENCES

Beattie, A. (1987) Making a curriculum work, in *The Curriculum in Nursing Education*, (eds P. Allan and M. Jolley), Croom Helm, London.

Bell, R. (1973) *Thinking about the curriculum*, Open University Press, Milton Keynes.

Bernstein, B. (1971) On the classification and framing of educational knowledge, in *Knowledge and Control: New Directions for the Sociology of Education*, (ed. M. Young), Collier Macmillan, London.

Bloom, B. (1956) *Taxonomy of Educational Objectives: The Classification of Educational Goals, Handbook One: Cognitive Domain*. McKay, New York.

Butterworth, C. (1993) *Introduction and Self-assessment Guide to Claiming APEL by Distance Learning*, University of Greenwich, London.

Davies, I. (1969) Education and Social Science. *New Society*, May 8th.

English National Board for Nursing, Midwifery and Health Visiting (1991) *Framework for Continuing Professional Education for Nurses, Midwives and Health Visitors: Guide to Implementation*, ENB, London.

English National Board for Nursing, Midwifery and Health Visiting (1993) *Regulations and Guidelines for the Approval of Institutions and Courses*, ENB, London.

Further Education Curriculum Unit (1985) *Multicultural Education*, FEU, London.

General Nursing Council for England and Wales (1977) *A Statement of Educational Policy*. Circular 77/19

Georgiades, N. and Phillimore, L. (1975) *The myth of the hero-innovator and alternative strategies for organisational change, Behaviour Modification with The Severely Mentally Retarded*, (eds C. Kierman and E. Woodford), Associated Scientific Publishers, London.

Gibbs, A. (1990) Curriculum innovation and the management of change. *Nurse Education Today*, **10**, 98–103.

Gronlund, N. (1978) *Stating Behavioural Objectives for Classroom Instruction*, Macmillan, New York.

Halpin, A. (1966) *Theory and Research in Educational Administration*, Macmillan, New York.

Harrow, A. (1972) *A Taxonomy of the Psychomotor Domain*. McKay, New York.

HMSO (1989) *Working for Patients, Education and Training, Working Paper 10*, HMSO, London.

Hogg, S. (1990) The problem-solving curriculum evaluation and development model. *Nurse Education Today*, **10**, 104–110.

Hoyle, E. (1972) *Problems of Curriculum Innovation*, Open University Press, Milton Keynes.

Hoyle, E. (1976) *Strategies of Curriculum Change. Unit 23, Curriculum Design and Development*, Open University Press, Milton Keynes.

Humphreys, J. and Quinn F.M. (1994) *Healthcare Education: The Challenge of the Market*, Chapman and Hall, London.

Hyland, M. (1981) *Introduction to Theoretical Psychology*, Macmillan, London.

Katz, E., Levin, M. and Hamilton, H. (1963) Traditions of research on the diffusion of innovation. *American Sociological Review*, **28**, (2)

Kerlinger, F. (1979) *Behavioral Research: A Conceptual Approach*, Holt, Rinehart and Winston, New York.

Kerr, J. (1968) Changing the curriculum, in *The Curriculum: Design, Context and Development*, (ed., R. Hooper), Oliver and Boyd, Edinburgh.

Krathwohl, D., Bloom, B. and Masia, B. (1964) *A Taxonomy of Educational Objectives: the Classification of Education Goals, Handbook 2: Affective Domain*, McKay, New York.

Lawton, D. (1983) *Curriculum Studies and Educational Planning*, Hodder and Stoughton, London.

Lewis, A. and Miel, A. (1972) *Supervision for Improved Instruction: New Challenges, New Responses*, Wadsworth, Belmont.

Loubser, J., Spears, H. and Moody, C. (1975) cited in *An Introduction to Curriculum Research and Development*, (ed. L. Stenhouse), Heinemann, London.

Mager, R. (1962) *Preparing Instructional Objectives*, Fearon, California.

Meleis, A. (1985) *Theoretical Nursing*, Lippincott, Philadelphia.

Miles, M. (1975) Planned change and organisational health, in *Curriculum Innovation*, (eds A. Harris, M. Lawn and W. Prescott), Croom Helm, London.

Quinn, F. (1988) *The Principles and Practice of Nurse Education*, 2nd edn, Chapman and Hall, London.

Saylor, J., Alexander, W. and Lewis, A. (1981) *Curriculum Planning for Better Teaching and Learning*, 4th edn, Holt, Rinehart and Winston, New York.

Scrimshaw, P. (1983) *Educational Ideologies. Unit 2 of Educational Studies*, Open University, Milton Keynes.

Simmons, S. and Bahl, D. (1992) An Integrated Approach to Curriculum Development. *Nurse Education Today*, **12**, 310–315.

Simpson, E. (1972) The classification of educational objectives in the psychomotor domain, in *The Psychomotor Domain*, vol 3, Gryphon House, Washington DC.

Skilbeck, M. (1984) *School Based Curriculum Development*, Harper and Row, London.

Stenhouse, L. (1975) *An Introduction to Curriculum Research and Development*, Heinemann, London.

Tanner, D. and Tanner, L. (1980) *Curriculum Development: Theory into Practice*, 2nd Ed, Macmillan, New York.

Tyler, R. (1949) *Basic Principles of Curriculum and Instruction*, University of Chicago Press, Chicago.

University of Greenwich (1992) *A Set of Standards for the Documentation of Pathways*, University of Greenwich, London.

Walker, L. and Avant, K. (1983) *Strategies for Theory Construction in Nursing*, Appleton Century Crofts, Norwalk.

Educational delivery systems 13

Since time immemorial, taught courses in educational institutions have been the predominant system of delivery for all types of education. However, there is a growing demand in education for flexible courses that are more relevant to the needs of individuals and their employers, and the advent of The Government White Paper *Working for Patients: Education and Training Working Paper 10* (HMSO, 1989) has given employers a major say in the process of educational contracting.

Traditionally, courses in British further and higher education have been based on a set of assumptions about the nature of learning and the role of students. One assumption is that the institution and its teachers know best what a student needs from a course. The educational provision was largely prescriptive, giving the student little or no control over attendance, length, content, process or assessment. Nurses undertaking continuing education courses found themselves repeating the same topics, especially in core subjects such as research or management. 'Concern has been expressed at the amount of apparently repetitious learning which currently takes place in continuing education' (ENB, 1990). Another assumption is that education is really about academic learning and the fact that nursing is very much a practice-based profession has tended to lower its credibility in the eyes of academics. Indeed, it was a common complaint that the registered nurse qualification did not even count as the equivalent of one GCE at Advanced Level!

The first part of this chapter discusses two delivery systems that, in the light of the foregoing discussion, have important implications for health-care education, i.e. CATS and open learning. This is followed by discussion of three other well-established delivery systems: personalized system of instruction, mastery learning, and programmed instruction.

CREDIT ACCUMULATION AND TRANSFER SCHEMES (CATS)

The CNAA National Credit Accumulation and Transfer Scheme was launched in 1986, and with the abolition of the CNAA in 1992 the Open University Validation Services (OUVS) has undertaken the provision of a national CATS service. Institutions are now designing their educational provision within a CAT framework

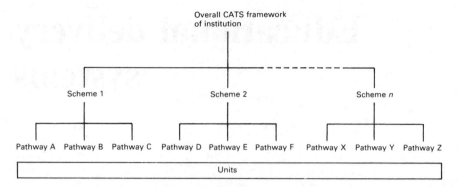

Fig. 13.1 Typical CATS structure in educational institutions.

Structure of CAT frameworks and schemes

The traditional structure of educational institutions was built around the concept of a course; a course consists of a clearly defined, self-contained curriculum leading to a specified academic and/or professional award. The term course was used for educational provision of varying length, from one- or two-day in-service courses, to those lasting three or more years. Courses within the same cognate area were administered through departments or schools, such as pre-registration nursing, or social sciences, and the teaching staff for a course were sited within the relevant department. With the advent of CAT schemes, this structure is undergoing radical changes that affect all aspects of the educational institution. Figure 13.1 illustrates a typical CATS structure in educational institutions.

Each institution will have an overall credit accumulation framework which lays down the principles and regulations for all credit schemes within the institution. A scheme is really a set of regulations and procedures for the operation of CATS, and institutions will typically have a varying range of schemes, each relating to a particular area of educational endeavour, e.g. in-service teacher education, health, science, etc. Within each scheme there are a number of pathways, each leading to a named academic award, and this term has replaced the term course. Within a health scheme, for example, there could be pathways leading to degrees in nursing, midwifery, physiotherapy, and health studies (Figure 13.2).

The key difference between pathways and courses is that pathways comprise many discrete, self-contained units of learning. Units of learning are termed modules of learning by some institutions, but for convenience the term unit is used in this chapter. From the foregoing it can be seen that, eventually, institutional provision will consist of many hundreds of units, some being specific to a given pathway and others being generic and therefore relevant to many pathways.

The major breakthrough in CAT schemes is the degree of unit choice available to students and the consequent opportunity this affords to both student and employer in terms of the professional relevance of the pathway. Pathways normally consist of compulsory or core units that

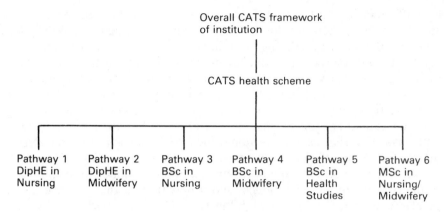

Overall CATS framework
of institution

CATS health scheme

Pathway 1	Pathway 2	Pathway 3	Pathway 4	Pathway 5	Pathway 6
DipHE in	DipHE in	BSc in	BSc in	BSc in	MSc in
Nursing	Midwifery	Nursing	Midwifery	Health	Nursing/
				Studies	Midwifery

Fig. 13.2 Typical structure of a CATS scheme for health.

define the nature of the award, and a wide range of option units from which each student may select those relevant to their own personal needs. The complete set of core and option units undertaken by a student is termed their programme of study for the pathway, and it can be seen that programmes of study will differ from student to student, according to the option units they choose. This is in marked contrast to a conventional course because each student in a CATS pathway may actually be doing a different 'course', but one that is tailor-made to meet their own unique professional needs and aspirations. The basic criterion for the inclusion of an option unit within a student's programme of study is that her or she must be able to demonstrate to the pathway leader the coherence and relevance of the unit to their overall programme of studies within the pathway. Let us take the example of a nurse working within the field of sexually transmitted diseases who is undertaking a post-registration degree pathway in nursing studies. This particular nurse may choose to study an option unit from a social science degree pathway on human sexuality, since this would be relevant to his or her particular professional needs and interests. Similarly, an option unit on personnel management from a diploma pathway in management studies may be undertaken so as to improve both knowledge and skills as a departmental manager.

The introduction of CAT schemes into institutions has major implications for organizational structures. Typically, each scheme has its own scheme board which has overall responsibility for the scheme. In addition, each pathway has a pathway committee which co-ordinates the day-to-day running of the pathway. In conventional courses, all teaching and assessment work was contained within the course team, whereas a CAT scheme deals with a range of units from across the entire institution. Normally, each unit leader in a CAT scheme is responsible for both teaching and the marking of assessments for the unit, but problems of compatibility can arise if different grading systems are used for pathways within an institution. The implication here is that institutions will need to adopt a standard marking/grading system throughout the institution if CATS is to be successfully implemented. The external examiner system is also affected, in that the traditional role has been one of attachment to a specific course, where the subject-matter is relatively generic. With CAT schemes, the pathway external examiners may have to scrutinize units that are totally outside their area of subject expertise, such as the option units on human sexuality and personnel management in the example cited earlier. The validity of the external examiner system may then be called into question, and institutions are tackling the problem by identifying external examiners for specific subject areas rather than for individual pathways. External examiners would then be responsible for unit assessments from across the entire institution in a given subject area. However, such a system makes it difficult for any external examiner to form a view of the overall student experience, and it may be that this aspect is given greater emphasis within annual pathway monitoring reports.

In CAT schemes, a specified number of credit points is awarded to the student on successful completion of appropriate learning. This learning can be gained in three ways: through formal study on a course, from existing qualifications, or by learning gained from professional or life experience.

The CATS system of credit points takes as its standard a three-year full-time undergraduate degree with honours course, which is credit rated at 360 credit points, 120 for each of the three years of the course. Each year represents a specific level of learning:

first year   =   level 1
second year =   level 2
third year   =   level 3

There is also a Level M for postgraduate study at masters degree level. Credit points gained from appropriate learning can accumulate towards a higher education award such as a diploma or degree, and the amount and level of credit normally required for these in England, Wales and Northern Ireland is shown below.

- *Certificate of higher education*: 120 credit points at level 1.
- *Diploma of higher education*: 240 credit points, 120 at each of levels 1 and 2
- *Unclassified degree*: 360 credit points, of which a minimum of 60 must be at level 3.
- *Degree with honours*: 360 credit points, of which a minimum of 120 must be at level 3.
- *Postgraduate diploma*: 70 credit points, of which a minimum of 50 must be at masters level
- *Masters degree*: 120 credit points, of which a minimum of 80 must be at masters level and the remainder at level 3.

The system in Scotland differs from that in the three countries above, in that there are four levels: SD1, SD2, SD3 and SD4. The first three levels equate with the certificate, diploma and unclassified degree as shown above, but the degree with honours requires 480 credit points, 120 at each of the four levels. Normally, units can be done in any order within a

Table 13.1 Typical components of a unit specification

Unit title:	Should be clear to students
Department:	
Credit points and learning time:	Proportion of a full-time year
Level:	CATS level 1, 2, 3 or M
Code:	For computer records
Co-ordinator:	Individual responsible for delivery
Pre-requisites and co-requisites:	Units that must be taken before or concurrently with the unit
Rationale:	Justifies the inclusion of the unit/module in the scheme
Aims:	Identify the overall purpose of the unit/module
Learning outcomes:	State what the student can do as a result of learning, e.g. 'Analyse the factors which influence the effectiveness of nurse–patient interaction'
Process of learning and teaching:	Range of activities to achieve learning
Assessment:	Means of testing achievement of learning
Indicative content:	List of key topics
Indicative reading:	List of representative texts

pathway, although some may be designated as pre-requisites for other units according to the nature of the pathway. Units are free-standing and self-contained, and the typical components of a unit specification are shown in Table 13.1. An example of a unit specification for a unit called 'Cognitive Psychology' is shown in Table 13.2.

Accreditation of prior learning (APL)

One of the fundamental principles of CAT schemes is that students who have been awarded credit points from one institution can transfer them to studies in another institution. The contribution of existing credits, gained outside the awarding institution, towards a higher education award is termed APL (accreditation of prior learning). In order for credit to count towards an award it must be relevant to that award, and be at an appropriate level. The length of time since the course was completed also affects its current relevance, so APL is normally confined to courses completed within the previous five years. There is a maximum percentage of APL that can be counted towards an award and this is normally between 50% and 75% of the total credit required for that award. In CAT schemes a distinction is made between general credit and specific credit, and the following vignette illustrates this.

> Tara was halfway through the second year of a degree in Nursing when her husband's company decided to transfer him to the north of England office. She contacted the university nearest to her new address who explained that there was currently no degree in nursing available, but that a degree in health studies was well established. Tara had earned a total of 240 credit points from her previous nursing degree studies, 120 at each of Levels 1 and 2. However, because the

Table 13.2 Example of a unit specification for cognitive psychology

Unit title:	Cognitive Psychology
Department:	Health and Social Science Dept.
Credit points and learning time:	15 credit points; 1 semester; 1/8th of a full-time year of study.
Level:	Level 1
Code:	9999
Co-ordinator:	A.N. Other
Pre-requisites and co-requisites:	Nil

Rationale: Cognitive psychology emphasizes the internal mental processes involved in perception, memory, thinking and language. This area of psychology has grown considerably over the past decade, particularly in the field of human information-processing, and the development of computer models of the brain. This unit provides an introduction to the principles of cognitive psychology.

Aims: The aim of the unit is to provide the student with a broad understanding of the nature of cognitive psychology with particular reference to the information-processing approach.

Learning outcomes:

1. Describe the components of an information-processing model.
2. Explain the processes involved in perception.
3. Describe the Atkinson–Shiffrin model of human memory.
4. Compare and contrast a range of approaches to the study of learning in both human and non-human species.
5. Discuss approaches to the study of thinking.
6. Explain the nature of psycholinguistics and its application to the understanding of speech disorders.

Process of learning and teaching: The learning and teaching activities will consist of lectures, seminars and laboratory work. The latter will include demonstrations and practicals. The proportion of lecture/seminars to laboratory work will be 50/50

Assessment: Assessment consists of two components:

1. a written assignment that demonstrates students' understanding of cognitive psychology with particular reference to the information-processing approach; and
2. a written record of practical laboratory work that the student has undertaken during the unit.

There is an attendance requirement of 70% for this unit.

Indicative content:

- *Information-processing model*: Newell and Simon.
- *Perception*: Selective attention, Gestalt principles, perceptual constancies, inference, illusions, cultural factors in perception, ESP.
- *Memory*: Atkinson–Shiffrin model, episodic and semantic memory, improving memory, theories of forgetting.
- *Learning*: insight learning, social learning, problem-solving, acquisition of psychomotor skills, transfer of learning, learning difficulties.
- *Thought*: concept formation, decision-making, convergent/divergent thinking, artificial intelligence.
- *Language*: linguistics and psycholinguistics, phonology, syntax, semantics, linguistic competence and linguistic performance, linguistic relativity hypothesis, Vygotsky's theory, Chomsky's theory, Skinner's theory, speech perception, reading, speech disorders.

Indicative reading:

Baddeley, A. (1990) *Human Memory: Theory and Practice*, Lawrence Erlbaum Associates.
Baron, J. (1990) *Thinking and Deciding*, Cambridge University Press.
Caron, J. (1992) *An Introduction to Psycholinguistics*, Harvester Wheatsheaf.
Eysenck, M. and Keane, M.T. (1990) *Cognitive Psychology: A Student's Handbook*, 2nd edn, Lawrence Erlbaum Associates.
McIlveen, R., Higgins, L. and Wadeley, A. (1992) *BPS Manual of Psychology Practicals*, British Psychological Society.

focus was nursing rather than generic health studies Tara was allowed to count only 80 of her Level 2 credit points towards the health studies degree.

Credit awarded to a student for specified learning in one institution is termed general credit and can be transferred to studies in other HE institutions. The receiving institution, however, may decide that only a proportion of this general credit is actually relevant to their course, and this proportion of the general credit is termed specific credit. If any specific credit matches the learning outcomes of a unit on the course to which the student is transferring, then or she can be given exemption from that unit. Hall (1994) introduces a third category of credit which he calls thematic credit. This is credit awarded within the level definitions of a particular educational theme, such as physics, nursing, or social science. Thematically based CAT schemes are administratively distinct from each other and are managed by staff from within the theme, giving ownership of the various unit curricula. In addition, development and change can be implemented quickly as necessary, without the inherent delays of a single monolithic CAT Scheme. Thematic credit also facilitates the production of a credit tariff of courses falling within a theme, and this brings about considerable savings in time and resources by avoiding the necessity of treating every APL claim as an individual entity. For example, within the theme Nursing and Midwifery, all participating pathway leaders share the same level definitions, against which they judge claims for APL. In addition, there is an agreed general credit tariff rating for all assessed courses in nursing and midwifery. This is taken as the minimum amount of credit a course is worth, and pathway leaders have discretion to increase the amount of credit in appropriate circumstances.

Course directors or pathway leaders in institutions are often faced with the task of deciding how much credit should be allowed for previous qualifications, and this is doubly difficult in the case of courses that do not carry a national credit rating. There are two aspects to be considered when examining sources of evidence about courses.

1. *Quantity of learning* This is based upon a full-time higher education academic year, with adjustment for variations in length of NHS courses.
2. *Quality of learning* In order to appraise the quality of learning it is necessary to scrutinize:
   (a) level of learning as defined in the scheme definitions – for example, the University of Greenwich Level 3 definition for health schemes is:

   Practitioners are specialists within their chosen areas, who have developed new professional skills, knowledge and understanding; who have utilized existing research; whose practice is enquiry based and who promote innovative practice.

   (b) apropriateness of the aims and outcomes of the course and the relationship between these and the definitions of learning;
   (c) appropriateness of the learning and teaching processes; and

(d) reliability and validity of course assessment in relation to (a), (b) and (c) above.

In 1989 the ENB, in collaboration with the CNAA, issued a tariff of credit ratings for nursing qualifications (CNAA, 1989). It is now generally acknowledged that this approach was over-cautious, in that it tended to undervalue the learning associated with nursing qualifications. A number of HE institutions therefore carried out their own credit ratings for these qualifications which generally resulted in a more equitable accreditation. The UKCC, the four National Boards for Nursing, and the Open University Validation Services have recently issued a joint statement on credit transfer from first-level nursing and midwifery qualifications to degree awards (UKCC, 1993). The aim of the statement is to serve 'as a guide to consistent and fair practice so as to facilitate credit transfer'. The statement applies to first-level nursing and midwifery courses undertaken after 1 January 1986, as the entry requirements for these was possession of five GCE/GCSE passes at grade C or above. The joint statement sees individual first-level courses as attracting a range of credit points; the lower end of the range attracting a credit rating of 60 credit points at Level 1, and the upper end 60 credit points at Level 2. The expectation is that the majority of courses will be credit rated at 120 credit points at Level 1. When considering awarding 120 credit points at Level 1, or additional Level 2 credits to a first-level registration course, institutions are advised to seek evidence of the quality of the learning environment in both college and clinical settings, the qualifications of staff, the quality of student assessments, courses designed for more highly qualified entrants, and well established quality assurance mechanisms.

Accreditation of prior experiential learning

Earlier, the concept of accreditation of prior learning was discussed. This was concerned with learning gained from previous qualifications, but prior learning can also be gained from the day-to-day experience of professional practice or of life generally, as in rearing a child or writing a book. It is important to note that experience alone is insufficient; the student must demonstrate how he or she has learned from the experience. A useful theoretical basis for APEL is given by Kolb (1984) in his experiential learning cycle. This is discussed in Chapter 3 (p. 83).

Credit points can be given for such experiential learning provided that it is relevant to the award which the student is seeking to achieve, and that a portfolio of evidence for such learning has been presented for accreditation to the awarding institution.

Butterworth (1992) describes two models of practice used to accredit prior experiential learning: the credit exchange model, and the developmental model. The widest application of the former is in the NVQ (National Vocational Qualifications) field, where the emphasis is very much on the production of satisfactory evidence of previous performance by the claimant.

In the developmental model, evidence of past achievements must also be produced by the claimant, but in addition he or she must produce an analysis of that evidence, including its significance to their professional development. This analysis must be supported by relevant theoretical perspectives. Butterworth argues that the developmental model is more appropriate for the accreditation of learning derived from professional practice.

Management structures for the operation of APEL

It was stated earlier that responsibility for the overall management of a scheme resides with the scheme board. A very important subcommittee of this board deals with all aspects of accreditation of prior learning, and is called the accreditation subcommittee. The subcommittee is responsible for monitoring the pathway leader's recommendations for the award of credit for APL and APEL, and is also responsible for accrediting courses from external providers. There are two roles that are essential in any APEL system, the APEL counsellor and the APEL assessor. The APEL counsellor's main role is to assist the claimant to formulate his or her learning claim in accordance with the procedures of the institution. Because of this close involvement in the process, the actual assessment of the claim is undertaken by the APEL assessor or gatekeeper, a different person who has had no previous involvement with the claimant in relation to the learning claim.

Problems with the concept of levels in CAT schemes

It was pointed out earlier that CAT schemes utilize the concept of levels of learning. Levels 1, 2, and 3 correspond to the first, second and third years of an undergraduate degree with honours, and level M is postgraduate masters level. In practice, however, it is difficult to identify precisely the characteristics of learning at each of these levels. Many institutions have devised level definitions and use these as a benchmark for judging claims for prior learning. These definitions often utilize the hierarchy suggested in Bloom's Taxonomy of Educational Objectives (Bloom, 1956), with greater emphasis on analysis, synthesis, and critical evaluation at the higher CATs levels. This approach can be seen in the ENB guidelines on the nature of diploma level for pre-registration courses (ENB, 1992). At diploma level, students are seen to have a greater depth of knowledge than certificate level, and the ability to apply this to practice. Students have 'some basis for informed critical comment and a level of thinking enabling them to progress into the third year of a degree course'. At diploma level, students have some understanding of the disciplines that contribute to nursing and their approach to the generation of knowledge. Students become 'analytical consumers of research results but are not yet capable of starting to do research'.

Further difficulty arises when considering pre-registration and post-registration courses in nursing and midwifery, in that the same definitions of levels tend to be applied in both cases. It is interesting to consider the example of two nurses with widely differing backgrounds, both of whom are studying units at Level 2. One is in the second year of a full-time, pre-registration, undergraduate degree course, whilst the other is a qualified and experienced ward sister who is undertaking a post-registration diploma in nursing. It is difficult to envisage a single definition of Level 2 that can reconcile the disparity in understanding and application to practice between that of a student nurse who is in the early stages of a course, and that of a qualified and experienced practitioner. A similar dilemma occurs when a registered nurse undertakes a further pre-registration course for a different part of the register. All pre-registration courses tend to be rated at the same level, usually Level 1 for non-Project 2000 courses, yet it is difficult to accept that the generic core abilities and skills acquired during the first registration course are not transferred largely intact into the new setting. It is interesting to compare this with the case of a qualified nurse who holds a first degree, and who wishes to undertake nurse teacher training. It is possible to take a postgraduate diploma course in education, which is rated at masters level, a level higher than the nurse's existing degree qualification, yet education is an entirely different discipline from nursing. It could be argued that there is much more likelihood of transfer of learning between courses for various parts of the register than there is between nursing courses and courses in education. The logical development would be that nurses undertaking a second registerable qualification would be awarded credit at a higher level than their first one.

Winter (1994) questions the validity of educational levels used in CAT schemes and NVQ. He studied the categories used to assess the work of students undertaking A level, undergraduate, and higher degree studies and found that many of the terms used to categorize A level assessments, such as logical coherence, critical evaluation, balanced synthesis, and originality, were also used in the assessment of undergraduate and postgraduate work in HE. Hence, these categories cannot be used to define the specific characteristics of educational levels, and there is no rational basis for the distinction between undergraduate foundation year (Level 1) and final year work (Level 3). Winter argues that the distinction between A level and HE lies in a shift in the role of the learner from dependence upon teacher control, to a more autonomous approach to study. This includes self-directed reading and the development of a mature personal stance towards their work. His analysis of postgraduate work also indicates a new role for the learner, in this case it is the student's commitment to a specialism and the external value of the student's work. For example, postgraduate work in nursing will specialize in some area of nursing, and the work would be of professional value to the organization. Winter suggests that assessment of students involves dimensions of learning that are common to all levels of education, and which include cognitive processes, values, commitment to learning, and emotional adjustments when integrating new experiences into existing knowledge. Winter proposes a new framework for credit accumulation in HE that attempts to overcome the problems inherent in the existing system. He suggests that units should consist of both unit-specific outcomes and general outcomes, the latter involving the general learning abilities that are common to all units of learning at all levels. Stage-related criteria, such as autonomous learning at undergraduate level, need not be included in every unit of learning, since this would be impractical. It should be sufficient that the student can demonstrate achievement of these in some units, as this constitutes evidence of overall achievement. Winter proposes that all awards should include an integrative unit, in which the students have to demonstrate their rationale for choice of units, and how these units form a coherent whole. He maintains that CAT scheme tutors should be able to specify pre-requisite and co-requisite units where appropriate in specific topic areas, and cautions against any built-in pre-requisites within the scheme, such as the insistence on students having to complete Level 2 units before proceeding to Level 3.

NATIONAL VOCATIONAL QUALIFICATIONS (NVQs)

The National Vocational Qualifications (NVQs) system is a different type of credit accumulation and transfer scheme which is concerned with awarding credit for the demonstration of competent performance. The NVQ Framework was designed to reform vocational qualifications by offering a coherent model of qualifications that facilitated comparison between vocational awards as well as facilitating transfer and progression within and between occupational areas (NCVQ, 1991).

NVQs are work qualifications based upon standards devised by industry lead bodies and are competence-based. We saw earlier that in CATS schemes learning is defined by learning outcomes, whereas in NVQs it is defined in terms of the learner's competence in a specified performance.

NVQ qualifications are classified according to the area of competence to which they refer, and also according to level. There are five clearly defined levels of achievement, Level 1 being the most basic, and Level 5 the most complex. There are also clear and flexible routes for progression through these levels. For example, Area 8 is called 'Preventing and treating ill health', and an example of an NVQ qualification in this area is 'Social care (residential, domiciliary and day care), Level 2'.

Each NVQ is composed of a number of units of competence that are relevant to the workplace setting. Each unit is in turn made up of elements, and performance criteria are defined for these. Satisfactory performance of each element leads to the award of credit for the unit, and credit can accumulate towards a full NVQ award. A recent development is that of General National Vocational Qualifications (GNVQ), termed the new 'vocational A levels'. Table 13.3 shows an example from NVQ in Care Level 2 (City and Guilds of London Institute, 1992).

Critics of the NVQ competence approach point out that it is concerned only with evidence of performance to the prescribed standard. There is little opportunity for the learner to propose variations from the required

Table 13.3 Example of NVQ in Care Level 2

Unit title:
  Z10:   Enable clients to eat and drink

Elements of competence:
  Z10.a   Enable clients to choose appropriate food and drink
  Z10.b   Enable clients to prepare for eating and drinking
  Z10.c   Assist clients with eating and drinking

Performance criteria for element Z10.a:
(NB Two examples only have been selected from the eight criteria for this element.)
  Z10.a1   The support required by the client is established with her/him
  Z10.a6   Supplementary foods are provided according to the specifications in the plan of care

competences, and this contrasts strongly with the student-centred, flexible approach of the CATS system. The splitting up of professional performance into large numbers of specific elements militates against an holistic approach to learning. The learning outcomes approach adopted by CAT schemes involves not only competence, but critical thinking abilities and attitudes, all of which are seen as important in professional education.

OPEN LEARNING AND DISTANCE EDUCATION

The demand for continuing professional education for nurses and midwives is greater today than it has ever been, and can be attributed to a variety of factors such as the rapid pace of professional change, fear of litigation, perceived threat of diplomate and graduate entrants to nursing, and the highly competitive job market. It is ironic that this increased demand has coincided with a drastic reduction in resources available for continuing education. Service managers are suffering severe budgetary constraints which have reduced the opportunities of funding and release for attendance on courses, with a consequent increase in competition for the limited resources available. Nurses and midwives often face a very long wait before obtaining support to attend a course. In a climate of diminishing resources, both employers and practitioners need a more flexible system of educational delivery, and are turning to open learning as a way forward. In turn, educational institutions have seen open learning as a way of expanding their provision beyond their immediate catchment area, and resources are being diverted into this type of delivery system.

Open learning is a flexible educational delivery system which is characteristically learner-centred and which utilizes multimedia learning materials, tutorial guidance and support. The notion of 'openness' is relative, given that educational programmes will vary widely in the degree of choice and control that students have over their learning. In open learning this student choice can encompass the whole spectrum of learning, including learning outcomes, content, teaching and learning methods and assessment. For example, open learning allows the student to study only those aspects of the learning materials that they need, avoiding repetition of previous learning. Above all, open learning attempts to remove any barriers that prevent an individual from gaining access to education or training, by offering flexible provision that takes into account the individual's needs and personal circumstances. Open learning can occur within educational institutions, or take place at a distance in the student's own home, and it is useful at this point to make the distinction between open learning and distance education, a closely related concept. Distance education is a term used to describe an educational delivery system that is planned on the basis of wide geographical separation of educational provider and student, and utilizing textual materials and other media such as radio and television broadcasts, videotapes, and telephone communication. It is common to find that open learning programmes utilize distance education, and vice versa, although, each system can stand on its own, and need not involve utilization of the other. In practice however, open learning programmes are mainly offered on a distance learning basis at national level, so the term distance learning is now being subsumed under the generic term open learning.

Types of open learning systems

Open learning can be operated in a number of different ways and it is possible to identify four types of system currently in use in British further and higher education (FEU/Open Tech, 1986):

1. *Flexible learning workshops*   In this system, students are able to have access to learning materials within a college setting, plus tutorial support as and when they need it. Thus, students can make appointments to visit the workshop, or simply drop in as required.
2. *Local systems*   Here the students are within reasonable travelling distance from the college and correspondence materials are supplemented by telephone communication and group seminars as required.
3. *Remote systems*   In the case of students who live a long way from the college, correspondence material is the main vehicle for tuition, but there may be residential blocks or weekends.
4. *Subcontracting systems*   In this scheme, students are registered with a particular institution, but can attend another institution that is close to their home for tutorial or other contact.

Flexible learning workshops

Flexible learning workshops allow students to drop in at a time convenient to them in order to study from specific learning resources, with the additional facility of tutorial guidance if required. Access to the learning workshop may constitute part of a student's normal timetable or simply be available for any learner when he or she happens to require its use. The notion of a learning workshop is different from the commonly encountered resource centre in that it offers more than simple access to learning materials. The tutorial backup needs a more sophisticated system of organization, with a nurse teacher designated as manager of the workshop; the role of the manager is to maintain records of the use of materials, to monitor the functioning of all aspects of the provision and to call upon the appropriate teaching staff to supplement students when required. There are important differences in the role of workshop tutors from the everyday role of a nurse teacher. In a workshop, the tutor is engaged in a one-to-one role as facilitator and consultant and therefore needs the skills of negotiation and diagnosis to be effective in this role.

The tutor must be able to use the learning materials available in the workshop, and effective management also involves the selection of materials for study. The manager needs to work closely with the library and media resources staff who can provide help with both the classification of materials and with one-to-one support of students. Kelly and Keeley (1992) describe the development of a flexible learning unit (FLU) for continuing education in nursing using the concept of a 'drop-in centre', which is situated close to a nursing library. The centre offers information, resources and guidance, and the opportunity for personal contact with centre staff. The FLU uses only commercially produced, off-the-shelf materials that have undergone rigorous testing.

Local, remote and subcontracting systems

Although each of these systems can operate independently, in practice open learning usually involves a combination of all three. One of the earliest examples of a national remote system is the British Open University, which offers undergraduate and postgraduate programmes in a wide range of subject areas. There is also an element of subcontracting within the Open University, with students having access to local educational institutions for tutorial, computing and other support. A number of institutions and private companies are currently producing open learning programmes in nursing, midwifery and health studies. The Continuing Nurse Education Programme of Barnet College, London, offers open learning modules on a variety of nursing topics as well as generic health topics. The Distance Learning Centre of the South Bank University, London, is another well-established provider of open learning materials for nursing and midwifery, and an example of an open learning programme on nursing resource management is *Using Information in Managing the Nursing Resource* (Rainbow Pack 1) by Greenhalgh and Company Ltd, Macclesfield. The University of Greenwich offers a Postgraduate Certificate in Education for initial teacher training of nurse teachers via a distance learning programme. One of the most comprehensive open learning systems for nursing is MacMillan Magazine's Nursing Times Open Learning (NTOL) programme. This originated as a professional development programme for second-level registered nurses conversion to first-level registration, and a unique feature is the inclusion of interactive educational material for the programme within the *Nursing Times* weekly magazine. In addition to the learning materials, students receive support within a local college of nursing and the programme carries approval as a conversion programme by all four National Boards for Nursing, Midwifery and Health Visiting. NTOL have since developed a credit accumulation scheme in partnership with the University of Greenwich, London, the first pathway of which is a Diploma of Higher Education in Post-Registration Studies for Nursing. Registered nurses from any part of the UK can access the programme, which utilizes open learning materials and tutorial support in local approved centres.

These examples demonstrate the flexibility of access and study conveyed by open learning, and the opportunities it offers to students to continue their professional education in a manner that is compatible with their lifestyle.

Clarke and Robinson (1992) make recommendations for good practice in open learning within nursing, midwifery and health visiting. They emphasize the importance of careful evaluation of open learning materials before deciding to include them in a particular course or programme. Planners must also ensure, where appropriate, that their programmes meet the requirements of national boards for courses with an open learning component. They also point out that course monitoring and evaluation for open learning programmes is more problematic than for conventionally taught courses.

Designing materials for open learning

The examples of open learning referred to in the previous section illustrative the diversity of the concept, from self-contained learning packages on a single topic, through to complete courses leading to academic awards. Despite this diversity, it is possible to identify generic principles involved in the production of effective open learning material, and Race (1989) offers useful guidance on these. Unlike books, which are content-centred, open learning materials are interaction-centred, focusing on student activities. The style of writing is user-friendly in order to capture the students interest, and aims to foster a sense of ownership of learning. Open learning materials undergo extensive editing and pre-publication testing on the target audience, which virtually eliminates errors and problems. Race (1989) offers guidance on writing open learning materials:

1. write in the first person, as this is more friendly;
2. leave white space for the student to write in;
3. ensure that visual information is included, and that students are asked to use it actively by doing something with it;
4. include questions and answers, so that students responses will highlight lack of understanding or errors quickly;
5. design information in manageable amounts;
6. include study skills advice;
7. include summaries, reviews and self-assessments; and
8. use visual symbols (flags) to indicate activities such as a pause for reflection, or a tea-break.

The term for a self-contained set of learning materials is a 'learning package'. This typically consists of a number of components organized in a logical sequence to help students achieve particular learning goals.

1. Rationale This consists of an introductory statement describing the package and its purpose. It provides an overview of the type of material to be studied and the reasons for such study.

2. Target population This identifies the stage of training or experience at which the package will be most suitable. For example, the package may have been designed for a student undertaking the Adult Branch of a DipHE Registered Nurse course.

3. Prerequisites If successful completion of the package is dependent on the learner having already achieved certain knowledge or skills, then this knowledge or skill is termed a prerequisite for the learning package. For example, a prerequisite for many nursing subjects will be a knowledge of normal structure and function.

4. Learning outcomes If the package is linked to a particular module or unit of study, then the learning outcomes will be derived from this. If the package is generic and free-standing, i.e. may be used for a number of units or modules, then appropriate learning outcomes will need to be formulated for the package.

5. Choice of learning activities If individuals differ in their learning styles, then it is logical to include more than one form of activity by which the learner may achieve the objectives. Activities such as reading, writing, listening, looking and doing should provide sufficient variety in one package to suit the needs of most individuals, who can then select the medium by which they learn best. Further variety can be introduced by the use of different media within these activities, for example the use of slides, audiotape and videotape. Activities need not be passive, but can actively involve the learner, such as in dissecting a specimen using instructions in a package.

6. Optional activities beyond the package Optional activities may be presented to the learner to enrich the learning experience, but which are outside the confines of the learning package. For example, one suggested activity from a package on 'Nursing the patient with a myocardial infarction' might be that the learner should take the opportunity to visit a patient who has suffered an attack and to discuss with the patient how the condition has affected him or her as a person. By this activity, the learner may develop insight into, and empathy with, such patients.

7. Tests The tests provide feedback to the learner and also serve as a diagnostic tool. They can be divided into three types.

(a) *Prerequisite test* This tests the prerequisite knowledge that the learner must possess before commencing the package.
(b) *Pre-test* This tests the actual content of the package to determine whether or not the learner needs to proceed through the package. If the pre-test is completed successfully, the implication is that the learner already knows the content of the package and can proceed to a higher level of study immediately.
(c) Post-test This is used to test the learner's achievement of the objectives following completion of the learning package.

The post-test is very commonly used as a pre-test, the learner initially attempting the test without success and then retaking it after completion of the package. The learner is usually successful the second time and this provides feelings of accomplishment from having visibly learned to pass the test.

8. Guidance concerning the next step Successful completion of the learning package should not be the final step; instead, the learner should be directed to the next component in the series, or given advice on the type of learning activities that they should now pursue.

9. Teacher's notes Every learning package should contain notes intended for the teacher. It may seem unusual to include these, but one must bear in mind that the intentions of the designer may not always be obvious to a teacher who has not been involved in the production. Such notes might contain details of the feedback received during the pilot study and guidelines for the interpretation of test scores.

The foregoing list of nine components can be considered as a basic list of 'ingredients' for a learning package, so it is useful to examine the 'recipe' for putting these components together.

The decision to produce a learning package will commit the teacher to a considerable amount of time and effort and if this expenditure is to reap its benefits, careful planning must be employed from the outset. Table 13.4 illustrates a planning sequence for producing an individualized learning package. This sequence follows a logical order of progression, with each stage designed to eliminate errors and omissions.

The costing of open learning raises interesting issues, and these have been addressed by Robinson and Clarke (1992). They contrast conventional taught courses, which are labour intensive and highly centralized, with open learning, which is technology intensive and decentralized. They suggest that costing is determined by the needs of three systems, the teaching technology, the tutorial system, and the administrative system, and that these need to be related to two phases, a developmental phase and a presentational phase.

Quality assurance of open learning

Quality assurance is a crucial aspect of open learning, particularly as it largely takes place at a distance from the main institution. The normal

Table 13.4 Planning sequence for producing a learning package

- *Explore the need* Does a similar package exist already? Is a learning package an appropriate medium?
- *Explore the feasibility of developing a package* Is the development feasible in terms of finance, personnel, resources and time?
- *Decide the target population* Pre-registration, post-registration or both? CATS level?
- *Decide the learning outcomes* Are they unit-specific, or generic to a number of courses/pathways?
- *Identify pre-requisites and co-requisites* Are there other packages/materials/units that should be studied first, or studied in conjunction with the package?
- *Decide the activities and media for the package* Reading? Writing? Audio-visual? Experiential? Sequencing? Instructions?
- *Decide any optional activities* For example, interviews with patients/clients/staff in relation to the theme of the package
- *Write the rationale for the package* Write a description of the purpose and structure of the package.
- *Decide format of pre-test and post-test if used* Teacher or student marked? Where will the answers be found?
- *Decide format of self-tests* How will student monitor his or her own progress through the package?
- *Decide content of teacher notes* Write any additional information that teachers might require, e.g. the theoretical assumptions underpinning the approach taken in the package.
- *Decide format of students' evaluation of the package* How will the user's opinion of the package be solicited?
- *Decide the contents list* Outline the sequence of content but omit page numbers until final draft completed.
- *Set production deadlines* Realistic, achievable deadlines, including time for any slippage, are needed.
- *Undertake draft production* Use Desktop Publishing (DTP) if available.
- *Undertake pilot study* Use a sample of the intended consumers, and obtain detailed feedback on all aspects of the package.
- *Modify draft package in light of feedback from pilot study* Note 'user-friendliness', clarity, interest and accuracy.
- *Produce final draft*
  - Text: DTP gives professional finish. Type of cover? Quality of binding? Size of print run? Copyright?
  - Information technology and audio-visual media: include instructions to user on how to operate the media.
- *Put package into full use* Include system of monitoring use of package plus evaluation by users.

mechanisms for taught courses need to be adapted to the special circumstances of open learning. Access to library and IT support facilities, for example, is an important aspect for distance learning, since the open learning materials need to be supplemented by further reading and inquiry. Whilst an institution can monitor the quality of its own libraries, it is more difficult when other institutions' provision has to be evaluated. Open learning can be a lonely experience for students, so it is important that networking is set up to help them meet and interact with other open learning students. If the system uses tutor/counsellors based within the student's locality, then staff development via workshops and meetings needs to be available. This also applies to systems that use local Colleges of Nursing to deliver open learning programmes. The University of Greenwich/Nursing Times Open Learning (NTOL) scheme, for example, uses the concept of 'approved centres' to offer its awards. Centre approval involves both scrutiny of documentation and a staff development visit to each centre in order to ensure that it meets the requirements of the scheme. In this case, quality assurance monitoring takes place on a national level throughout the UK.

PERSONALIZED SYSTEM OF INSTRUCTION (PSI; KELLER PLAN)

This system of instruction is commonly known as the Keller plan after its originator F.S. Keller (1968) and is based upon Skinner's theory of operant conditioning (see Chapter 4, p. 93), with its emphasis on feedback and reinforcement. The two main characteristics of the system are self-pacing and mastery and these decide to a large extent the format of the system. The concept of self-pacing is incompatible with the use of lecture methods and so lectures are only used as motivators and as a vehicle for developing group contact.

Keller emphasizes the importance of interaction with teachers during progress through the system. The concept of mastery of the material implies regular testing to see if objectives have been achieved and the usual format for a PSI system consists of written unit material, objectives for the student, methods by which the objectives can be achieved and tests by which achievement is assessed. However, the methods used in instruction need not be only the written word and the use of practical work and problem-solving exercises has been reported. The testing procedure can involve both self-tests during progress through the unit and also a terminal test of mastery of the material.

When students feel they have mastered the material in a particular unit, they then present themselves for testing; if successful, they proceed to the next unit, if not, they go back to the previous unit to study it again. PSI also utilizes the concept of the 'undergraduate tutor', i.e. another student peer who has already mastered the unit in question; this tutor can mark the tests of other students and can teach the material during the process of feedback. This has the added advantage that the 'tutor' must know the material well in order to teach it effectively, a phenomenon known to all practising teachers.

Incentives are available in the form of course credits for those acting as 'tutors'. PSI allows the student the freedom to choose the pace at which he or she will progress through the units, but procrastination can be a problem, with students putting off doing the material until nearly the end of the course.

MASTERY LEARNING

This method was devised by Benjamin Bloom (1968) and is based upon Carroll's 'model of learning', which asserts that all tasks can be learned by students provided they are given sufficient time. This key notion of the time taken to learn a task forms the basis for a sequence of instruction called 'mastery learning'. The amount of time taken to learn a task is seen as being dependent on a number of variables:

- the complexity of the task,
- the student's aptitude and experience,
- the ability to understand the material,
- their perseverance, and
- the quality of instruction.

Mastery learning takes the view that individual differences in the achievement of students are not inevitable and the sequence is designed to ensure that virtually every student will reach the same level of achievement, i.e. mastery level or grade A. The sequence for mastery learning is as follows.

1. The subject or topic is divided up into a number of units, each of one or two weeks duration.
2. Learning objectives are prescribed for each of the units.
3. The subject-matter of the unit is taught.
4. Formative tests are administered at the end of the unit and are used to identify the successful and unsuccessful students.
5. If students do not achieve mastery, then remedial teaching is given.
6. When a student has completed all the units, a summative test is given to test mastery of the course, which equals a grade A.

There has been a phenomenal spread of mastery learning over the past decade, including the United States, Korea and Indonesia. Its use has spread to a wide range of classes and subjects in education and a number of adaptations have emerged. Mastery learning can be used for competency-based learning, humanities and self-development and it aims to create equality in society by making it possible for all students to attain excellence

There are, however, a number of problems associated with mastery learning, in particular, the use of specific behavioural objectives and the increased amount of time and resources required for its implementation.

PROGRAMMED LEARNING (PROGRAMMED INSTRUCTION)

Programmed learning is based upon behaviourist psychology and the fundamental notions are those of reinforcement and 'chaining'. Programmed learning requires specially prepared materials, which students use for individual study of particular topics. There are two kinds of programme, linear and branching, which differ in a number of respects from each other.

Linear programmes

This kind of programme was devised by B.F. Skinner and consists of a series of closely linked boxes of information called 'frames'. The students are presented with information in frames and are required to supply a missing word at the end of each frame; they can check whether their answer is correct or not before going on to the next frame. The linear programme thus offers information in very small steps, with immediate reinforcement in the form of feedback of correct answers. Each frame is designed to contain material that overlaps with the previous frame as well as the succeeding one, forming a chain of stimulus–response connections. Since it is correct answers that are reinforcing, errors are reduced to a minimum by careful piloting of the programme prior to production.

Branching programmes

In contrast to linear programmes, these provide the student with a series of choices rather than allowing the student to supply missing words. In this multiple-choice situation, the student is required to select the answer to a question raised in each frame from a choice of answers supplied. When an answer has been selected, the student is directed to a particular frame, depending on whether the was correct or not; if the answer was incorrect, the student will be directed to a frame that gives remedial information. It can be seen that this kind of programme has a series of branches that the student follows in his or her progress through the programme, the slower students taking in more branches than the brighter ones.

Programmed learning can take the form of printed texts such as books, or electronic machines that contain a window and a series of buttons for choosing responses, or computer programs. Branching programmes are rather cumbersome when used in book form, since the reader has to move backwards and forwards through the book in order to follow the branching frames. Students tend to like the programmed-learning format, particularly for topics with largely factual material; the careful formulation of goals for the student and the small steps in learning make it a useful, if sometimes boring, way of studying.

REFERENCES

Bloom, B. (1956) *Taxonomy of Educational Objectives: The Classification of Educational Goals, Handbook One: Cognitive Domain*, McKay, New York.

Bloom, B. (1968) Learning for mastery. *Evaluation Comment*, **1**(2). Center for the study of evaluation of instructional programs, University of California, Los Angeles.

Butterworth, C. (1992) More than one bite at the APEL: contrasting models of accrediting prior learning. *Journal of Further and Higher Education*, **16**(3).

CNAA (1989) Academic Credit for Professional Qualifications in Nursing, Midwifery and Health Visiting, Press release, CNAA, London.

City and Guilds of London Institute (1992) 3033 Care Level 2, City and Guilds of London Institute, London.

Clarke, E. and Robinson, K. (1992) *Good Practice in Open Learning Within Nursing, Midwifery and Health Visiting, Monograph No.3*, ENB, London.

ENB (1990) *Framework for Continuing Professional Education and Training for Nurses, Midwives and Health Visitors: Summary Report for Educationalists*, ENB, London.

ENB (1992) *Additional Guidelines for the Development of Pre-Registration Nursing Courses Leading to Parts 12–15 of the Professional Register and DipHE*, Circular 1992/09/RLV, ENB, London.

FEU/OPEN TECH (1986) *Implementing Open Learning in Local Authority Institutions*, FEU/Open Tech Unit of MSC.

Hall, D. (1994) A strategy for awarding students credit for prior experiential learning whilst protecting academic standards. *Journal of Further and Higher Education*, Vol 18, No 1, 1994

HMSO (1989) *Working for Patients: Education and Training, Working Paper 10*, HMSO, London.

Keller, F. (1968) Goodbye teacher. *Journal of Applied Behavioural Analysis*, **1**, 79–98.

Kelly, J. and Keeley, P. (1992) *Flexible Learning in Post Registration Nurse Education, Monograph No. 1*, ENB, London.

Kolb, D.A. (1984) *Experiential Learning: Experience as the Source of Learning and Development*, Prentice-Hall, London.

NCVQ (1991) *NVQ Briefing Pack Portfolio*, NCVQ, London.

Race, P. (1989) *The Open Learning Handbook*, Kogan Page, London.

Robinson, K. and Clarke, E. (1992) *Costing Open Learning: Factors for Consideration, Monograph No.4*, ENB, London.

United Kingdom Central Council for Nursing, Midwifery and Health Visiting (1993) *Registrar's Letter*, **13**, UKCC, London.

Winter, R. (1994) The problem of educational levels part 2: a new framework for credit accumulation in higher education. *Journal of Further and Higher Education*, **18**(1).

Course and pathway management $\boxed{14}$

The purpose of nurse education is to provide quality education and training that meets the needs of service providers for an appropriately skilled nursing workforce, that meets the needs and aspirations of the students, and that facilitates the development of the nursing profession. The quality of education and training does not reside solely in the teaching and learning processes, but is also dependent upon the organization and administration of the course or pathway. This chapter focuses on the overall nature and processes of course and pathway management, and more detailed discussion of some of the issues raised can be found in Chapters 12, 13 and 15.

With the widespread adoption of credit accumulation and transfer (CAT) structures, the term 'course' is being replaced by 'pathway', but the principles of management apply equally to both concepts. For convenience, the term pathway is used throughout this chapter.

PATHWAY DIRECTOR AND PATHWAY COMMITTEE

The key role in relation to pathway management is that of pathway director, who is responsible for the day-to-day running of the pathway. The typical responsibilities of the role are:

1. organization of recruitment and selection;
2. organization of staffing, timetabling, rooming, teaching, tutoring, pastoral care;
3. ensuring up to date pathway documentation;
4. organization of examination procedures;
5. production of pathway statistics;
6. pathway monitoring and annual pathway monitoring report; and
7. academic leadership of pathway tutors.

This 'sharp-end' role can be one of the most rewarding in education, as the incumbent has considerable scope to influence the development of the pathway and the students' experience of it. Within the HE sector, management structures tend to be less hierarchical than those found in Colleges of Nursing and Midwifery, and the role of pathway director may be undertaken by academic staff of varying grades and is not necessarily linked with formal positions of seniority nor with line-management responsibility. It is common to find that the role is held for some four to five years before being assigned to another member of the academic staff. This helps to avoid complacency and staleness, and encourages new ideas and approaches. The pathway director is assisted in his or her task by a pathway committee, the typical composition of this committee being:

- appropriate senior manager (Chair),
- pathway director,
- representatives of staff teaching the course,
- representative from library/resources, and
- normally one student from each year of the pathway.

The basic structure of pathway management applies to all pathways regardless of the number of students, and whether or not attendance is full time. However, very large pathways will require one or more deputy pathway director roles to cope with the greater administrative workload. The role of the pathway committee is to:

- develop new units/modules as required;
- review and develop teaching and learning strategies;
- review and develop assessment strategies;
- review pathway recruitment;
- monitor student progress;
- assist the course director with preparation of annual pathway monitoring report;
- provide a formal route of communication between teachers and students; and
- address issues raised by the pathway director, senior managers or relevant committees.

ADMISSIONS

It is common in HE for departments to have admissions tutors who are responsible for admissions procedures for one or more courses or pathways. They liaise closely with the pathway director and the Academic Registry, and their role involves making arrangements for recruitment and selection of students. Admissions policies differ markedly between pre-registration and post-registration education in nursing and midwifery; the former tend to be mainly full-time, and the latter part-time. HE uses the Universities Central Admissions System (UCAS) for general undergraduate admissions, whereas applications for nurse training are dealt with by the Nurses Central Clearing House (NCCH).

There are two categories of student who can access units and modules: registered students and associate students. Registered students are those who have registered with the institution to undertake a pathway leading to an academic award. Associate students, on the other hand, simply undertake one or more units that they need for some specific staff development purpose, e.g. counselling skills. They receive the appropriate credit for the unit or module on successful completion, but they do not register for an academic award.

Admissions regulations

Each pathway will have its own admission regulations within which recruitment and selection will operate. One very important aspect of this is equal opportunities, in that recruitment and selection processes must be compatible with the equal opportunities policy of the institution. Admissions regulations normally contain a statement on equal opportunities, and the following is a typical example:

> This institution operates an equal opportunities policy and invites applications from suitable candidates regardless of race, gender, age, disability, religion, political affiliation, or sexual orientation.

Another important aspect is that of access. Pathways will vary in their degree of openness of access according to the nature of the pathway and the ideology of the institution. For example, pre-registration pathways would normally have specific admission requirements such as a minimum of five GCSE passes, whereas post-registration pathway requirements tend to be more general, e.g. a minimum of two years post-registration experience in nursing or midwifery. Some pathways may have completely open access, with candidates being required solely to demonstrate that they can benefit from undertaking the pathway.

Publicity and recruitment

Students find out about pathways from a variety of sources such as the institute's prospectus, recommendations from friends, direct marketing by the institution, such as mail-shots, careers advisors, and advertising in journals and newspapers.

Desktop publishing (DTP) enables departments to produce sophisticated publicity materials in-house for mail-shots and other distribution. Advertising can reach much greater numbers of people, but the cost is relatively high. A quarter-page advertisement in a journal can cost several hundred pounds when VAT and production costs are included.

Pathway enquiries from prospective candidates are dealt with by the Registry, who send out an information pack about the pathway, including an application form. The information is compiled by the pathway director, and it is helpful to give the candidates as much information as possible to assist them in making a decision about the suitability of the pathway for their own needs. It's useful to include a document of the form 'Your Questions Answered' in the pathway information pack, containing answers to all the likely questions that a candidate might have about the pathway. If the selection procedures involve a face-to-face interview, this type of document makes the interview much more efficient by cutting down information-giving, thus allowing the interviewer more time to focus on the candidate. The key headings for such a document might be as follows:

- What is a credit accumulation and transfer (CATS) scheme?
- How many credit points do I need for the degree?
- What is meant by CATS levels?
- What are my existing qualifications worth?
- What are core units?
- What are option units?
- How is the pathway assessed?
- What tutorial support will I receive?
- When does the pathway run?
- How many units can I take at one time?
- How much does a unit cost?
- How long will I take to complete the pathway?
- How can I get credit for experiential learning?
- What will my interview be like?

The selection interview

Although interviewing has been the subject of widespread criticism on the grounds of the subjective nature of the decision-making process, the technique is well-established in health care education generally. Ideally, an interview should give the candidate and the institution the opportunity to explore the match between the candidate's needs and the given pathway under consideration, and also to clarify any questions or issues on which either party is unclear. In reality, it can easily become an ordeal for the candidate if the style of the interview is that of an inquisition, so interviewers need to be aware of the basic requirements for conducting interviews.

Preparing for the interview

Wherever the interview is held, there are certain requirements that must be met, namely privacy and freedom from interruption. This implies the cancellation of all incoming telephone calls for the duration of the interview and the use of 'Do Not Disturb' signs on the door. An informal arrangement of room, with no desk intervening between the candidate and the interviewer – and using chairs of the same height – attempts to make the interview appear as normal as any other social meeting, so that the candidate feels at ease.

There is no consensus of opinion with regard to the number of interviewers present, but if one agrees with the aim of the interview as outlined above, then it becomes obvious that the more people who are involved, the less 'normal' the situation becomes from the candidate's point of view. This might imply that a single interviewer is best. On the other hand, if two interviewers are present, one can observe the candidate closely whilst the other is engaged in conversation.

Courtesy is the watchword for interviewing, however challenging and probing the interview becomes. Candidates should be given an indication of the time of their interview, and the availability of refreshments made clear. It is the responsibility of the interviewer to have read the candidate's application form thoroughly before the interview, so that the impression gained can be extended and modified according to the candidate's response. It is debateable whether or not the interviewers should have access to references prior to the interview; there is the possibility of a positive or negative halo effect if they are seen beforehand.

Conducting the interview

There are a number of approaches or plans for interviewing; two of the better-known ones are considered here.

The seven-point plan (National Institute of Industrial Psychology, 1970)
This consists of seven main headings, but these are not ranked in any particular order. The headings are really questions that the interviewer(s) ask themselves when conducting the interview.

1. *Physical make-up* This deals with any physical defects or health problems that might affect job performance. In addition, it includes appearance, manner and speech.
2. *Attainments* This involves education attainment as well as occupational training. Consideration should be given to achievement in relation to circumstances, rather than in isolation. For example, a candidate may have obtained five GCSE passes despite lack of interest by parents.
3. *General intelligence* This is a difficult concept to measure without using specific tests.
4. *Special aptitudes* There is often confusion with regard to the importance of special aptitudes in relation to nursing. Thus, interviewers may ask about a candidate's ability to perform fine motor abilities, such as sewing or dressmaking, or playing a musical instrument. This is then extrapolated to the fine motor skills of nursing, such as removal of sutures. However, the mere presence of these abilities in a candidate must not be taken as evidence of special aptitude. Aptitude is best measured by specific aptitude tests.
5. *Interests* These give an indication of whether they are primarily mental, physical, practical, etc., and may guide the interviewer in rating other attributes.
6. *Disposition* This concerns personality, character and temperament, and may indicate qualities of self-reliance, etc.
7. *Circumstances* This involves the candidate's background and opportunities.

The Fear method This method consists of a number of stages (Fear, 1978), of which the main ones are outlined below.

1. *Helping the candidate to talk spontaneously*   This is designed to ensure that the candidate feels at ease, and so will volunteer information freely. It is facilitated by use of social skills such as pleasant greetings, facial expression, use of small-talk and giving encouragement by minimizing reactions to unfavourable revelations.
2. *Exploratory questions*   These are used to prompt candidates from time to time, to encourage them to reveal more information. Comments are usually more effective for stimulating conversation, and they are less like interrogation. The main skill in using these is to keep the candidate at the centre of attention, with the interviewer remaining unobtrusive.
3. *Controlling the interview*   Control is a delicate mechanism, for if it is overused the candidate will become less spontaneous. An interview guide sheet helps to keep the interview going in the right direction, but skill is required in its use.
4. *Interpretation*   Every statement which is made by the candidate is interpreted by the interviewer, and it is through this process that a picture is built up. It is useful to make a mental list of assets and liabilities during the interview. These should be so well documented in the interviewer's mind that they can be written down when the candidate leaves the room.

Making a decision

After the interview has been concluded, a decision must be reached as to whether or not the candidate is acceptable. This is done by weighing the positive and negative aspects, including the results of any special tests, such as aptitude or trainability tests. The information is then conveyed to Registry, who send out the standard letters that either offer a place on the pathway, or reject the candidates application. Once the target recruitment figure has been reached, Registry is instructed to notify any further applicants that the pathway is full.

TIMETABLING, ROOMING AND STAFFING

Once a decision has been made to run the pathway, it is necessary to undertake timetabling and rooming. As part of the pathway planning process the pattern of attendance will have been established, including semesters, day(s) and times. Most institutions have a central system of room booking, and it is important that the pathway director is able to make a case for any special requirements such as lecture or laboratory space. Evening sessions require the availability of late catering facilities, but this may not be cost effective if only small numbers of students are involved.

Since it is unusual for a pathway director to have direct responsibility for allocation of staff, he or she needs to make the teaching staff and technician requirements known to the appropriate senior manager. The staffing requirements for a given pathway are largely determined by the amount of resource that is generated by the student numbers, and this will vary according to the funding arrangements of the pathway in question. Institutions vary in the formulae they use to calculate staffing, but the following rule of thumb may be helpful. In order to calculate the teacher hours generated by a given number of students, it is necessary to understand three concepts:

1. Full-time student equivalent (FTE), also termed whole-time equivalent (WTE): a part-time student may count as less than half a full-time equivalent.
2. Staff-to-student ratio (SSR) of the department or institution: if the SSR is 1:20, this means that for every teacher there are 20 students.
3. Teacher contact time: this is the amount of actual contact with students, excluding administration, that a teacher is contracted to undertake in a week. In HE it is typically around 17 hours a week.

If we assume that the SSR is 1:20, the calculation is fairly straightforward for a group of 20 full-time students, in that they generate one teacher, i.e. 17 hours of student contact time per week. This means that the pathway director has a maximum of seventeen hours per week to devote to the pathway, and this must include not only the actual teaching, but tutorials and administration time. If we take a group of 25 part-time students, the calculation is very different, as part-time students equate to 0.4 of a full-time equivalent; 25 times 0.4 equals 10 FTE, and with a ratio of 1:20 these 10 FTEs generate only half a teacher, i.e. 8.5 hours of student contact per week. Hence, this part-time pathway, although it has more students, generates only half the hours of the previous example. The pathway director has to work with this figure when timetabling and staffing the pathway. The apportioning of the available hours needs careful consideration by the pathway team, as it is important to strike an appropriate balance between face-to-face teaching and individual tutorials. There is a general feeling in education that students have been over-taught, and this has led to a reduction in class contact and a shift towards more individual study time and personal tutorials. In my own pathways, unit teachers are required to keep two meetings free of normal unit content, and to undertake individual tutorials on the assessment requirements of the unit during this class time. This ensures that every student has the opportunity to discuss assessment ideas with the unit teacher on at least two occasions during the course of the unit.

In HE it is common practice to use visiting lecturers (VLs) as well as full-time teaching staff, and this is likely to become more common as institutions try to reduce their staffing costs. VLs are given a contract for a certain amount of specified teaching, such as a unit or module, and the rate of pay includes preparation, teaching and marking of coursework and assessments. The use of VLs has certain advantages from a managerial point of view; their use makes it possible to adapt quickly to demands for new provision, while at the same time avoiding the risk of the new provision drying up, and being left with a permanent member of staff who is surplus to requirements. However, it can be argued that the use of VLs is not good use of resources, since their contract contains no provision for them to contribute to the overall academic development and administration of the department. VLs need careful induction and briefing if they are to undertake their teaching in the most effective way, and it is good practice to pay them for attending induction sessions prior to the arrival of students.

INDUCTION OF STUDENTS

The first stage in the induction of students is the mailing of joining instructions for the pathway. These should contain details of the date, time and venue of the induction meeting of the pathway. The joining instructions should also contain details of the induction programme, and a typical example is shown in Table 14.1.

At the induction meeting, students are issued with their own copy of the *Students' Pathway Handbook* for the current academic year. This handbook is of major importance to students, since it sets out the regulations and procedures for all aspects of the pathway. Typical contents of a Students Pathway Handbook are shown in Table 14.2.

One of the problems that arises within CAT schemes is the very wide range of option units from which students choose their programme of study. There is great potential for chaos if the organization of choices is left until the induction day, as it is virtually impossible to negotiate with each individual on the day. It is preferable to send out a questionnaire to both new and continuing students before the end of the previous academic year, to ascertain their unit preferences, so that they can be allocated to units in advance of their arrival. There is still some opportunity for students to adjust their preferences on the induction day, but there should be relatively few who need to do this. Another idea which may prove useful during the induction programme is to distribute a 'Guide to Successful Study and Assessment'. Regardless of whether the pathway is pre- or post-registration, students often experience difficulty in adjusting

Table 14.1   A typical pathway induction programme

Pathway:	BSc Honours degree in Nursing Studies (Post Registration)
Date:	1 October 1994
Venue:	Williams Lecture Theatre, Thornhill Hall Campus, University of Melchester

Programme:

1400	Welcome and Introduction to Pathway	Pathway Director
1410	Outline of Units for First Semester	Unit Leaders
1500	Registration	Registrars
1600	Resources for Learning	RFL Team
1630	Individual Consultations	Pathway Team
1730	Cheese and Wine Reception	Pathway Team
1900	Conclusion of Induction	

Table 14.2 Typical contents of a student's pathway handbook

BSc Honours degree in Nursing Studies
Student's Pathway Handbook 1994/95
Contents

1. Introduction to the pathway
2. Summary of key information:
    (a) Semester dates 1994/95
    (b) Assessment handing-in deadlines
    (c) Procedure for handing-in assessments
    (d) Return of marked assignments
    (e) List of units for 1994/95
    (f) Tutorial arrangements
3. Key personnel
4. Aims of pathway
5. Pathway structure and process
6. Accreditation of prior learning
7. Assessment regulations
8. Board of Examiners
9. Pathway committee
10. Quality assurance
11. Equal opportunities

Appendices
A: Grounds and procedures for appeal: the University of Melchester
B: Statement on cheating and plagiarism: the University of
    Melchester
C: Unit specifications for Academic Year 1994/95
D: Tariff for nursing and midwifery qualifications

to the level of work required for a diploma or degree course, and also in organizing their study effectively. Some post-registration students have not undertaken formal study since their initial qualifications many years ago, and often experience great difficulty, especially in relation to the writing of assessment work. A written guide can help these students to approach their studies more effectively, and the contents of such a guide are given in Table 14.3.

ONGOING PATHWAY MANAGEMENT

The pathway director is responsible for the day-to-day running and trouble shooting of the pathway and this involves a variety of tasks. For example, attendance registers must be available for unit teachers to complete at each meeting of the unit, since it is common to find that pathways have a percentage attendance requirement regulation. In order to pass a unit, students have to attend a certain percentage of classes e.g. 75%, and the unit registers provide evidence of this attendance. Pathway directors usually offer a personal tutorial service to students which complements any unit specific tutorials offered by the unit tutors. At these tutorials, the pathway director can advise students on general aspects of the pathway such as accreditation of prior learning, and deal with requests for extensions to assessment deadlines, and other pathway issues.

Table 14.3 Contents of a guide to successful study and assessment

Introduction
1. Studying at honours degree level
2. Planning your studies
3. Undertaking a unit
   (a) Pre-reading and follow-up reading
   (b) Note-taking
   (c) Participation in unit activities
   (d) Choosing an open unit
4. Application to professional practice
5. Planning your assignments for unit assessment
6. Reading for your assignment
7. Writing your assignment
   (a) Designing the structure
   (b) Achieving the right level
   (c) Editing for the final draft
   (d) Handing-in the assignment
8. Making the most of tutorials
9. Tackling the research project
10. Further reading

Pathway committee meetings

Meetings can be the bane of most nurse teachers' lives if the conduct is not well regulated, especially where one or two individuals are allowed to go on and on without any attempt by the chairperson to check them. Meetings are extremely costly in terms of the time occupied by individuals; a meeting lasting one and a half hours with fifteen members of the teaching staff is extremely costly in staff salaries. It can be seen that a poorly managed meeting is extremely wasteful of resources, as well as acting to demotivate the members present. The principles of running an effective meeting are straightforward, and involve adequate prior planning, effective group and leadership skills and a good sense of timing. Most committees need a secretary to take minutes and it is worth considering the use of a member of the non-teaching staff for this as they tend to be more efficient at recording proceedings and might even enjoy the chance to be involved in something different from the day-to-day administration.

Prior planning

The chairperson is responsible for requesting agenda items from members of staff and subsequently drawing up the agenda in an appropriate order. All substantive items on the agenda should be accompanied by a paper addressing the item, so that members of the committee are given the opportunity to read and digest the issues in good time before the day of the meeting. Only rarely should the chairperson allow tabled items to be included, since this precludes the proper study of such items prior to the meeting. The room in which the meeting is to be held needs to be booked in advance and made ready for the meeting. It is good practice to ensure that tables are available, plus note-pads and pencils for each committee member. It is also important to provide glasses and jugs of water, and to maintain a no-smoking rule at all committee meetings. The latter point is extremely important, since every individual should have the right to conduct his business in an atmosphere that is conducive to discussion and thinking. Some chairpersons choose to take a vote on whether smoking should be permitted, but this should not be a subject for democratic voting: only one objection should ensure that the no-smoking rule applies.

Effective chairmanship

The role of the chairperson is to ensure the smooth running of the committee and to make an accurate recording of the business that takes place. Chairpersons differ in the degree of formality they prefer; on the one hand they may insist that all the correct procedures and formalities are observed, such as raising the hand before being given permission to speak and addressing all comments through the chair. Alternatively, some chairpersons allow a degree of informality by letting discussion flow more spontaneously rather than insisting on each remark going through the chair. This can make the meeting less rigid and more interesting, but there is always the danger of total confusion if everyone tries to make a point at the same time. A good sense of timing is crucial to the effective running of meetings; so often a great deal of time is spent on the first one or two items, leaving little time for the rest of the agenda. An effective chairperson will allocate a block of time for each substantive item, and should be prepared to move on, even if discussion is still proceeding. Some people may feel that this is undemocratic, yet it is no more undemocratic than allowing one item to dominate the agenda at the expense of all the others. One major facet of committees is the system of voting, in which members vote for or against a particular motion. This ensures a democratic system in which the majority decision carries the motion, but its use needs careful consideration. The chairperson needs to ensure that voting is reserved for crucial issues in which there is genuine division of opinion about the merits of a motion. It needs to be borne in mind that a manager is appointed to manage, and although he or she may have a course committee to assist, the final responsibility rests with the manager. If the committee is to be run on majority-vote lines, it begs the question as to why the manager is there in the first place.

EXAMINATIONS AND ASSESSMENT

This is the area of pathway management that has the greatest potential for problems. Fortunately, the pathway assessment regulations provide a safeguard, and should be followed to the letter if difficulties are to be avoided. The first difficulty arises when students ask teachers to comment on an initial draft of their unit assignments. The danger here is that the

Table 14.4 Typical procedure for handing-in assignments

- Students collect a carbon-copy assignment form from the Department office, Thornhill Hall Campus, well before the final meeting of the unit.
- Students agree the title and content of the assignment with the unit tutor, complete the relevant sections of the form, and ask the unit tutor to sign that this is the agreed assignment.
- Students hand in to the Department office the completed assignment by the date specified, ensuring that the secretary who accepts the assignment signs and dates the form, and gives the student a copy as a receipt.

NB   UNDER NO CIRCUMSTANCES SHOULD STUDENTS GIVE ASSESSMENTS DIRECTLY TO UNIT TUTORS.

teacher may influence the subsequent draft to such an extent that the assessment is no longer the student's own work, but a collaborative effort of both student and teacher. The dilemma can be resolved by asking the student to give a brief verbal outline of their ideas, and offering helpful general comments as appropriate. This approach needs to be adhered to by all unit teachers to ensure fairness in the assessment process.

Handing-in of assessments

Another key area is that of the handing-in procedures for unit assessments. Students must be made aware of the correct procedures for handing in their assessments, and no deviations should be allowed. Pathways will vary in their handing-in procedures, and a typical example is given in Table 14.4.

Extensions to the deadline for submission of assessment

Students may request an extension to the unit assessment deadline in the case of prolonged illness, bereavement, severe domestic problems or other exceptional circumstances. Requests should be made in writing to the course director in advance of the submission deadline, giving the reasons for the request and providing supporting evidence e.g. medical certificate. If a request for extension is not granted, students should note that work submitted after the deadline will lead to the assessment being referred. They should also note that everyday pressure of work would not normally be grounds for an extension. Following the deadline for submission of unit assessments, the pathway director has to sort them out and forward them to the appropriate marking teachers along with marking guides and deadlines for return of marked work.

Marking and moderation of students' assessment work

The pathway director is responsible for distributing the assessments to the appropriate members of the team for marking, and they should be accompanied by a deadline for the return of the marked work. When the work has been returned the pathway director will need to organize an internal moderation meeting at which the range of assessment work is sampled and scrutinized by the pathway team. Of course, it is important that markers avoid moderating their own work.

When internal moderation has been completed, a sample of assessments should be sent to the external examiner for further scrutiny. Normally, all refer/fail papers and all first-class or distinction papers would be sent plus a sample of the range of grades awarded. The pathway director needs to ensure that the external examiner has a timescale sufficient for adequate scrutiny of the papers.

Board of Examiners' Meeting

It is the pathway director's responsibility to organise meetings of the Board of Examiners, and this includes drawing up the agenda in consultation with the Chair, producing results lists and pass lists in conjunction with the Academic Registrar, and ensuring that arrangements are made for room booking and catering. All marking grades are provisional until the Board of Examiners has agreed the results, and there may be alterations to the proposed grades at the meeting. Students should be given written information regarding this point, and also notice of when their work is likely to be available for collection.

Further details on the marking, moderation and role of external examiner and Boards of Examiners are given in Chapter 11.

QUALITY ASSURANCE

The main formal mechanism for quality assurance of pathways is the annual pathway monitoring report. This is prepared by the pathway director in consultation with the pathway committee, and typically consists of a commentary on the following aspects of the pathway for the previous academic year:

1. overall view of the delivery of the pathway;
2. statistics on student achievement;
3. analysis of students' evaluation of pathway units
4. pathway director's response to the external examiners' reports;
5. views of employers about the pathway, where appropriate;
6. an action plan for the next academic year; and
7. any other issues.

The annual monitoring report goes to the faculty board, where issues raised by the report are discussed. Some institutions use a scrutineer system, in which a member of staff from another department in the faculty acts as a scrutineer of the report, offering the pathway director advice about aspects of the report. Subsequently, the scrutineer leads the discussion at faculty board about the monitoring report. Annual pathway monitoring is addressed further in Chapter 15.

LEADERSHIP

The terms formal and informal leader are often used to distinguish types of leader; the role of pathway director is one of formal leadership. On the other hand, an informal leader is one who most closely embodies the group's norms. The formal leader is often described by the term 'headship' to signify the nature of the leadership position, but it is not necessarily the formal leader who has most power in a group.

It is probably fair to say that there is no such thing as an ideal leadership personality or style; leadership is very much dependent on relationships within the group and the particular purpose for which the group exists. An individual may be an effective leader in one setting but of little use in another; it would be hard to imagine an army officer, who is a capable leader of his men, functioning effectively as leader of an encounter group because of the very different style and context in which it operates. There are, however, certain characteristics that leaders possess such as sociability, extraversion, intelligence and self-confidence (Gaskell and Sealy, 1976). The classic study of leadership that formed the beginning of experimental approaches to social groups was that by White and Lippit (1960). They used real-life groups of boys who attended an after-school club to carry out model-making and other handicrafts. The boys were allocated to three groups, each led by an adult who adopted a pre-determined style of leadership:

- in the 'autocratic' groups the leader imposed work on the boys, remaining friendly but aloof from them;
- in the 'democratic' groups the leader discussed the work with the boys, and functioned as part of the group, allowing them to decide what to do;
- the 'laissez-faire' groups were left to their own devices to do what they wished, with the leader offering no help unless requested.

The results of the different styles of leadership were evaluated after several weeks with striking differences being found. The autocratic groups showed aggression towards the leader or to a scapegoat within the group and were resentful and hostile. The work rate was good, but dropped off when the leader left the room. In contrast, the democratic groups were more cohesive, the leader was popular, the work was better and they continued to work when the leader was absent. The laissez-faire groups did very little work, showed some aggression and were uncontrolled whether or not the leader was present.

This study is often quoted as supporting the superiority of democratic leadership and the importance of self-imposed discipline, and certainly gives food for thought in terms of educational management.

The leadership role is important for many reasons, but it also has a crucial bearing on the resolution of conflict within the college.

CONFLICT

Conflict is a very emotionally charged term that implies a clash or disagreement between opposing issues or persons. Interpersonal conflict occurs whenever an action by one person prevents, obstructs or interferes with the action of another person (Johnson, 1983). Conflict is normally thought of as a negative phenomenon, but it can have many positive effects; change arises out of conflict, and much useful material can come out of disagreement among a group. Indeed, the whole notion of committees requires a measure of disagreement as the starting point, so that useful ideas and alternatives are generated. Conflict can also be exciting, provided that energy is not expended on wasteful aspects such as power confrontation and it can also serve to 'clear the air' when minor interpersonal irritations occur.

De Bono (1985) suggests that people disagree for four fundamental reasons:

1. *Differences in perception* Individuals differ markedly in their perception of situations or events and this means that each individual is convinced that their perspective is the right one.
2. *They want different things* People differ in their personal goals and needs, as well as in their values. Conflict of values is a common problem, often referred to as 'a matter of principle'.
3. *Thinking style encourages them to disagree* DeBono claims that our thinking style favours the principle of contradiction, in which two ideas are seen to be mutually exclusive. This explains the intractability of a dispute between two people and needs to be substituted for a way of thinking that allows the possibility of both ideas being possible.
4. *They are supposed to disagree* Society is largely attuned to the notion of conflict and newspaper headlines attest to this by their warlike descriptions of events.

Marsh (1979) sees conflict in terms of two management approaches: the human relations viewpoint and the realistic viewpoint.

The human relations viewpoint Conflict is seen as an abnormal disturbance of a relatively stable situation, which is caused by disruptive behaviour of individuals, or by lack of the exercise of authority or discipline. Conflicts should be resolved, according to this view, by use of authority, power or compromise. In organizations which subscribe to this, conflict tends to remain hidden or suppressed.

The realistic viewpoint Conflict is seen as an inevitable aspect of normal life, as power is sought and changes in this resisted. The causes of conflict are seen to be frustration and aggression of individuals, lack of balance in group members' needs and conflict between aspects of the organization such as functions and levels. Resolution of conflict is achieved by constructive, integrated solutions to problems, and the conflict is out in the open. The more rigid and hierarchical the organization is, the more difficult it is to bring conflict out into the open and to discuss the solutions. Internal conflict within individuals can arise as a result of many factors, and has a profound effect on their behaviour. Conflict can be created in an individual whenever there is a threat to his or her needs, status or prestige, but the most common source is that of power relationships between group members and between members and leader. This conflict stimulates mental-defence mechanisms for coping, and the result is such things as aggression, withdrawal and rationalization. An adaptive group meets conflict by discussing the issues and adapting goals, whereas a maladaptive group may fragment into small, competing elements.

REFERENCES

De Bono, E. (1985) *Conflicts: A Better Way to Resolve Them*, Penguin, Harmondsworth.

Fear, R. (1978) *The Evaluation Interview*, McGraw Hill, New York.

Gaskell, G. and Sealy, P. (1976) *Groups, D305*, Open University Press, Milton Keynes.

Johnson, D. (1983) *Reaching Out*, 3rd edn, Prentice-Hall, New Jersey.

Marsh, D. (1979) Conflict resolution. Coombe Lodge Working Paper, Information Bank Number 1402.

National Institute of Industrial Psychology (1970) *The Seven Point Plan*, NIP, London.

White, R. and Lippit, R. (1960) *Autocracy and Democracy*, Harper and Row, New York.

Educational quality assurance $\boxed{15}$

Educational quality assurance (QA) is a process for monitoring and evaluating the efficiency and effectiveness of educational provision, and to institute corrective action where appropriate. Institutions develop their own systems and mechanisms for QA but the overall purpose remains the same. Quality is best conceptualized as 'fitness for purpose', in that it has meaning only if it relates to the mission and aims of the organization. It is useful to distinguish QA from a related industrial concept, quality control (QC). This is a technique which involves the sampling of products to check them against a specification, those failing to meet the specification being rejected. QC is a much more limited concept than QA; QA emphasizes prevention as well as detection.

Within the HE sector there are a number of organizations concerned with issues of quality. The Higher Education Quality Council (HEQC) consists of three divisions: the Division of Quality Audit (DQA), which is responsible for undertaking quality audit of HE institutions throughout the UK, the Division of Credit and Access (DCA), which is responsible for quality assurance of credit ratings, and the Division of Quality Enhancement (DQE), which is responsible for gathering and disseminating information. HEQC works closely with the Quality Assessment Committees of the three Higher Education Funding Councils. The Quality Support Centre (QSC) was created out of the now-defunct CNAA research, development and information services, by the Open University, and provides information on quality issues to staff working in HE.

This chapter will explore performance indicators, educational audit, course-related quality assurance, standards, including BS 5750, total quality management (TQM) and quality circles.

PERFORMANCE INDICATORS (PIs)

Within the literature of quality assurance there is little consensus with regard to the definition of performance indicators. However, it is possible to identify some of their characteristics from the numerous interpretations available. The term 'performance indicator' itself gives an impression of something tentative, rather than precise or exact measures, that are used to guide decisions about quality. Balogh, Beattie and Beckerleg (1989) state that PIs 'express relationships between input and output via intermediate throughput or activity'. Cave, Hanney and Kogan (1991) define a PI in HE as 'an authoritative measure, usually in quantitative form, of an attribute of an HE institution, which may be ordinal or cardinal, absolute or comparative'. A cardinal measure would be of fundamental or primary importance, whereas an ordinal measure would be of a specified order within a series of measures. The Morris Report of the Committee of Enquiry of the now-defunct Polytechnics and Colleges Funding Council (PCFC) defines PIs as 'statistics, ratios, costs and other forms of information which illuminate or measure progress in achieving the mission and corresponding aims and objectives of the PCFC or of a college or polytechnic which it funds (Morris, 1990). PIs are usually classified as the three 'E's – efficiency indicators, effectiveness indicators, and economy indicators – and these are applied to educational inputs, processes, and outputs. Donabedian (1980) has described a similar triad of components to the latter, i.e. structures, processes and outcomes.

Performance indicators, then, are used help judge the quality of education within an institution and are applied to a wide range of general attributes of the system. Table 15.1 gives a range of general attributes under the headings inputs, processes, and outputs, for which performance indicators may be developed.

It can be seen from Table 15.1 that while some of the general attributes, such as examination success rates, lend themselves to quantitative measurement it is apparent that others, such as teacher/student relationships, would be very difficult to quantify. Another difficult PI is the concept of 'value-added' as an output measure. Traditionally, students' attainment has been judged by their qualifications or degree classifications, and has taken no account of the differences in individual students' abilities at the start of their course. Many educationalists believe that the real importance of education lies in the value it adds to the student as a result of undertaking it. The concept of value-added can therefore be applied even if the student fails to complete the programme. One measure of value-added is the relationship between input, i.e. entry qualifications and output, i.e. degree classification. However, further research is required before valid PIs for value-added can be developed.

Cave, Hanney and Kogan (1991) highlight some of the problems in using PIs in HE. Those PIs that are difficult to measure may be given a lower priority; for example, teaching is a much more difficult activity to measure accurately than is research, and this could lead to a shift in emphasis from teaching towards research. PIs may also result in pressure upon academics to publish material in journals, possibly resulting in quantity rather than quality of publications.

EDUCATIONAL AUDIT

An educational audit is a quality assurance mechanism for monitoring and evaluating the quality of educational provision, and performance indicators provide a tool for this. Table 15.1 gave the general attributes of an educational system, and this can form the basis for educational audit.

Table 15.1 General attributes of an educational system as a basis for performance indicators

A. Inputs

1.	College organization and policy	Quality of leadership Institutional philosophy Mission statement Vision Management structure Relationships with staff Financial management Staff development policy Public relations and publicity Equal opportunities policy Quality assurance systems

2.	Personnel	Teaching staff and library/support staff
		   qualifications
		   motivation
		   morale
		Staff–student ratio
		Staff development opportunities
		Individual performance review

3.	Library and support services	Adequacy of book stock and periodicals Opening hours Student support Information technology and media resources Secretarial and administrative support
4.	Enterprises	Teaching accommodation Halls of residence Security arrangements Ground maintenance Catering Car parking Recreation Child-care
5.	Students	Admission and access Entry qualifications Motivation

B. Processes

6.	Curriculum	Relevance Employer-focus Planning Validation, monitoring and review
7.	Teaching	Preparation Delivery Assessment Teacher–student relationships Support for new teachers
8.	Research and consultancy	External funding Publications in refereed journals Citations Client satisfaction with consultancy
9.	Student guidance and counselling	Guidance and counselling by teachers Availability of a college counselling service

C. Outputs

10.	Student achievement	Assessment/examination success rates Employment rates Progress to further study Value-added
11.	Course monitoring/evaluation	Annual monitoring reports Quinquennial review

The English National Board for Nursing, Midwifery and Health Visiting has produced detailed guidelines for educational audit (ENB, 1993). There are seven audit areas and each is further subdivided into specific categories within which dimensions and focus are identified. Each area has a quality statement relating the area to the institution, and evidence of performance is described for each category.

Area 1   Efficiency

The quality statement is 'the institution demonstrates efficient management and utilization of resources', and there are seven categories:

> financial management,
> manpower,
> staff/student ratios,
> use of staff time,
> courses/programmes,
> learning resources, and
> accommodation.

Area 2   Effectiveness: goal achievement 'fitness for purpose'

The quality statement is 'the institution demonstrates a clearly identified purpose and progress in working towards its mission statement', and there are seven categories:

> organizational development,
> student academic development,
> student career development,
> student personal development,
> faculty academic development,
> faculty career development, and
> faculty personal development.

Note: The term faculty refers to staff.

Area 3   Effectiveness: resource acquisition

The quality statement is 'there is evidence that the institution is systematically analysing market forces and responding to identified needs', and there are five categories:

> income generation,
> market forces – students,
> market forces – faculty, community relations, and
> skill mix.

Area 4   Effectiveness: participant satisfaction

The quality statement is 'there is evidence that the institution is beginning to establish mechanisms to identify customer/consumer/staff satisfaction and acceptability', and there are five categories:

students,
faculty,
higher education,
region, and
service providers.

Area 5   Effectiveness: social justice

The quality statement is 'the institution is committed to maximize accessibility to potential recruits, both staff and students', and there are seven categories:

accessibility,
equality of opportunity,
availability,
awareness,
responsiveness,
extensiveness, and
appropriateness/relevance.

Area 6   Effectiveness: internal processes

The quality statement is 'the institution is committed to effective communication, effective course delivery and course development through efficient management information systems', and there are six categories:

communication structures,
human resources,
evaluation styles,
counselling support structures,
management/leadership styles, and
curricular policies.

Area 7   Effectiveness: practice placement

The quality statement is 'the institution is committed to the provision of effective clinical learning experiences to ensure the achievement of competencies to enhance the quality of patient care', and there are six categories:

student learning experience/evaluation,
academic staff perspective,
service provider unit staff perspective,
RHA purchaser/other purchaser requirements,
environment, and
quality assurance mechanisms.

COURSE-RELATED QUALITY ASSURANCE

This section deals with those aspects of quality assurance that relate directly to courses and pathways, such as validation and review, monitoring and evaluation, role of external examiner, and annual monitoring reports.

Course validation and review

Validation is the process by which a proposal for a new course or pathways is examined to assess its suitability for inclusion in the institution's portfolio, and/or to meet the criteria of a validating body. Review is a periodic investigation to see if the course or pathway is still meeting its objectives, and whether appropriate monitoring and evaluation is taking place. To ensure the quality of these events membership of the panel is drawn from a wide range, including members from the proposing institution, subject experts from other institutions, members from the relevant industry or profession, and members with understanding of the processes of HE. The purpose of validation and review is to ensure that the course or pathway is of a standard comparable to similar awards elsewhere within HE. The procedure involves initial scrutiny by panel members of the course or pathway documentation prior to the validation or review event, so that key issues can be identified and conveyed to the chair of the event for inclusion in the agenda for the meeting. During the event, the panel will engage the course or pathway team in dialogue and debate on the issues identified, and at the end of the meeting a decision will be made on whether or not the course or pathway should be approved to run. A report of the meeting and decisions is circulated to the course or pathway team shortly after the event. The composition of the panel should provide a rigorous examination of the course and the course team, thus ensuring the quality of the course.

Course evaluation and monitoring

This involves the continuous appraisal of the course or pathway by the course director and course team, and the production of an annual course or pathway monitoring report for the institution. There are a number of facets to course evaluation, which are now considered.

Evaluation of teaching

Teaching has always been seen as the pivotal activity in any educational system, although nowadays there is increasing emphasis on learning as well. The evaluation of teaching is an important part of educational quality assurance and there is a variety of techniques for carrying it out.

Competency-based evaluation

This is used within a competency and performance-based teaching system and consists of evaluating the teacher on the competencies identified as being important for the role of teacher (Tuxworth, 1982). These competencies are identified by analysis of the field of teaching and they are stated in behavioural form, e.g. 'set up an overhead projector for use in classroom teaching'. Each of the competencies that have been identified are then linked to criteria for performance; these criteria are usually stated as a five- or six-point scale that ranges from a weak description of the competency to a strong one. For example, a weak criterion might say, 'can perform the skill in a partial fashion, requiring supervision and assistance periodically'. A strong criterion would be, 'can perform the skill without supervision, with initiative and flexibility'. The basic documentation is the master chart of competencies, on which are set out the entire descriptions for each competency and each criterion. The evaluator then simply ticks the appropriate cells for the given competency. Competency-based evaluation can assist in identifying areas of weakness in teachers, but the behavioural nature of the system renders it prone to the same criticisms as those levelled at behavioural objectives, namely, trivialization and rigidity.

Questionnaires and checklists

A standard technique in all forms of evaluation, questionnaires require respondents to answer questions about the teacher. These respondents may be the teacher, students of the teacher or colleagues of the teacher and this approach can provide very useful feedback to the teacher. An example of a teacher-evaluation form to be used by colleagues is given in Table 15.2.

It is also very important to ascertain students' opinions of teaching, but it is more useful to ask them to evaluate a course of lessons rather than individual ones (provided that the teacher has had more than one encounter with the students). There are two reasons for this, the first being that it would be boring to have to complete a large number of evaluations, and second the teacher then obtains a more average response to their teaching rather than the specific points from a single session. A different form is needed for the learner's evaluation, since the colleague's one is much more related to a professional educationalist's view of teaching. An example of a teaching evaluation form to be completed by students is given in Table 15.3.

Classroom observation of teaching

One obvious way of evaluating teaching is for an observer to sit in on a class or sample of classes to observe what the teacher does. Interaction analysis is a generic term for this and can range on a continuum from highly structured, systematic observation (SO) to more open, impressionistic observation and participation.

The best-known system of systematic observation is that of Ned Flanders, called Flanders Interaction of Analysis Categories, or FIAC, which uses a number of categories of 'teacher talk' and 'pupil talk' (Flanders, 1970). The observer has been trained to use the ten categories in Flanders system and these are shown in Table 15.4.

Table 15.2 Checklist for self and peer evaluation of teaching

Item	Highly satisfactory			Weak
A. Lesson plan				
1. Learning outcomes defined	1	2	3	4
2. Organization and sequence	1	2	3	4
3. Variety	1	2	3	4
4. Student activity	1	2	3	4
5. Learning aids	1	2	3	4
6. Learning checks	1	2	3	4
7. Timing	1	2	3	4
B. Delivery of lesson				
8. Audibility of voice	1	2	3	4
9. Clarity of speech	1	2	3	4
10. Expressiveness of voice	1	2	3	4
11. Speed of delivery	1	2	3	4
12. Use of pauses	1	2	3	4
13. Confidence	1	2	3	4
14. Enthusiasm	1	2	3	4
15. Warmth	1	2	3	4
16. Psychological safety	1	2	3	4
17. Sense of humour	1	2	3	4
18. Non-verbal communication	1	2	3	4
19. Accuracy of content	1	2	3	4
20. Content up to date	1	2	3	4
21. Research quoted	1	2	3	4
22. Clarity of explanations	1	2	3	4
23. Level of lesson appropriate	1	2	3	4
24. Quality of media resources	1	2	3	4
25. Technique for using media resources	1	2	3	4
26. Use of questioning	1	2	3	4
27. Student participation	1	2	3	4
28. Opening of lesson	1	2	3	4
29. Closing of lesson	1	2	3	4

There are eight categories for teacher talk and only two for student talk and the underlying philosophy is that the better teachers use a more indirect influence.

When the lesson begins the observer starts recording the teacher and student behaviours on an analysis sheet, entering a tick in the appropriate category every three seconds, according to who is speaking and in what category. At the end of the lesson the data is analysed to show the interaction patterns during the session and a whole range of ratios can be calculated. One of the great drawbacks is that so much of the richness of the classroom is lost during the process of reduction into categories. In addition, it has been argued that the categories are too over-inclusive. For example, the category for teacher questions does not distinguish between the type and level of question. Another problem is that the schedule contains only two pupil categories, which puts the emphasis very much on the teacher talk; this approach has been criticized by some commentators,

Table 15.3 Teacher evaluation form for completion by students

The purpose of this questionnaire is to help me to adapt my teaching to your needs as a student. Please indicate your opinion of my teaching during the course you have just completed by putting a tick in the appropriate box.

	X applies	*Marked tendency to X*	*Some tendency to X Y*	*Marked tendency to Y*	*Y applies*	
Content relevant to nursing						Content not relevant to nursing
Organization of subjects good						Organization of subjects poor
Subjects made interesting						Subjects made rather dull
Presented with clarity						Presented in a confusing manner
Audibility and speech good						Audibility and speech poor
Speed of delivery ideal						Speed of delivery too fast or too slow (underline appropriate one)
Amount of information ideal						Amount of information too much or too little (underline appropriate one)
Level of subject ideal						Level of subject too high or too low (underline appropriate one)
Visual presentation good						Visual presentation poor
Good rapport with class						No rapport with class
Good student participation						No student participation
A lot of learning took place						Very little learning took place
Good feedback given on student progress						No feedback given on progress

Irritating and distracting mannerisms (please specify)

Comments:

Table 15.4 Categories of FIAC

Teacher talk	Indirect influence	1.	*Accepts feeling*: accepts and clarifies the feeling tone of the students in a non-threatening manner. Feelings may be positive or negative. Predicting and recalling feelings are included.
		2.	*Praises or encourages*: praises or encourages student action or behaviour. Jokes that release tension, not at the expense of another individual, nodding head or saying 'uh huh'?' or 'go on' are included.
		3.	*Accepts or uses ideas of student*: clarifying, building, or developing ideas or suggestions by a student. As teacher brings more of his or her own ideas into play, shift to category five.
		4.	*Asks questions*: asking a question about content or procedure with the intent that a student answer.
	Direct influence	5.	*Lectures*: giving facts or opinions about content or procedure; expressing own ideas; asking rhetorical questions.
		6.	*Gives directions*: directions, commands, or orders with which a student is expected to comply.
		7.	*Criticizes or justifies authority*: statements intended to change student behaviour from non-acceptable to acceptable pattern; bawling someone out; stating why the teacher is doing what he or she is doing, extreme self-reference.
Student talk		8.	*Student talk-response*: talk by students in response to teacher. Teacher initiatives the contact or solicits student statement.
		9.	*Student talk-initiation*: talk by students, which they initiate. If 'calling on' student is only to indicate who may talk next, observer must decide whether student wanted to talk. If he or she did, use this category.
		10.	*Silence or confusion*: pauses, short periods of silence, and periods of confusion in which communication cannot be understood by the observer.

as it overlooks the importance of pupil talk as a classroom variable. The use of FIAC is really only suitable for the classical type of lesson in which the teacher talks at the class from the front; it is not readily adaptable for group work. In addition, in order to make the findings reliable, observers have to undergo training in the use of categories and this may impose artificial constraints on their perceptions.

The underlying philosophy of FIAC is that of the direct versus the indirect style of teaching; the former implying authoritarian ways and the latter much more freedom and choice. Many may not agree with these categories, since Flanders equates direct with 'bad' and indirect with 'good' teaching style!

An alternative observation strategy is that called 'ethnographic' or 'participant' observation; in this system the observer or researcher attempts to see things from the point of view of the students by involving themselves in whatever is happening in the classroom. The observer can ask questions, observe events, listen and so on, the idea being that more of the richness of the classroom environment can be captured. This is obviously a much more qualitative evaluation as opposed to quantitative.

Course or pathway evaluation

Although evaluation of teaching contributes useful information it is insufficient in itself as an indicator of course quality, since it does not cover other aspects such as organization and resources. Overall course evaluation is particularly important in CAT schemes, where pathways consist of many units. In this case, unit evaluation will not provide evidence of the overall aspects of the pathway, so provision needs to be made for this before students leave the pathway. Institutions may have a standard format for course evaluation forms, or they can be designed specifically for the course in question. Table 15.5 shows an example of a course evaluation questionnaire specifically designed for a Stress Management Course for GP Referrals.

EXTERNAL EXAMINER AND QUALITY ASSURANCE

The external examiner system plays a key role in educational quality assurance by bringing in an external, objective perspective to the assessment system. The role involves scrutiny of students' assessment work to ascertain if the standards are comparable with students on similar courses throughout. In addition, the external examiner can comment on the consistency and standard of internal marking, and make suggestions for improvements to the assessment system. The role of the external examiner is discussed in more detail in Chapter 11 (p. 264).

ANNUAL COURSE/PATHWAY MONITORING REPORTS

The pathway director and pathway committee are responsible for the production of an annual pathway monitoring report which is sent to the college or department faculty board or equivalent. The annual monitoring report is one of the key mechanisms for quality assurance, and provides data about a range of aspects of educational delivery.

Scrutineer system for annual monitoring reports

Some institutions use a scrutineer system for annual monitoring. A scrutineer is a member of academic staff assigned to a particular course or pathway, and who scrutinizes the annual monitoring procedure. There is dialogue between the scrutineer and the course director about the draft monitoring report and how it might be made more effective. The

Table 15.5 Example of a course evaluation from a stress management course for GP referrals

---

EVALUATION OF STRESS MANAGEMENT PROGRAMME

Dear Participant,
As the leader of the Stress Management Programme you have just completed, I would be very interested to know your opinion of the programme. This questionnaire is designed to evaluate the programme, and I would be most grateful if you could kindly take ten minutes or so to complete it, and to return it to me at the Health Centre in the envelope provided.

DELIVERY OF THE PROGRAMME

1. How adequate was the pre-course information?
2. How satisfied were you with the venue used for the programme?
3. How well-suited to your lifestyle was the time of day for the programme?
4. What are your feelings about the length of each session?
5. What did you feel about the social interactions within the group of participants on the programme?
6. What did you think about the overall standard of teaching on the programme?
7. What did you feel about the manner and approachability of the programme leader?
8. What did you think about the way in which the information was explained?
9. What did you feel about the exercises and activities you participated in?
10. How useful do you think the programme has been in reducing your level of stress?
11. Have you any suggestions about how the programme could be made more effective?

Thank you very much indeed for taking the time to complete this questionnaire.

---

scrutineer also speaks to the report at the Faculty Board, and the system provides added rigour to the process of quality assurance.

Aspects of the annual course/pathway monitoring report

Typical aspects of an annual monitoring report, based on University of Greenwich procedures, are given in Table 15.6.

DEVELOPING STANDARDS

Within nursing and midwifery practice the development of standards of care is well-established, and the aim is to provide patients/clients, their representatives, and other health professionals with information about the quality of care delivered by the relevant service provider. Standards are desired and achievable levels of performance against which actual practice is compared. Standards, whilst conforming to regional guidelines, will reflect the special needs of a particular client group or practice area.

Table 15.6 Typical categories for annual course/pathway monitoring report

1. OVERALL VIEW OF THE DELIVERY OF THE COURSE/
   PATHWAY
   This section should comment on the extent to which the action plan for
   the previous year has been implemented. It should also comment on the
   highlights and problems of the year and how these were addressed.

2. HOW WELL THE STUDENTS DID
   This section should contain a summary of assessment statistics and
   comments on overall student performance.

3. WHAT THE STUDENTS THOUGHT OF THE UNIT/COURSE/
   PATHWAY
   This section should contain summary information from students'
   evaluations of the units, and the overall course/pathway. Details and
   examples of the techniques used to obtain student feedback should be
   included.

4. RESPONSE TO EXTERNAL EXAMINER'S REPORT
   This section should comment on the proposed action to be taken in
   response to criticisms and suggestions made by the external examiner.
   Any special commendation should be highlighted. External examiners'
   reports should be attached to the annual monitoring report.

5. WHAT EMPLOYERS THINK OF THE COURSE/PATHWAY
   This section should comment on employers' perceptions of the value of
   the course/pathway, and include examples of the techniques used to obtain
   employer feedback.

6. ACTION PLAN FOR THE NEXT YEAR
   This section should indicate the key objectives to be implemented or
   explored during the next academic year. This should include the timescale
   for each objective, and a named person who is responsible for
   implementing each one.

7. OTHER ISSUES FOR THE REPORT
   This section is for reporting on any issues or concerns identified.

Standards have also been developed for nurse education which aim to
inform college staff and service providers about the quality of education
delivered by the college.

Standards are composed of the following components:

1. Standard statement
   This describes the goal or outcome to be met.
2. Criteria
   These are systems and mechanisms necessary to achieve the standard, and
   are usually written under the headings structure, process and outcome.

Table 15.7 gives an example of a standard for student placement in the
community (North Hampshire Loddon Community NHS Trust, 1992)

BS5750 standards

The British Standards Institute BS5750 is the standard for quality
assurance systems in the UK. Although designed for manufacturing

Table 15.7 Standard for student placement in the community

STANDARD STATEMENT: Within 48 hours of arrival students have a negotiated programme for community experience designed to help them meet community placement and personal objectives.

CRITERIA:

A. Structure

Health visitors will have:		
	1.	notification of a student placement, preferably to plan a year ahead;
	2.	up-to-date information on local services;
	3.	time and space for a student;
	4.	written objectives for community placement, and
	5.	blank outlines to record student programmes

B. Process		
	1.	Student contacts assigned HV in the fortnight prior to placement.
	2.	HV and student appreciate the constraints on each other by open discussion of difficulties.
	3.	Negotiation occurs about experience during placement.
	4.	Failure to achieve objectives is explored together to help current and future students.

C: Outcome		
	1.	An agreed programme is written in duplicate. Student knows the arrangement he or she has to make.
	2.	Learning objectives and outcomes are documented.
	3.	HV retains a copy of each student's programme, noting its strengths and weaknesses.
	4.	Students have their own programme copy which includes documented outcomes.

industries, it is capable of adaptation to meet the requirements of education and training. BS5750 has three standards:

- Part 1: Specification for design/development, production, installation and servicing for organizations
- Part 2: Specification for production and installation
- Part 3: Specification for final inspection and test

Freeman (1993) acknowledges that the 20 separate standards contained in BS5750 are difficult to relate to education and training, but he suggests that Part 1 applies to education and that twelve of the standards are highly relevant to the teaching process:

Management responsibility
Quality system
Contract review
Design control
Purchasing
Purchaser supplied product
Process control
Control of non-conforming product

Corrective action
Quality records
Internal quality audits
Training

If an educational institution wishes to have its QA system recognized it must approach a Certification Body which will assess its system against the BS 5750 standards.

TOTAL QUALITY MANAGEMENT (TQM)

There is a growing interest within HE in total quality management (TQM). TQM is a system that aims to meet the needs of the market, to develop competitiveness, and to constantly monitor and achieve the highest quality without consuming more resources. Its greatest strength is its principle that every employee is responsible for continuously monitoring quality by participating in problem-solving. TQM emphasizes the importance of producing design specifications that can be delivered, rather than ideal or expensive designs that cannot be implemented, and standards are constantly upgraded. TQM is very much a market concept, and educationalists might feel that its application to education is inappropriate. However, with the advent of contracting for education within the NHS, competition becomes a real issue, hence the interest in TQM from nurse educators. TQM is applied in practice by using quality circles.

QUALITY CIRCLES

Quality circles is a strategy that involves group problem-solving in order to enhance the quality of the service. The group should consist of between three and twelve people from similar areas of work who meet together for an hour per week during the working day. The group should be trained in problem-solving skills and they focus on problems occurring within their work. Their solutions are implemented directly by them or via management. 'Quality activities are targeted at the consumer in realizing a service which is safe, reliable, economical and effective' (Hutchins, 1985). This could easily be implemented in the college of nursing using a group of nurse teachers who tackle common problems.

REFERENCES

Balogh, R., Beattie, A. and Beckerleg, S. (1989) *Figuring Out Performance*, ENB, London.
Cave, M., Hanney, S. and Kogan, M. (1991) *The Use of Performance Indicators in Higher Education*, Jessica Kingsley, London.

Donabedian, A. (1980) *The Definition of Quality and Approaches to its Assessment*, Health Administration Press, Ann Arbor.

English National Board for Nursing, Midwifery and Health Visiting (1993) *Guidelines for Educational Audit*, ENB, London.

Flanders, N. (1970) *Analysing Teaching Behaviour*, Addison-Wesley, Reading, Mass.

Freeman, R. (1993) *Quality Assurance in Education and Training*, Kogan Page, London.

Hutchins, D. (1985) *Quality Circles Handbook*, Pitman, London.

Morris, A. (1990) Performance Indicators: Report of a Committee of Enquiry Chaired by Mr Alfred Morris, London, PCFC.

Tuxworth, E. (1982) *Competency in Teaching*, FEU, London.

North Hampshire Loddon Community NHS Trust (1992) Standards for Health Visiting.

Teaching study skills 16

In the UK, nursing, midwifery and health visiting education has developed a close relationship with the higher education (HE) sector and is therefore being exposed to a different educational culture. Traditionally, nurse education has been largely institution-controlled, with a strong emphasis on the delivery of teaching. Student contact time with teachers was commonly twice that required by HE courses, with little or no time available for independent study. The validation process in HE, on the other hand, requires all courses to provide substantial periods of time each week for independent study. Nurse teachers will therefore need to help students to adopt a more enquiry-based approach to learning, and although taught inputs will remain useful, they will function more as an adjunct to the main learning resource, the library. The pre-eminence of study skills is nicely captured in the following quotations:

'The most socially useful learning in the modern world is the learning of the process of learning' (Rogers, 1969).

'No educational objective is more important for students than learning how to learn, and how to function as an independent, autonomous learner' (Howe, 1984).

COGNITIVE STYLES (LEARNING STYLES)

Nurse teachers need to be aware that there are important individual differences in students' approach to study. Nisbet and Shucksmith (1986) make a distinction between study skills and study strategies, the latter being at a higher level than the former. Strategies can best be seen as higher-order skills such as planning, monitoring, checking, revising and self-testing. A number of terms are employed to describe the preferred ways of learning or processing information that characterize an individual, namely learning styles, cognitive styles, learning strategies and study strategies. An outline of the main categories of learning styles is given below.

Field dependence and field independence

These terms refer to ways in which individuals perceive and order the world around them; some people tend to see patterns as wholes, whereas others focus on particular parts. Witkin and his colleagues (Witkin, 1977)

Table 16.1 Characteristics of field dependent and field independent students

Field dependent	*Field independent*
Need structured materials	Impose own structure on material
May have difficulty reorganizing material already organized in another way	Can break down material and reorganize it
May need clear instructions on how to solve problems	Likely to solve problems without specific guidance
May need to learn to use mnemonics	
Are better at learning and remembering social information	May need assistance with materials containing social information
Are likely to work in social careers such as psychiatric nursing or social work	Are likely to work in sciences or practical things like mechanics or surgical nursing

have carried out extensive research into this phenomenon using tests that involve the separation of figure from background or context. Individuals who are higher on one dimension than another are not better or worse because of it, since field dependence or field independence are not value-laden. Table 16.1 shows the main differences between the two types of cognitive style.

Reflective and impulsive styles

These styles refer to an individual's tendency to either produce an answer to a problem very quickly, or to spend some time in reflection before giving an answer. The kind of test used in this situation is called the 'matching familiar figures test' (Kagan, 1965) and consists of a number of pictures of familiar objects that the individual has to match with another picture. There are two styles of answering the problem; some people answer very quickly and others take time to answer. Kagan considers the former to be impulsive and the latter reflective, taking only the speed variable into account. Thus, whether or not a person is accurate is not relevant to the test. Students can be taught to become more reflective by the use of self-instruction and scanning strategies.

Kolb's learning style inventory (LSI)

Another approach to cognitive style is Kolb's learning style inventory (Kolb, 1976). Kolb's experiential learning theory is discussed in Chapter 3, and the learning styles inventory utilizes concepts from the theory. There are two dimensions measured by this approach, concrete to abstract, and action to reflection, and four types of learning styles are identified.

1. Converger

The converger is so-called because they tend to do best in situations requiring a single correct answer or solution. Convergers excel in the application of ideas to practical situations, and their dominant learning abilities are abstract conceptualization (AC) and active experimentation (AE). Persons with this style tend to prefer things to people, and often work in engineering and other physical sciences.

2. Diverger

Divergers, as the name implies, are the opposite of convergers. They tend to do best in situations requiring generation of ideas, and they tend to excel in the use of imagination and the organization of concrete situations into meaningful wholes. Their dominant learning abilities are concrete experience (CE) and reflective observation (RO). Kolb suggests this style is characteristic of people with humanities and liberal arts backgrounds, and also counsellors and personnel managers.

3. Assimilator

Assimilators tend to do best at creating theoretical models and inductive reasoning, and are less interested in practical applications. Their dominant learning abilities are abstract conceptualization (AC) and reflective observation (RO). People with this style tend to be found in basic maths and science, and in research and planning departments.

4. Accommodator

Accommodators tend to do best at carrying out plans and experiments. They tend to be risk-takers more than the other styles, and they excel in situations where they need to accommodate and adapt to the specific circumstances. Their dominant learning abilities are concrete experience (CE) and active experimentation (AE). People with this style tend to be found in action-oriented positions such as marketing or sales.

Serialist and holist strategies

In a series of experiments (Pask and Scott, 1972; Pask, 1975; Pask, 1976) on learning strategies, Pask and his co-workers found that subjects could be classified into two categories, serialist and holist. He used a system of classification for imaginary Martian animals as the learning task and found that subjects approached the problem in very different ways. Those subjects using a serialist strategy tended to proceed in a step-by-step manner, whereas the holists adopted a more global approach to what was to be learned. Pask suggests that these strategies reflect basic learning styles; holist strategies reflect a comprehension learning style and serialist strategies an operation learning style. Some students are able to employ both serialist and holist strategies as appropriate and this learning style is referred to as versatile. Pask has related specific learning pathologies to the two strategies. The holist is prone to the pathology called 'globetrotting', which involves a tendency to overgeneralize from insufficient evidence and to use inappropriate analogy. Serialists, on the other hand, are prone to improvidence, which means that they may not build up an overview of how the sub-components of the topic interrelate, nor utilize important analogies. In an experiment that matched and mismatched holist and serialist students with holist and serialist teaching styles, there was a clear superiority for students whose learning style matched the teaching style, but the sample size was small.

Deep approach and surface approach

Marton and his co-workers at Gothenburg focused on how students read academic articles (Marton and Saljo, 1976). Students were given an academic article to read and were then interviewed afterwards to ascertain their approach to the article. These interviews were recorded and the audiotapes transcribed and analysed in terms of level of understanding and approach to learning. The latter showed a clear-cut distinction between deep approaches and surface approaches. Those adopting a deep approach commenced with the intention of understanding the article, relating it to their own experience and evaluating the author's evidence. Those adopting a surface approach concentrated on memorizing the important points and were guided by the type of questions they anticipated being subsequently asked. The researchers suggest that these approaches are indicators of the students' normal approach to study.

Lancaster inventory of study strategies

Entwistle and his colleagues at Lancaster also studied how students read academic articles (Entwistle, Hanley and Hounsell, 1979; Entwistle, 1981) and this culminated in the development of the Lancaster Inventory of Study Strategies. The inventory contains the following scales:

1. *Achieving*: relates to competitiveness and organized methods
2. *Reproducing*: relates to surface approach and the syllabus-bound concept
3. *Meaning*: relates to deep approaches and intrinsic motivation
4. *Comprehension*: reflects a holist strategy
5. *Operation*: reflects a serialist strategy
6. *Versatile*: indicates a versatile approach to learning
7. *Pathological*: indicates pathological symptoms in learning
8. *Overall academic success*: prediction for success

Honey's learning styles

Honey (1982) developed a scheme of learning styles involving a questionnaire of 80 items. Learning styles are classified under four headings – activists, reflectors, theorists and pragmatists – and the questionnaire data reveals the subject's scores on each of these variables.

- *Activists* are characterized by openness to new experiences and a sociable nature, albeit rather egocentric and impulsive.
- *Reflectors*, on the other hand, tend to be cautious people who like to explore things carefully before coming to a decision. They are observers rather than participants.
- *Theorists* are logical, rational people who like theories and systems; they are unhappy about subjective impressions and ambiguity.
- *Pragmatists* like very much to apply things in practice and to experiment with ideas; they tend to be impatient and like to get going with new ideas.

Syllabus-bound and syllabus-free students

Malcolm Parlett (1970) classifies students into two types, syllabus-bound (sylbs) and syllabus-free (sylfs). The terms are largely self-explanatory. Sylbs tend to accept the system and are very much examination-oriented and like to know exactly what is required of them in assignments. Sylfs, on the other hand, find the confines of the syllabus very limiting and wish to explore much more widely than that. They are happy to find things out for themselves and take responsibility for learning.

Dunn and Dunn's four learning styles

Dunn and Dunn (1978), Dunn, Dunn and Price (1984) have identified four preferred learning styles of students, as outlined in Table 16.2. An inventory based on these learning styles has been devised, which enables teachers to arrange the environment so that students' preferences are catered for.

Cognitive styles and nurse education

Given the foregoing outline of selected cognitive styles the nurse teacher may well ask 'this is all very interesting, but how can I use it to make my teaching more effective?' Since there are some 20 such classifications of cognitive styles in the literature, it follows that each student could well differ on the dimensions of every one of these! Hence, attempting to match teaching style to these would be impossible. The problem is further compounded when one considers the likelihood of a student's cognitive style being to some extent dependent upon the particular learning context. Let us take the example of a student nurse undertaking a clinical placement visit during the early stages of a pre-registration course. If this is perceived as a potentially threatening learning environment the student may adopt a 'reflector' learning style in which he or she demonstrates caution and a tendency to approach things carefully before making a decision. However, during the final year of a course, the same student

Table 16.2 Dunn and Dunn's four learning styles

Environmental conditions		
Needs quiet	——	Tolerates sound
Needs bright light	——	Needs dim light
Needs cool environment	——	Needs warm environment
Needs formal design of furniture	——	Needs informal design
Emotional and motivational states		
Self-motivated	——	Unmotivated
Persistent	——	Not persistent
Responsible	——	Not very responsible
Needs structured learning	——	Needs little structure
Sociological preferences		
Prefers learning	⎱	Alone With one peer With two peers With several peers With adults Through several ways
Physical characteristics and needs		
Prefers:	⎱	Auditory Visual Tactile Kinaesthetic
Requires food intake	——	Does not require food
Functions best in:	⎱	Morning Late morning Afternoon Evening
Needs mobility	——	Does not need mobility

may well approach clinical placements with a 'pragmatist' learning style, eager to apply things in practice and to experiment with ideas. The validity of attempting to match teaching styles with learning styles is criticized by Tennant (1988) on the grounds that it would produce harmonious viewpoints between teacher and student, but that educational growth is more likely to occur when the student has to move outside the confines of his or her own learning style. In other words, a degree of challenge or conflict may well result in more creative learning. Tennant goes on to suggest that teachers should use the theories of learning styles to assist students to understand how they may approach learning, to facilitate expansion of their learning styles, and to provide a learning climate in which diversity is encouraged.

CHARACTERISTICS OF UNDERGRADUATE LEVEL STUDY

The links between nurse education and HE range from university validation of courses within Colleges of Nursing and Midwifery, through to the complete incorporation of colleges into universities or institutions of

HE. Whatever the nature of the link, it means that eventually all pre-registration and post-registration courses will be taught at undergraduate or postgraduate level.

The essence of undergraduate level study is that it aims to help the student to acquire or develop a range of characteristics (CNAA, 1989):

1. the development of intellectual and imaginative powers, understanding, judgement, and problem-solving skills;
2. the ability to see relationships in what is learned and to perceive the field of study in a broader perspective;
3. the capacity for sustained independent and high quality work;
4. the ability to engage in critical thinking, enquiry and analysis, including research skills; and
5. the development of self-awareness and the ability to reflect upon professional practice.

At degree level students must be much more autonomous in their learning and must not expect to be 'spoon-fed' with information by the tutors. They must also be much more critical of the information they encounter, taking care to analyse and evaluate it rather than just accepting it as valid or 'true'. How then can the nurse teacher help students to achieve autonomy in their study skills? Simply putting in the odd lecture on the topic will not suffice; what is needed is a structured programme that includes diagnosis of needs as well as information about study strategies and learning resources. Since one of the main characteristics of undergraduate and postgraduate study is the ability of the student to work independently, the library is the single most important educational resource for this. If they are to benefit from their studies, students need to develop a thorough understanding of all the facilities afforded by a library.

USING THE LIBRARY

Library registration usually takes place at the same time as general registration for a course or pathway, and library cards are issued. In HE it is common practice for the library to provide an induction programme for new students, complemented by written guides to the various library facilities. The induction covers such aspects as the opening hours, the borrowing rights of students, any system of fines that may be in operation, and photocopying facilities. In addition, it should be pointed out that no food or drink is allowed into the library, and conversation reduced to the bare minimum to avoid disturbing other people's study. Most libraries in HE have a security system which is activated if a book is taken out of the library without the appropriate authorization. Multidisciplinary libraries are common within the health service and combine the resources for a wide range of health professions such as nursing, midwifery, medicine, and the professions supplementary to medicine. The periodicals or journals stock is usually very extensive in multidisciplinary libraries.

Classification systems

The Dewey classification scheme (Dewey decimal system) is the system favoured by HE libraries to classify resources. It is divided into ten main classes:

000 Generalities
100 Philosophy and related disciplines
200 Religion
300 Social sciences
400 Language
500 Pure sciences
600 Technology
700 Arts
800 Literature
900 General geography and history

Within this main classification there are more specific ones, for example, nursing is classified at 610, anatomy and physiology at 612, psychology 150–159 and education at 370. The Dewey classification is used not only for the main book stock, but for reference books, periodicals, oversize materials, pamphlets, and audio-visual media. When searching for specific subjects students tend to concentrate on books, and may need reminding to look at the other resources shelved in different areas of the library. An alternative system that may still be used in some Colleges of Nursing and Midwifery is the National Library of Medicine classification. This was developed from the classification of the Library of Congress, Washington and the following are examples under the heading 'Medicine and Related Subjects':

WE Musculo-skeletal system
WF Respiratory system
WG Cardio-vascular system
WH Haemic and lymphatic systems
WI Gastrointestinal system
WJ Urogenital system
WK Endocrine system
WL Nervous system

Nursing is classified as WY and if this classification were used without adaptation, then every book in the nursing library would be under the same category. Thus, college of nursing libraries usually employ the categories of the body systems, classifying the related nursing books under these. For example, they might include cardio-vascular nursing under WG.

The catalogues

HE libraries, and many college of nursing and midwifery libraries, use an on-line public access catalogue (OPAC). This computer system offers a range of options when searching for resources; for example, keyword search allows the student to enter keywords such as bereavement, and the computer will display a list of titles to match the keyword. Author search is used if the name of the author is already known, and the computer displays a list of titles under the author's name. Title search works in a similar way if the title is already known. The quickest search of all is quick author/title search if both are known. In institutions not yet using OPAC, catalogues are usually on microfiche, which employs an electronic device that enlarges the image from a microfiche film. The author catalogue is compiled using the author's surname and is arranged alphabetically. The subject index is also alphabetical and the class of each subject is given next to the name. The classified catalogue contains all the stock on a given subject, arranged according to the classification numbers. Some libraries also have a title catalogue.

Books

Although the majority of the book stock of a library is available for loan, there are some categories that have restricted access. A short loan collection consists of books that are in very great demand, and the loan period for these is only one or two weeks in order to maximize their availability to all readers. A counter text collection also contains popular books as well as other materials, and is available for use in the library only. The reference collection contains materials that are not available for loan, including statistical sources, encyclopaedias, dictionaries and directories. If the library does not stock a particular book or other resource, it can be obtained via the inter-library loan service, and a charge may be levied for this service.

Periodicals

The term periodical applies to any journal, newspaper or magazine, and these are a valuable source of reference, particularly as they contain material that is published long before it reaches the textbooks. Current editions of periodicals are usually displayed prominently in the library, with back copies stored under the appropriate classification.

Databases

Most libraries will have a range of computer databases stored on CD-ROM (Compact Disc – Read Only Memory). A compact disc can hold the equivalent of a quarter of a million pages of A4 writing, with very fast access to indexes and abstracts. One of the most frequently used in nursing is the Cumulative Index of Nursing and Allied Health Literature (CINAHL), which contains citations from a large number of journals. MEDLINE is the database of the National Library of Medicine, USA, and NERIS is a British educational database. BIDS (Bath Information and Data Services) Inside Information Service is a British Library product that gives access to the recent contents of the 10,000 most popular journals held by the Document Supply Centre. The service is accessed over the JANET (Joint Academic Computer Network).

Other library resources

In addition to books, periodicals and databases, libraries hold syllabuses, prospectuses from educational institutions, student dissertations, and audio-visual materials such as videotapes.

Searching the literature

The quickest and most efficient means of carrying out a literature search is by CD-ROM.

Before the search

1. Decide exactly what it is you want to know, i.e. the subject. Use dictionaries or encyclopedias if unsure of definition, and check synonyms and related terms.
2. Decide on the limits of the search, for example how far back will it go? Will it be restricted to certain areas or aspects? How long will it take?

During the search

3. Consult the OPAC and/or other catalogues for the material held by the library on your subject.
4. Consult relevant bibliographies on your subject.
5. Consult relevant abstracts and indexes on your subject.
6. Consult the relevant CD-ROM databases on your subject.
7. Locate each of the references, using inter-library loan as appropriate.
6. Read this material, noting the quality. For example, is there any obvious bias? Does it contain a bibliography? What is the quality of the index? Have there been previous editions? It is easier to start with the latest material first, proceeding to the earlier material.
9. Complete a separate reference card for each reference, using a standard format such as the Harvard system.
10. Complete reference cards for further references which might be given in the sources you locate.

Bibliographies

There are two main types of bibliography, each of which contains references to work in a given subject area. The first kind is the retrospective bibliography, which gives a list of references up to a particular date, for example, Thompson's Bibliography of Nursing Literature 1961–70. The second kind is the serial bibliography, which is published at regular intervals, for example, Nursing Bibliography (monthly) and Current Literature on Health Services (monthly). The British National Bibliography is published weekly and contains every publication in Britain since 1950.

Abstracts

These consist of summaries of publications in certain fields, for example Hospital Abstracts, Nursing Research Abstracts, Research into Higher Education Abstracts.

Indexes

Indexes contain references for articles on a particular subject, culled from a variety of journals, for example International Nursing Index, British Education Index.

Bibliographic citations

Students should be encouraged to use a standard format or citation style in their work, such as the Harvard System, for books and journal articles. For the following essential information is needed to assist the reader:

Author's surname and initials
Year of publication
Title
Edition
Publisher
Place of publication

For example:

Humphreys, T.J. and Quinn, F.M. (1994) *Healthcare Education: The Challenge of the Market*, Chapman and Hall, London.

For journal articles, slightly different details are needed for the reader to locate the information:

Author's surname and initials
Title of article
Title of journal in full
Volume number or date
Page numbers of article/extract (first and last)

For example:

Suppiah, C. (1994) Working in partnership with community mothers, *Health Visitor*, **67**(2), 51–3.

Further examples of the style of reference appear at the end of each chapter of this book.

EFFECTIVE READING

The student may gain a great deal of information by simply handling a book and noting some of the features of it. An idea of its content can be ascertained from reading the publicity description found on the back of the book or the flaps of the dust jacket. In addition, a preface or foreword will indicate the target audience and often the aim of the author, but it should be remembered that a foreword by an eminent writer, although usually a good recommendation, should not be taken as the sole criterion of the excellence of a book.

A glance at the bibliographical page will indicate the author, title and date of publication and if the book is into a second or subsequent edition, this may indicate success. The contents page can be scanned for an idea of the main sequence of the book and it is important to examine the index to see the kind of content included. The use of references by the author may give a guide to the standard of a book, particularly the dates of these, if few recent ones are mentioned.

Pre-reading and follow-up reading

It is very useful for students to do some relevant reading prior to each meeting of a class or unit, if at all possible. They will be in a much better position to contribute during the session, and will also have a good insight into the topic under discussion. It is equally valuable to do some follow-up reading each week after the unit meeting, as this will help them to consolidate their learning and also offers further perspectives on the topic.

Processing texts

Understanding of written texts can be thought of as a constructive process in which the reader first tries to classify the information into fact, narrative and so on. Two levels are then identified, microstructure and macrostructure (Kintsch and Van Dijk, 1978): microstructure is the structure of sentences, propositions and words, and macrostructure is the global meaning of the text, which is obtained by combing the microstructure. There are four rules for isolating the macrostructure:

1. *Deletion*: the taking out of irrelevant properties.
2. *Generalization*: Substitution of lower-order concepts by higher-order ones, e.g. substituting furniture for tables and chairs.
3. *Selection*: removal of properties already stated in the text, i.e. removal of repetitive ideas.
4. *Construction*: the creation of a general concept where none is apparent.

These rules are under the control of schema; these are said to be the basic building blocks of the human information-processing system and can be defined as 'large, complex units of knowledge that organize much of what we know about general categories of objects, classes of events and

Table 16.3 Examples of algorithm procedures for reading texts

SQ3R procedure (Robinson, 1946)
SURVEY: student tries to get an overview of the main points in chapter.
QUESTIONS: each main point stated in form of a question.
READ: student reads the passage to find out answer to questions.
RECITE: answer recited out loud without using the book.
REVIEW: whole chapter reviewed to give overall impression.

MURDER procedure (Dansereau, 1978)
MOOD: getting the right mood for study.
UNDERSTANDING: reading for understanding.
RECALLING material.
DIGESTING material.
EXPANDING knowledge by self-enquiry.
REVIEWING mistakes.

types of people' (Anderson, 1980). When attempting to understand text, students try to select appropriate schema that will account for the material under consideration. The end result of these rules is that a summary or gist of the material is made and this equates with understanding it. These rules can be taught to students to help them to process texts in nursing and the teacher can test each stage to monitor progress.

Another helpful approach to reading texts is to teach students to use procedures or algorithms, two of which are outlined in Table 16.3.

Readability tests

It is useful to apply tests of readability to textual materials as a rough guide to their difficulty or otherwise, one of the most common being the 'Flesch formula for reading ease' (Flesch, 1974). This consists of testing a random sample of passages from the text and applying a formula to calculate reading ease. The formula is:

$$RE = 206.835 - 1.015SL - 0.846WL$$

where RE is the reading ease, SL is the average sentence length and WL is word length. The procedure is as follows:

1. Test a minimum of three, randomly selected passages of 100 words each, avoiding introductory ones and beginning with a new paragraph.
2. Calculate the SL by taking the number of words in the sample and dividing by the number of sentences.
3. Calculate the WL by counting the number of syllables in each word of the 100-word sample.

The reading ease score is interpreted as in Table 16.4

EFFECTIVE NOTE-TAKING

There are both advantages and disadvantages in taking notes during a unit as detailed in Table 16.5. On balance, though, note-taking is to be

Table 16.4 Interpretation of reading ease score: Flesch formula

Level of material	Reading ease score
Very easy	90–100
Easy	80–90
Fairly easy	70–80
Standard	60–70
Fairly difficult	50–60
Difficult	30–50
Very difficult	0–30

Table 16.5 Advantages and disadvantages of note-taking

Advantages	Disadvantages
Provides a permanent record for later review.	May be inaccurate.
Material is encoded in student's own words.	Student may miss parts of lesson whilst writing notes.
Material is actively processed by student.	May inhibit student's own processing activities if structured by teacher.

recommended if it is done effectively, i.e. recording the key points rather than trying to write down everything word-for-word. At degree level, it is more important to note key references given in the unit, so that the original source can be accessed later, avoiding reliance on secondary sources.

Some teachers prefer to give notes in the form of handouts, so that accuracy is ensured and nothing is missed during the lesson. On the other hand, giving printed notes means that the students do not have a chance to encode material in their own words, a major disadvantage. It also means that students' own unique processing activities are suppressed. Perhaps the best compromise is for the teacher to use incomplete handouts that contain the key headings and sub-headings of the lecture, but with sufficient space for the student to write in their own notes.

If students wish to take notes from lessons, there are a number of systems for this. The standard system consists of writing down the key headings and sub-headings, with outline descriptions under each one as in Table 16.6.

The 'pattern' system uses only main concepts, which are connected by lines showing the interrelationships, as in Figure 16.1.

The Cornell University system

This system is best used with loose-leaf A4 size paper, on which the student rules a two-inch margin on the left-hand side. The system uses five Rs, namely record, reduce, recite, reflect, review. Notes are recorded

Table 16.6   Standard system of note-taking: bronchial carcinoma

Aetiology	(i) Males:females = 4:1; age 50–75
	(ii) Cigarette smoking; urban living; asbestos
Pathology	Squamous; small-cell; large-cell; adenocarcinoma
	Narrowing, obstruction and infection
	Spread via pleura, lymphatics, mediastinum, brachial plexus
Clinical features	General: weight loss, lassitude or metastases
	Local: chest pain, cough, haemotysis, Horner's syndrome
Investigations	Radiology, sputum cytology, bronchoscopy, biopsy
Treatment	Surgery (only about 20% operable)
	Pnemonectomy or lobectomy
Prognosis	30% five-year survival

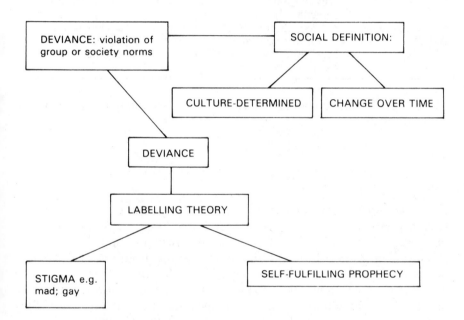

Fig. 16.1   Pattern system of note-taking: labelling theory.

during the lecture, using only the right-hand side of the paper. As soon as possible afterwards, the learner underlines the key words in the notes and then enters cues in the left-hand column, which will stimulate recall of the ideas in the notes. It is often a difficult exercise to think of appropriate cues, so the learner is required to reorganize and work through the material, which in itself encourages remembering. The third component is reciting the main material, using the cues in the left-hand column. The main material is kept covered and the learner recites out loud their own version of the lecture material. After this, the learner reflects on the content of the lecture and at this stage may add their own ideas and conclusions. The final stage is review, which should be done at regular intervals to assist long-term retention. An example is given in Table 16.7.

Table 16.7 Cornell system of note-taking: proliferative glomerulonephritis

Cues	Notes
Immune Streptococcus	*Aetiology*: Usually immune response following beta-haemolytic streptococcus infection 3 weeks before.
Swelling Antigen-antibody	*Pathology*: Affects glomerular capillaries, with swelling and proliferation of cells; deposits of antigen-antibody complexes on basement membrane.
Youngsters Febrile, Urine Oedema	*Clinical Features*: Children or young adults; oliguria, haematuria, proteinuria, facial oedema, pulmonary oedema, fever, headache, malaise, hypertension.
Urinalysis Biochemistry	*Investigations*: Urinalysis, renal function tests
Fluids, diet Pencillin	*Treatment*: Fluids restricted to 500 ml plus volume of previous day's output; diet; low protein 40 grams, low salt; penicillin; bed rest.
Rest ADL	*Nursing*: Bed rest until hypertension and haematuria disappear; assistance with activities of daily living i.e. hygiene, mouth care, movement, social contact, independence, etc.

This system has the advantage of avoiding the rewriting of notes, which is wasteful of time.

PARTICIPATING IN GROUP DISCUSSION AND SEMINARS

A key aim of units at undergraduate and postgraduate level is to foster students critical thinking abilities, and one way of doing this is to encourage them to participate actively in discussion and debate. They should be encouraged to venture opinions to the group, even if they are not entirely sure of their knowledge. The value of participation lies in stimulating other members of the group to challenge contributors' ideas, and students should try to keep an open mind about the issues they confront, even if they feel strongly one way or the other; this will allow them to evaluate the issue more objectively.

Not everyone likes group work, and students may feel that the same few people always dominate the discussion, so that others cannot get a word in. Unit leaders need to be alert to this, and be prepared to take steps to encourage the more silent members to contribute. Students must be encouraged to participate in group discussions during the units; it really is important that they experience the process of constructive criticism.

Seminar presentation involves speaking to the group on a particular topic, either chosen by the student or allocated by the tutor. Students may feel that this is a nervewracking experience, especially if they have not done anything like it before! Tutors can give guidance and tips to help students with seminar presentations as follows.

1. Prepare your material carefully, i.e. ensure that any visual materials are written large enough to be seen.

2. Make a brief plan of the presentation, so that you have the sequence in front of you (it is very disconcerting for you to lose your place).
3. Ensure that you have thoroughly understood the content of your material, you may be questioned about it by group members!
4. Prepare the classroom carefully beforehand, i.e. make sure that everyone can see the chalkboard/screen, etc.; ensure that the overhead projector is aligned carefully, with a full-sized image on the screen (if unsure how to do this, ask your tutor).
5. Remember, the aim of the seminar is that the group *learns* something from your presentation, i.e. do not bombard them with masses of information; use overhead projector or handouts for key points; allow sufficient time for note-taking.
6. Allow opportunities for *discussion*, i.e. the seminar is *not* about giving information, but should stimulate thinking and debate; keep formal information to a minimum; posing questions for the group to answer can stimulate debate.
7. Try to make your presentation serve two purposes, i.e. for the seminar and also as the basis of your unit assessment. This will ensure that you take the necessary care over the reading and preparation of the topic

PLANNING TO STUDY

Organizing the environment for study

It is important that books and materials can be left lying in the same place, since having to put them away and then take them out on another occasion can be very demotivating. A comfortable chair is crucial, with good support for the lumbar spine and the room should be at a comfortable temperature with adequate ventilation to offset fatigue. Daylight is the best form of illumination, but in the evenings it is good to have two light sources with adequate shading to prevent glare. Many students automatically switch on music when commencing study, as this makes the task less of a chore. However, music is a source of distracting input that will interfere with studying, so it is better to save music for the five-minute breaks in studying every hour or so.

Planning study time

Like most other activities in life, studying is facilitated by planning. A carefully prepared plan of study can eliminate the somewhat haphazard approach that tends to be common among students. To be really effective, study must be seen as a natural part of the student's life, just like meal times and other routines. Another aspect is the temptation to escape from the chore of study by using certain devices that may or may not be unconscious. For example, day-dreaming is a common occurrence during study and also frequent trips to make coffee, or some other ploy that takes one away from the 'unpleasant' situation. Boredom is another problem against which the student must fight, and it is good advice to suggest that he or she uses a pencil to make notes at regular intervals, thus aiding concentration and providing a feeling of 'getting somewhere'. Joining with a small group of students to examine a common problem can be a motivating activity from time to time and gives different perspectives to an aspect of study.

When planning for study it is important to include regular breaks so that fatigue is avoided. Stretching one's legs every hour or so will help keep concentration and make the subsequent study more efficient. It is unlikely that a period of study longer than about three hours will be useful at any one time and even this length may prove difficult. An interesting suggestion is given by Bandura (1977), which he terms 'self-reinforcement'. It involves setting oneself certain study goals and allocating a reward that is conditional upon attainment of these goals. For example, students might decide to study a particular section of a textbook until they could describe its content in their own words. The reward that they allocate could be a walk in the park, which can be taken only when the objective has been achieved.

METACOGNITIVE STUDY STRATEGIES

Metacognition is another word for reflection; it involves knowledge about one's own internal cognitive processes. We engage in metacognition when we realize that we are, for example, having difficulty remembering something, and there are certain strategies of metacognition that can help us to learn and study better.

Rehearsal

This is the silent repetition of sentences or words over and over again as a way of remembering them. It is a particularly important metacognitive strategy for retention of material and there are two closely related concepts that need to be considered also. Review involves going back over material that one has previously read and recitation is actually saying the material out loud.

Mnemonics

These are memory aids that involve mental strategies, the best-known ones involving rhymes such as 'Thirty days hath September . . .'. The cranial nerves have been remembered by generations of students using a rhyme beginning 'On old Olympus' towering tops . . .'

Table 16.8 shows the classification of disease and its application to the causes of haematuria. A very useful mnemonic for remembering the classification of disease is CTINMADII, pronounced 'see, tin, mad, eye-eye'. Each letter stands for a cause of disease and is often called the 'pathological sieve'. It can be seen that any disease or disorder can be recalled using this device, provided the student can remember the examples of each condition.

Table 16.8 Classification of disease and an example applied to haematuria

Cause	Definition	Application to haematuria
Congenital	Present at birth	Haemophilia
Traumatic	Injury	Ruptured kidney
Infectious	Due to microorganisms	Cystitis
Neoplastic	Tumours	Papilloma of bladder
Metabolic	Disorder of metabolism	Renal calculus
Allergic	Due to hypersensitivity	Glomerulonephritis
Degenerative	Due to ageing	Not applicable
Iatrogenic	Doctor-induced	Anticoagulants
Idiopathic	Cause unknown	Haematuria of unknown origin

Mnemonics can be visual, as in the case of imagery. Evidence suggests that by forming a mental picture or image we can remember items much better. For example, one can picture items associated with aspects of the home; one item may be hanging in the hall, another on the sofa. A more practical example in nursing is the use of images of patients one has nursed in the past. The student should try to recall a patient who had nursing problems and picture the care given. Narrative is a closely related idea, which consists of making up a story that links all the words one wishes to remember. In the example given above of classification of disease, the narrative might go as follows: 'A man went to SEA in a TIN because he got MAD when he and his partner didn't see EYE to EYE.'

SELF-ASSESSMENT

Self-testing can be a useful strategy for increasing retention of material and evidence for this is offered by Rothkopf (1970); Rothkopf and Johnson (1971). Rothkopf maintains that learning from written materials involves two processes, the first one being the study and inspection behaviours of the student. He calls these 'mathemagenic behaviours', i.e. behaviours that give birth to learning. The second process is the actual acquisition of learning of the subject matter. Rothkopf maintains that the study habits of students are fluid and can be constantly modified during study. He tested these ideas in a series of experiments involving the use of inserted questions into texts and found that the greatest facilitative effect on learning occurred when the questions were inserted after the material to which they related, i.e. post-questions. The implications for students are that the regular testing of study materials by the use of post-questions may well enhance learning.

ASSESSMENT TECHNIQUES

It is probably true to say that most students experience some mild anxiety over the course assessment requirements, and this is no bad thing if it motivates them to do well.

Approaching coursework assessment tasks

The most important single step in tackling the assessment is to read the assessment specification carefully. It is, unfortunately, a relatively common occurrence to find that a student has been referred on an assignment because he or she has not conformed to the assessment specification for that unit. No matter how scholarly or erudite an assignment is, it will not gain a pass grade unless it meets the specification for the unit. It is no good having 'the right answer to the wrong question'. When a student has thoroughly understood the assignment brief (if in doubt, it can be checked with the unit leader), they should ask themself the following questions:

1. Assuming that there is a choice of assignments, is it sufficiently motivating to pursue in preference to other relevant topics?
2. Is it manageable in terms of time and resources available to meet the deadline for handing in?
3. Are there sufficient references available to be able to demonstrate skilful use of the literature?

Reading for the assessment

When writing assignments it is vital to demonstrate the ability to use the literature with insight. Textbooks are a good starting point by providing an overview of the topic. Students should always check the date of publication, especially in books that have been reprinted several times. It is easy to misinterpret a current reprint date and assume that the book is quite new, whereas it may be several years old and therefore possibly out of date. Journals offer up to date articles on specific aspects of a topic, and usually contain an abstract from which the students can quickly tell whether or not the article is relevant to their study. Journal articles are also important as a source of criticism of other articles or theories. Journals often run consecutive editions containing 'blasts and counter-blasts' from contributors with opposing viewpoints, and these provide fascinating insights into critical, analytic argument. The literature of philosophy is often overlooked by nursing students, but can be extremely useful in providing insights into issues such as values, beliefs, judgements, freedom of choice, etc. The mass media is also a useful source of reference, i.e. newspapers, radio and television. There are many excellent articles/programmes relating to health matters, and these tend to address current, controversial issues.

Writing coursework assessments

It is the coursework assessments, along with clinical assessments and examinations, that enable students to demonstrate achievement of the learning outcomes of their course units. Most students will require some help with the formulation of their assignments, particularly if they have not had recent experience of study.

Composing an essay-type assignment

Composing an essay involves four main processes (Humes, 1983):

1. *Planning* This takes more time than any other process, and includes not only the initial planning before commencement of writing, but the constant planning that goes on throughout the composition. Planning includes the organization and generation of content and the sequencing of goals.
2. *Translating* This is the transformation of thoughts into written form and consists of complex mental activities such as attending to syntax and structure.
3. *Reviewing* Writers engage in retrospective activities to check if their written ideas are actually what was intended. It also serves to re-orientate the writer for the next section.
4. *Revising* This covers editing of the written material and usually results in the production of a second draft, although much editing can occur during the initial draft.

Essay-type assignments vary enormously in their approach, from the standard essay question to case studies and problem-centred assignments. However, it is possible to draw a few general guidelines for students to consider. Essays must be written in prose, not in note form, with sentences of appropriate length and the sensible use of paragraphs. Great store is attached to legibility and clarity of expression in all educational systems, so careful planning is required beforehand. Even under examination conditions it is important to do a brief plan before attempting to write an answer to ensure that all the main aspects have been considered for inclusion. The length of an assignment must be clearly indicated by the teachers and any minimum and maximum length strictly adhered to. It is quite unfair to state that an assignment has a maximum of 3,000 words and then to accept ones that are perhaps twice this long. Students who stuck to the limit are then, in effect, penalized as the others will have included much more material in their work. Strict attention must be paid to the wording of the assignment; there is an ever-present temptation to interpret the question or title in the way the student would like it to be phrased, rather than how it actually is phrased. Students should use fluorescent highlighter pens to identify the key words in the question or title, since these dictate the form of response required. Table 16.9 gives a list of common terms and their meaning.

It is well worth spending time initially on designing the overall structure of the assignment, as a good assignment can be weakened by a poor or incoherent structure. Whilst there is no ideal or standard structure, it may be helpful to offer the student a basic pattern as shown in Table 16.10.

Word processing is the answer to students problems when editing the final draft for submission. With this technology they can move paragraphs

Table 16.9 Common terms used in assessment

ANALYSE	Literally, breaking-up the issue into its constituent parts and describing them in detail.
ASSESS	Estimate the pros and cons of the issue and give a judgement on these.
COMPARE AND CONTRAST	Show the similarities and differences between the concepts
DEFINE	Show the exact meaning of the concept
DESCRIBE	Give a picture of an object or event without judgement.
DISCUSS	Give viewpoints from both sides and then round off with own conclusion based on these.
LIST	Write down in tabular form with minimum words.
OUTLINE	A general overview without fine detail.
STATE	Present the points briefly without elaboration.

Table 16.10 Typical structure of an essay assignment

1. Title
2. Introduction
   - Focus of assignment
   - Problem or issue
   - Context
   - Literature review
3. Main body
   - Description
   - Analysis/argument
   - Synthesis/argument
   - Evaluation
4. Conclusions
   - Review of issues
   - Student's opinions in the light of the foregoing discussion
   - Recommendations if appropriate
5. References
   - Use standard system of referencing, e.g. Harvard
6. Appendix   Useful for documents that could not be included fully in the text for want of space, but which would provide useful information for the reader.

around, or insert and delete until they are happy with the result. Handwritten assignments do not easily allow for alterations without a great deal of re-writing, so it might be worth their while to acquire word processing skills. Tutors can offer useful advice and tips on editing:

1. Check the number of words (do a spellcheck on WP); it is normal to accept 'plus or minus 10%' of the required word length, i.e. if the assignment is 2500 words, then an acceptable range would be 2250–2750 words. If you go outside these boundaries you may well find that your marks are adversely affected. It is more difficult to write concisely, and therefore students would be unfairly advantaged if they were allowed to exceed the word length by a significant amount.

2. Avoid 'padding' your assignment with materials that are not strictly relevant to the topic. Students are often tempted to include material in the appendix just because it is readily available from their institution. Any material in the appendix must be referred to in the main text, and must have a substantial contribution to make to the assignment.
3. Carry out a final check against the unit assessment specification to ensure that all aspects have been addressed.
4. It is imperative that careful attention is paid to the procedures for handing-in of your assignment.
5. Always keep a copy of the assignment. In the very best systems there is always the possibility of a mishap, and an assignment may occasionally go astray. It is heartbreaking if this occurs and you have not kept a copy.

Revising for examinations

Examinations are virtually confined to pre-registration programmes in nursing and midwifery education, and are often perceived by students as the most stressful aspect of a course. It is crucial that students commence revision as early as possible if stress is to be minimized, and the regular review of lecture notes will help. Again, planning is the key to effective revision, with objectives and deadlines for each week, but in the case of examination revision, motivation is of paramount importance. The use of study groups for revision can provide excellent motivation and in addition, the presence of other students who feel equally ignorant can be very reassuring. Frequent changes of stimulus can help combat staleness and the use of a learning resources centre with audio-visual aids may provide a welcome change from reading. It cannot be over-emphasized that cramming is a very inefficient and risky business, as the high levels of stress that develop close to the examination act to impair the learning performance.

Examination technique

Sitting for an examination requires a degree of self-control, since panic can so easily undermine an otherwise well-prepared candidate. If the examination consists of an unseen paper, the candidate will not be allowed to take any resources into the examination room other than those for writing and drawing. The instructions for filling in the answer book should be noted. On the first scan of the paper, the student should carefully note the number of questions to be answered, the parts from which they should each be selected if relevant, and the amount of time to be allocated to each. It is wise to allocate an equal amount of time to each question, including an allowance at the end of the examination to go back over and check the answers. The students should be advised to scan the questions and to select the one which they feel most confident about. Once writing begins anxiety levels should fall, and the students will be able to choose subsequent questions in a more rational frame of mind. Students should be advised to make a brief plan before commencing a question, as this can ensure that all necessary elements of the answer have been considered. This plan can then act as a prompt when the writing begins to flow. It is important that a careful watch is kept on the time, as it is all too easy to overrun on the easier questions, leaving a shortfall for the more difficult ones. During the last five minutes or so, the student should read through all answers, adding brief points that were missed the first time. As a final check the student should ensure that all papers are properly identified according to the instructions.

Undertaking objective tests

Objective tests seem to have gone out of fashion over the past few years, but some institutions may still use them. Students should be given careful guidance about how to approach objective tests:

1. Read the instructions for the test carefully, especially those concerned with completion of the answer sheet.
2. Check the procedure for changing an answer.
3. Check if the test has a correction-for-guessing built into the marking, as this will make it advisable to avoid guessing.
4. Work quickly through the test, completing only those items which can be answered easily.
5. Return to the beginning and attempt the next level of difficulty, again leaving the items which require a great deal of thought.
6. Finally, spend the remaining time on the difficult items; keep a careful watch for negative items, as these may easily be overlooked.

REFERENCES

Anderson, J. (1980) *Cognitive Psychology and Its Implications*, Freeman, San Francisco.

Bandura, A. (1977) *Social Learning Theory*, Prentice-Hall, Englewood Cliffs, New Jersey.

CNAA (1989) *CNAA Handbook*, Council for National Academic Awards, London.

Dansereau, D. (1978) The development of a learning strategies curriculum, *Learning Strategies*, (ed. H.F. O'Neil), Academic Press, New York.

Dunn, R. and Dunn, K. (1978) *Teaching Students through their Individual Learning Styles: A Practical Approach*, Reston Publishing Co, Reston Va.

Dunn, R., Dunn, K. and Price, G. (1984) *Learning Style Inventory Research Manual*, Lawrence, PO Box 3271, Kansas.

Entwistle, N. (1981) *Styles of Learning and Teaching*, John Wiley, Chichester.

Entwistle, N., Hanley, M. and Hounsell, D. (1979) Identifying distinctive approaches to studying. *Higher Education*, **8**, 365–80.

Flesch, R. (1974) *The Art of Readable Writing*, Harper and Row, New York.

Honey, P. (1982) *The Manual of Learning Styles*, Honey and Mumford, Maidenhead.

Howe, M. (1984) *A Teacher's Guide to the Psychology of Learning*, Blackwell, Oxford.

Humes, A. (1983) Research on the composing process. *Review of Educational Research*, **53** (2), 201–16.

Kagan, J. (1965) Reflection-impulsivity and reading ability in primary grade children. *Child Development*, **36** (3), 188–90.

Kintsch, W. and Van Dijk, T. (1978) Toward a model of text comprehension and production. *Psychological Review*, **85**, 363–94.

Kolb, D. (1976) *The Learning Style Inventory: Technical Manual*, McBer and Co, Boston.

Marton, F. and Saljo, R. (1976) On qualitative differences in learning. 1. Outcome and process. *British Journal of Educational Psychology*, **46**, 4–11.

Nisbet, J. and Shucksmith, J. (1986) *Learning Strategies*, Routledge and Kegan Paul, London.

Parlett, M. (1970) The syllabus-bound student, in *The Ecology of Human Intelligence*, (ed. Hudson), Penguin, Harmondsworth.

Pask, G. (1975) *The Cybernetics of Human Learning and Performance*, Hutchinson, London.

Pask, G. (1976) Styles and strategies of learning. *British Journal of Educational Psychology*, **46**, 128–48.

Pask, G. and Scott, B. (1972) Learning strategies and individual competence. *International Journal of Man–Machine Studies*, **4**, 217–53.

Robinson, F. (1946) *Effective Study*, Harper, New York.

Rogers, C. (1969) *Freedom to Learn*, Charles Merrill, Ohio.

Rothkopf, E. (1970) The concept of mathemagenic activities. *Review of Educational Research*, **40**, 325–36.

Rothkopf, E. and Johnson, P. (1971) *Verbal Learning Research and The Technology of Written Instruction*, Teachers College Press, New York.

Tennant, M. (1988) *Psychology and Adult Learning*, Routledge, New York.

Witkin, H. (1977) Field dependent and field independent cognitive styles and their educational implications. *Review of Educational Research*, **47**, 1–64.

17 Teaching biology and psychology in nursing and midwifery

The biological and social sciences are significant contributory disciplines to the study of nursing and midwifery, and are mainly represented in curricula by human biology, microbiology, pathology, pharmacology, medicine, surgery, psychology and sociology. In Colleges of Nursing these subjects have been taught almost entirely by the transmission mode of teaching. In the past two or three years, however, the linking or incorporation of Colleges of Nursing and Midwifery with HE has given access to biology and psychology laboratories, along with the services of specialist lecturers and technicians. This opens up opportunities for teaching biology and psychology in the same way that professionals of these disciplines have studied it, namely, by practical experiments, research and enquiry. By definition, enquiry involves active participation by the student, one of the hallmarks of experiential learning as outlined in Chapter 7. Over-reliance on didactic techniques of information giving leads the student to believe that the information contains fixed, immutable truths and this does little to prepare them for changes in knowledge as science advances.

THE NATURE OF BIOLOGICAL CONCEPTS

An overview of the nature of concepts was given in Chapter 3 (p. 47) and the principles will be applied to biology in this section.

Modes of representation

Concepts are acquired as a result of interaction with the environment and are the basis of knowledge. It is suggested that there are three ways of knowing something (Bruner, Olver and Greenfield, 1966) and that these ways emerge during childhood development in a given order. The first of these is called the 'enactive mode of representation' and involves 'knowing by doing something', such as manipulating objects in the environment. The second is the 'iconic mode', which involves making images either visually or via the other senses and storing these in the

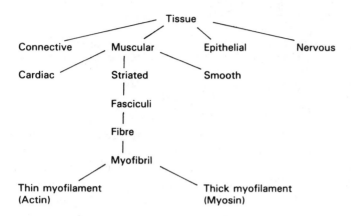

Fig. 17.1 Hierarchy of the concept 'muscular tissue'.

mind. The third mode is called the 'symbolic mode' and as the name suggests, is concerned with the symbols of language as a means of making sense of the world. Bruner, Olver and Greenfield suggest that these three modes continue to be used throughout life as a means of representing knowledge.

A principle can be defined as a relationship between two or more concepts (Klausmeier, 1985) and is also termed a rule. In order to understand a principle, it is necessary to understand its constituent concepts.

Concepts form hierarchies, with the most general, inclusive ones at the top and the more specific ones beneath. Figure 17.1 illustrates this, taking the concept 'muscular tissue' as an example. This concept clusters with similar concepts of tissue, i.e. 'connective', 'epithelial' and 'nervous' tissues at one level and the hierarchical nature of the concept is shown by the ever-increasing detail of each successive subordinate concept. Thus 'striated muscle' is a more general concept than 'fasciculi', which in turn is more general than the concept 'fibre'.

There are three stages in learning a concept (Gagne, 1985): discrimination, generalization and abstraction.

1. Discrimination The student must first 'discriminate' between two stimuli, one that is an example of the concept and one that is not. In the Operating Department, a nurse may have to learn the concept 'retractor' and the discrimination phase involves showing the nurse a retractor and a pair of tissue forceps until he or she can identify the retractor correctly.

2. Generalization The second stage involves presenting the nurse with a number of other surgical instruments, all of which differ from retractors and asking him or her to discriminate between the original retractor and these other instruments. This is generalization of the original discrimination learning.

3. Abstraction In the final stage of concept formation, a number of different retractors are presented along with a variety of non-retractors

Table 17.1 Sequence for teaching a concept by deductive method

1. Define the concept to the student.
2. Show an example of the concept, or a representation of it.
3. Give two different examples of the concept along with two non-examples and check the student's discrimination.
4. Help the student to identify the critical attributes of the concept.
5. Give novel examples to check concept attainment.

and the student's ability to identify which are retractors shows that he or she has 'abstracted out' the relevant qualities of the concept. To check on the concept attainment, we now present the nurse with a new example of a retractor that has not been seen before. If the nurse can identify this, we can say that he or she has acquired the concept of 'retractor'.

Inductive and deductive teaching

There are two main ways of teaching concepts, deductively and inductively. When teaching a concept deductively, the teacher begins by giving a definition of the concept and then follows this up with a number of examples. Thus, when teaching the concept of 'cell' a definition would be given, followed by a number of examples of various cells such as nerve cells, epithelial cells and so on. Examples would also be given of non-cells to aid discrimination of the concept. Table 17.1 summarizes the sequence for teaching a concept by the deductive method.

When teaching a concept inductively, the teacher first gives a number of examples of the concept and then draws out from the student the definition of the concept. The teacher might begin with descriptions of a number of patients, some grossly overweight, some extremely thin, others with specific nervous disorders. The students then try to ascertain any factors common to all the examples, eventually coming up with a definition of the concept 'malnutrition'. Much of the subject matter of the biological sciences involves higher-order concepts such as osmosis and homeostasis, so it is first necessary for the teacher to break these down into their constituent subordinate concepts. This 'analysis of the concept' is a crucial stage in preparation for teaching, without which the teacher cannot hope to simplify the explanation. A useful way of doing this is to use 'concept-mapping', in which the central concept is represented diagrammatically with the relevant related concepts pictured around it as in Figure 17.2.

THE LECTURE METHOD

Although probably overused as a strategy for teaching biological concepts, lectures still have a place in the facilitation of meaningful learning. However, the points made in Chapter 6 about lecturing should be borne in mind when planning the session, particularly with regard to sequencing

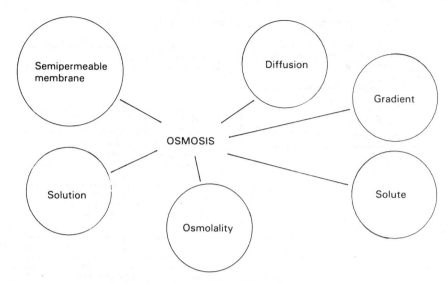

Fig. 17.2 Concept-mapping for a lesson on osmosis.

and interaction. Sequencing needs careful planning in order to lead the students from one concept to another in a logical order and the use of flow diagrams such as Figure 17.3 can be very useful.

Lecturing by the 'structure and related function' approach

This approach involves an inductive style of lecturing, which draws out the students' existing knowledge and stimulates thinking skills. It has a certain crossword type of appeal and can be used to teach a topic for the first time, or for revision and consolidation prior to examinations.

Table 17.2 shows the basic matrix for this approach, which can be used to study any organ of the body. If the subject is being introduced to a class for the first time, then the teacher may wish to provide the information in a normal lecture manner for the column headed 'Structure'. The related functions can then be elicited from the students using inductive techniques and these functions can often be worked out even though the students have no prior knowledge of them. This has the effect of making the students discover, by reasoning, the related functions of an organ. These are written down in the 'Related function' column, opposite the structure to which they refer. Table 17.3 is an example that shows the matrix being applied to study of the heart. The section on macroscopic structure only has been completed to give the reader an idea of how the matrix works.

Use of this approach is also beneficial to the teacher, as it quickly reveals any weaknesses in their own knowledge of the subject. It also provides a basis for the students' individual study of an organ. It can be varied by transposing the columns and asking the students to work out how the structure is designed to carry out each function. For example, the following questions might be asked during the study of the heart: 'What properties would you include in a design for the lining of the heart? What

Blood flow through any vessel is determined by two main factors:

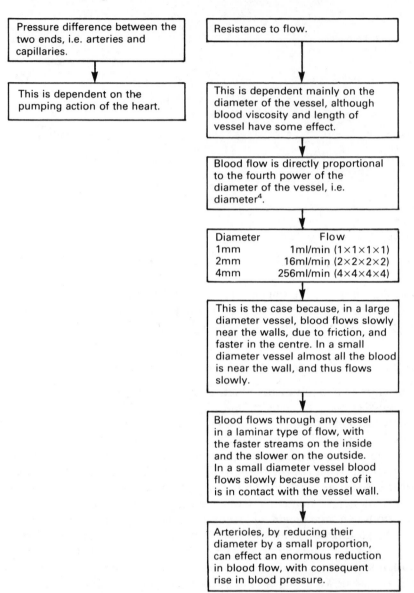

Pressure difference between the two ends, i.e. arteries and capillaries.	Resistance to flow.
↓	↓
This is dependent on the pumping action of the heart.	This is dependent mainly on the diameter of the vessel, although blood viscosity and length of vessel have some effect.

Blood flow is directly proportional to the fourth power of the diameter of the vessel, i.e. diameter^4.

Diameter	Flow
1mm	1ml/min (1×1×1×1)
2mm	16ml/min (2×2×2×2)
4mm	256ml/min (4×4×4×4)

This is the case because, in a large diameter vessel, blood flows slowly near the walls, due to friction, and faster in the centre. In a small diameter vessel almost all the blood is near the wall, and thus flows slowly.

Blood flows through any vessel in a laminar type of flow, with the faster streams on the inside and the slower on the outside. In a small diameter vessel blood flows slowly because most of it is in contact with the vessel wall.

Arterioles, by reducing their diameter by a small proportion, can effect an enormous reduction in blood flow, with consequent rise in blood pressure.

Fig. 17.3 Flow diagram for sequencing a lesson on haemodynamics.

materials would you use?' This will hopefully elicit such things as smoothness, anticoagulant properties and simple squamous epithelium.

Lecturing by the 'inductive build-up' approach

This is quite a useful approach, particularly for revision purposes, when a variety of applied anatomy and physiology needs to be consolidated. It is

Table 17.2 Matrix for 'structure and related function' approach

	Structure	Related function
Organ		
Position and boundaries		
Macroscopic structure		
Microscopic structure		
Blood supply		
Lymphatics		
Nerve supply		
Anatomical relations		

Table 17.3 Section of completed matrix for heart

	Structure	Related function
Macroscopic	MYOCARDIUM: middle layer of cardiac muscle; contains areas of specialized cardiac muscle	Acts as a syncytium, cells all contract as one; has property of myogenic rhythm
Microscopic	SINU-ATRIAL NODE: in right atrium, called pacemaker ATRIO-VENTRICULAR NODE: in right atrium; very small diameter fibres	Has fastest rate of self-excitation; initiates impulse. Delays passage of impulse down bundle until atria have contracted

almost entirely done by inducing from the students their knowledge, except when the teacher has to clarify or correct a statement. An example of this approach is that of the renal blood supply and its application to nursing. I begin by drawing the abdominal aorta on the chalkboard, with the renal artery branching off it. From this point the students are invited to contribute the subsequent branches from the hilum to the entire kidney and back again. The renal blood supply is not too difficult to understand, but surprisingly enough tends to be ignored in many curricula, apart from the glomerular components. Thus the interlobar, arcuate and interlobular

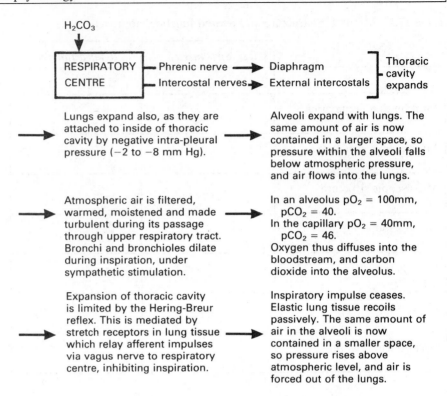

H_2CO_3

RESPIRATORY CENTRE — Phrenic nerve → Diaphragm ⎤ Thoracic cavity expands
— Intercostal nerves → External intercostals ⎦

Lungs expand also, as they are attached to inside of thoracic cavity by negative intra-pleural pressure (-2 to -8 mm Hg). → Alveoli expand with lungs. The same amount of air is now contained in a larger space, so pressure within the alveoli falls below atmospheric pressure, and air flows into the lungs.

Atmospheric air is filtered, warmed, moistened and made turbulent during its passage through upper respiratory tract. Bronchi and bronchioles dilate during inspiration, under sympathetic stimulation. → In an alveolus $pO_2 = 100$mm, $pCO_2 = 40$. In the capillary $pO_2 = 40$mm, $pCO_2 = 46$. Oxygen thus diffuses into the bloodstream, and carbon dioxide into the alveolus.

Expansion of thoracic cavity is limited by the Hering-Breur reflex. This is mediated by stretch receptors in lung tissue which relay afferent impulses via vagus nerve to respiratory centre, inhibiting inspiration. → Inspiratory impulse ceases. Elastic lung tissue recoils passively. The same amount of air in the alveoli is now contained in a smaller space, so pressure rises above atmospheric level, and air is forced out of the lungs.

Fig. 17.4   Sequence for 'inductive build-up approach' as applied to respiration.

arteries are often omitted, yet this complexity of supply is very important for the understanding of such questions as 'Why does the kidney undergo acute tubular necrosis when a patient becomes severely hypotensive?' and 'Why do the surgeons perform a nephrectomy for a ruptured kidney?' Application to the clinical setting can be elicited at each stage of the build-up and many misapprehensions clarified. For example, I commonly find that students draw both the afferent and the efferent arterioles the same size, whereas the glomerular filtration pressure can only be maintained if the efferent vessel is of smaller calibre.

This approach works quite well with the respiratory system to illustrate the sequence of events during respiration. The technique is similar, in that the students are invited to contribute their ideas about the sequence, commencing with the cells of the respiratory centre in the medulla responding to the level of carbonic acid in the blood perfusing them. Figure 17.4 shows this sequence as it might appear at the end of such a session, on the chalkboard or overhead projector roll. Again, I find that the fine detail helps to clarify any mistaken ideas. The fact that the bronchi and bronchioles dilate during inspiration and constrict during expiration provides the explanation as to why the patient with bronchial asthma has more difficulty breathing out than breathing in. The normal constriction during expiration is accentuated by the triad of spasm, oedema and secretion.

Lecturing using interspersed questions

The work of Ernst Rothkopf was outlined in Chapter 16 (p. 391) in connection with study skills and the following is an account of an experiment I carried out on student nurses, using the notions suggested by Rothkopf's work (Quinn, 1984). The study concentrated on a class of 53 student nurses in their first year of training as registered general nurses. The students were randomly assigned to one of three experimental groups and given a lecture entitled 'Shock and Haemorrhage'. The first group received the traditional lecture only; the second group received the lecture plus interspersed questions at the end of each subsection of the topic; the third group received the lecture plus an 'advance organizer' at the beginning. A test of 'delayed retention of general understanding and detailed knowledge' about the lecture was administered three weeks later and results showed a significantly higher score for the group who were given interspersed questions during the lecture.

Table 17.4 shows the outline lesson plan for the group given interspersed questions. The superior scores for this group tend to support the notion of Rothkopf that inserted questions following sections of prose text facilitate learning. On the other hand, it is possible that novelty may account for the superiority in scores, or the effect of having students review each subsection may be the main reason. What is important, though, is that the role of questioning during a lecture needs to be looked

Table 17.4 Outline lesson plan on shock and haemorrhage, showing interspersed questions

Introduction
This afternoon we are going to look at shock and haemorrhage. At several points in the lecture I am going to ask you questions. Please don't shout out the answers: think about the answers and I will invite one of you to share it with us.
Definition of shock syndrome   *OHP*

Three major groups of causes
(i) Cardiac   (ii) Venous pooling   (iii) Hypovolaemic
Further details of each   *OHP*
Question 1   How would a myocardial infarction cause shock?
Question 2   A patient returns from theatre to the ward. What class of
                  haemorrhage might occur within the next twelve hours?

Stages of shock
Compensatory; progressive; irreversible   *OHP*
Question 5   How does the body cope in the compensatory stage of shock?
Question 6   In the progressive stage, what damage occurs in the body?

Patient management and care
Observations; treatment; nursing   *OHP*
Question 7   How is shock generally treated?
Question 8   What observations would lead you to believe that a patient was
                  developing shock?

at very carefully by the teacher and more detailed planning done for this element.

Lecturing using 'advance organizers'

In Chapter 3 (p. 65) an outline of the work of David Ausubel was given and his notion of an advance organizer was described (Ausabel *et al.*, 1978) In my experiment referred to above, one of the variables was the use of an advance organizer. The third group of student nurses was given the traditional lecture, preceded by an advance organizer formulated in accordance with Ausubel's principles. An advance organizer must contain all the concepts that will follow in the lecture, but at a much greater level of generality and inclusiveness. It is like an abstract of the key points of the lecture, but in addition, it must contain specific links with the student's existing knowledge about the topic. In order to show the advance organizer, it is necessary to show the subject-matter sequence from which the organizer is designed.

Table 17.5 gives the sequence of subject-matter notes as written on the overhead projector for the lecture. This sequence of material for the lecture forms the basis of the advance organizer. I had already given some lectures to the entire group on the normal structure and function of the circulatory system and this knowledge was used in the organizer to bridge the gap between what they already knew and the new information to be given in the lecture. The advance organizer in Table 17.6 is in the form which it was given to the students.

It can be seen that the advance organizer contains material that links what the student already knows to the new information given in the lecture. This should serve as scaffolding for the detailed information that will follow in the lecture. In the aforementioned study, the group given the advance organizer did not do significantly better than the control group on the test of delayed retention. The efficacy of advance organizers has not been fully established. Barnes and Clawson (1975) reviewed 32 studies involving the use of advance organizers and found that 12 reported significant effects and 20 were non-significant.

BIOMEDICAL TERMINOLOGY

One of the most daunting aspects of biological science confronting the student nurse is the incredibly complex language of biomedical terminology. Dallas (1981) suggests that it is like being confronted with a totally unintelligible form of communication out of reach of the vocabulary of ordinary people in society. This 'language of the priesthood' must be mastered by student nurses before they can understand the concepts upon which their practice is based. However, a student may also know the word for something without understanding the concept it represents. The role of the nurse teacher is to make this unfamiliar language meaningful to the student so that it can be remembered and recalled when required. The

Table 17.5 Sequence of subject-matter for a lecture on shock and haemorrhage

Definition of shock syndrome
General inadequacy of blood flow throughout the body leading to tissue damage.

Three major groups of causes
1. Cardiac shock: due to failure of the heart-muscle pump
2. Venous pooling shock: due to blood pooling in the veins
3. Hypovolaemic shock: due to loss of blood volume

Further details of causes
Cardiac shock: acute heart failure e.g. myocardial infarction, causes fall in blood pressure and cardiac output. This in turn reduces oxygen to the heart causing further weakening – a vicious circle!
Venous pooling shock: blood volume is normal but veins lose their tone; this results in dilatation and pooling of blood so that there is insufficient venous return to the heart. Fainting and anaphylaxis are examples of this type of shock.
Hypovolaemic shock: blood volume is decreased due to burns or haemorrhage.

Haemorrhage
Severity depends upon amount of blood lost and speed with which it occurs.
Haemorrhage can be: acute or chronic;
                     arterial, venous or capillary;
                     primary, reactionary or secondary.

Stages of shock
Compensatory stage: veins constrict and reservoir of blood maintains normal venous return to heart; patient is not in imminent danger as condition will correct itself.
Progressive stage: if shock becomes severe, then it promotes more shock by damaging the heart, vital centres, small blood vessels and enzymes in tissues.
Irreversible stage: here extreme damage has occurred because shock has been present for a long time; no amount of treatment will save the patient's life.

Patient management and care
Observations: pulse and blood pressure – regular observation for rising pulse and falling blood pressure; respirations rapid; appearance is pale and clammy; falling central venous pressure.
Treatment: according to cause, but general principles are intravenous fluid or blood transfusion; drugs such as dopamine hydrochloride.

Nursing care
Assistance with all activities of daily living.

Table 17.6 Advance organizer for lecture on shock and haemorrhage.

In previous sessions you have examined the components of the circulatory system. These are the heart, blood and blood vessels. Effective circulation is necessary for adequate functioning of tissues and organs. Ineffective circulation can arise from disorders of any of the three components of the system, and is termed 'shock'. Shock can lead to specific damage to tissues and organs. It is not a static condition but can progress through a series of stages which, if untreated, can lead to death. Management of the patient involves careful observation, administration of intravenous fluids, and the use of drugs.

Table 17.7 Biomedical terms and their literal meanings

Graeco-Roman word	Literal meaning
Physiotherapy	healing by nature
Physiology	science of nature
Epithelium	upon the nipple
Pupil	little doll
Nausea	seasickness
Atheroma	porridge-like tumour
Syndrome	running together
Scaphoid	boat-shaped
Lumen	light
Acetabulum	vinegar cup
Epididymis	upon the twins
Eosinophil	dawn, to love
Ectopic	out of place
Sagittal	arrow
Coronal	crown
Trochanter	to run
Ischaemia	to check
Sesamoid	sesame seed
Coccyx	cuckoo-beak
Reticulum	little net
Hemiplegia	blow to half
Collagen	glue
Decubitus	lie on one elbow
Pathology	science of suffering
Malaria	bad air
Hypochondriac	below the cartilages
Hysteria	womb
Fontanelle	little fountain
Hypercapnia	high level of smoke (CO_2)

best way to help students remember material is to link it to what they already know, but the problem with biomedical terminology is that there may be no existing knowledge with which to link the new terminology. One way to overcome this problem is to use the literal meanings of the Graeco-Roman terms as a link to their everyday lives. The word 'acetabulum' has no meaning to a student in its existing form, but its literal translation is 'vinegar cup' which conjures up a meaningful picture in the students' minds related to acetic acid in vinegar. Table 17.7 gives a list of biomedical terms and their literal translation, which might give students a more meaningful way of remembering the terms. It may also give a glimpse of the richness of language in the dim-and-distant past, alas now largely forgotten.

LABORATORY ACTIVITIES

The importance of practical biology sessions cannot be over-emphasized. They provide opportunities for students to become actively involved in their own learning and also help to foster a spirit of enquiry about the subject-matter. Practical sessions can be very motivating, particularly when students are using their own bodies as in blood-grouping experiments; few people in life have the opportunity to examine their own blood cells under a microscope and to see these for the first time is a unique experience in itself. Dissection of animal organs provides a three-dimensional perspective totally different from that in two-dimensional textbook pictures; it also allows learning by touch, which is particularly insightful in the case of the smooth endocardial lining of the heart.

The linking of nurse education with HE means that the opportunity now exists for practical work in biology laboratories equipped and serviced for this function. The practical biology activities described below are much less sophisticated than those in HE, and are included only for those institutions that have no alternative access to laboratory facilities.

Organizing laboratory activities

The most important factor here is the Health and Safety at Work Act and the teacher must ensure that all the necessary precautions have been taken to make the environment safe for the students. Protective clothing must always be worn and blood-contaminated materials must be disposed of in the proper manner and in accordance with the regulations concerning prevention of transmissions of Acquired Immune Deficiency Syndrome (AIDS). The maximum number of students per teacher is about twelve to allow for adequate supervision.

Teaching by dissection of animal organs

Animal organs such as heart and kidneys are easily obtainable from commercial butchers, but superior specimens for dissection are best obtained from specialized biological suppliers. It is worth asking students before doing dissection if anyone has objections from an 'animal rights' point of view. Table 17.8 gives guidelines for the dissection of a sheep heart.

Practical haematology

Making a blood film

This can be a very motivating activity for students because it involves them in looking at their own blood cells under a microscope. Before commencing the film, students must be taught how to use a microscope, with emphasis on the use of high- and low-power magnification and the fine and coarse adjustment of focus. Table 17.9 gives guidelines for conducting a session on blood films. Of course blood-letting must always be an optional activity, with no coercion.

Table 17.8 Dissection of a sheep heart

Requirements
Trays, dissection forceps, scissors, cannulae for coronary arteries, syringe, probe or orange sticks, container of water, disposal bags.

Procedure
The following procedure can be given as a list of instructions to the students.

1. *Observe* the external appearance of the heart, noting visceral pericardium.
2. *Ascertain* the anterior surface of the heart.
3. *Locate* the right and left atria and ventricles.
4. *Identify* the mitral and tricuspid valves.
5. *Identify* the aorta and pulmonary artery.
6. *Locate* the mouths of the coronary arteries.
7. *Cannulate* the coronary arteries, injecting 5 ml of water forcibly into artery, noting the course of the coronary arteries over the surface of the heart.
8. *Introduce* water into each atrium. Holding the heart in palm of hand, squeeze gently at base in a rhythmical fashion. Note the opening and closure of the atrio-ventricular valves.
9. *Open* the right atrium with scissors, cutting along the lateral border. Note the following: atrial appendage, opening of coronary sinus, pectinate muscle, orifices of superior and inferior venae cavae, fossa ovalis, endocardium.
10. *Open* the right ventricle, cutting down lateral wall. Note: pulmonary valve, tricuspid valve, chordae tendinae, papillary muscles, trabeculae carnae, moderator band.
11. *Open* the left atrium, comparing it with the right atrium. Note entry of pulmonary veins.
12. *Open* the left ventricle, cutting down lateral wall. Note: interventricular septum, thickness of muscle wall, mitral valve, chordae and papillary muscles, trabeculae carnae.

Students should be encouraged to bring textbooks to the dissection, looking up any structures which they cannot identify from memory. Details of pathology can be discussed in relation to the structure identified.

Table 17.9 Making a blood film

Requirements
Glass slides, with one corner cut off, 70% meth, lancets, Leishmann stain, distilled water, microscope.

Procedure
Place a small drop of blood at one end of the slide.
Spread the blood evenly by drawing a second glass slide backwards and forwards over the first slide. (The missing corner allows some white cells to remain in centre of slide.) Allow the slide to dry in the air, then stain with Leishmann stain for one minute. Wash in distilled water and blot dry on filter paper.
The student is requested to identify the various cells on the slide under low and high power. This could form the basis of small-group discussion on the types and proportion of blood cells in the body.

Blood grouping

The concept of blood groups and compatibility is one of the most difficult ones to teach in the whole of biological sciences, so the use of practical activities can be of great help in promoting understanding. The simplest way of doing practical blood-grouping is to use commercially-available blood-grouping kits, consisting of cards impregnated with anti-serum plus pipettes, lancets and alcohol swabs. The teacher need only provide de-ionized water and follow the instructions contained in the kits. Students work in pairs, one using the swab and lancet to obtain three drops of blood from the other. A drop is placed on each of three circles on the card, and mixed carefully with the stick provided. The three circles are impregnated respectively with anti-A serum, anti-B and the third is a control. Students can then see if agglutination occurs in one or more of the circles.

The follow-up to this activity is important, as it is here that the students must work out what their blood group is. I use a series of cards backed with magnetic tape for use on a metal board, to represent the normal state of agglutinogens and agglutinins in the plasma. Each card represents an agglutinogen or an agglutinin and is shaped so that they fit into each other to indicate agglutination. Students can manipulate these concrete representations until they have worked out their group and can continue to work out the effects of different kinds of blood transfusion on any given donor. Figure 17.5 illustrates this system.

When students have the opportunity to manipulate these cards they can use the enactive mode of representation to make sense of the complex concept of blood grouping. The key to understanding transfusions and compatibility is contained within one key principle as follows: 'In blood transfusions it is the *plasma* of the *recipient* that affects the *corpuscles* of the *donor*.' This statement is necessary to explain the direction of the reaction, as students are invariably confused by the two-way nature of incompatibility. Very rarely the opposite reaction occurs, as in a massive blood transfusion where the amount of plasma in the donated blood may cause agglutination of the recipient corpuscles.

Using physiological experiments

These are designed to encourage enquiry on the part of the student and Table 17.10 shows examples of simple experiments that require little or no equipment.

Using 'gaming' techniques

There is a variety of gaming techniques available in teaching biological concepts, most of them marketed commercially. Card-games and board-games concerned with such topics as the functions of the liver can be a novel way of learning factual material. Quiz competitions may also provide an element of novelty whilst using competition as a motivator.

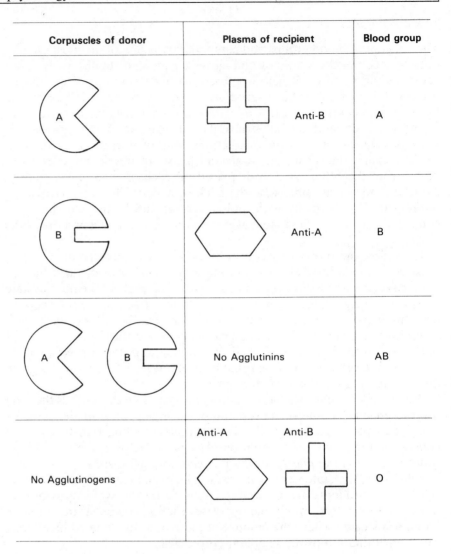

Fig. 17.5 Concrete representation of classical blood groups.

One such strategy is 'University Challenge'. I have found the use of this type of quiz useful for revision sessions prior to important examinations. The game is played with rules similar to the television game. Two teams of four students play each other, with a question master providing the questions and with starters and bonuses being available. Picture starters can be given in the form of slides, that have to be identified, but the main difference from the game on television is that any question that is not answered, or answered incorrectly, is offered to the audience. It is part of the question master's role to clarify and explain any points of confusion.

The rationale for using this strategy is that students are often in a state of anxiety in the weeks preceding important examinations, and this method provides relief of tension, while at the same time providing

Table 17.10 Simple respiratory and cardio-vascular experiments

There are a number of experiments which require no equipment, but which can assist the student to apply knowledge gained in lectures to the normal working of the human body.

   The role of the teacher in these experiments is to explain the procedure, but not to disclose the purpose. The student is required to draw his or her conclusions, using the facts given during lectures or study. They are fun to do, and the students usually find them highly motivating.

A. Breaking point
Student inspires deeply and holds breath. The period of time taken to reach breaking point is recorded. After resting for one minute the student breathes in and out as deeply as possible for six respirations, holding his or her breath on the seventh. The time taken to reach breaking point is again recorded. Student is asked to explain the results in terms of normal physiology.

B. Blood pressure and hyperventilation
Student is asked to lie down, and blood pressure is recorded. The cuff is left in position, and the student is asked to hyperventilate six times. The blood pressure is again recorded.

C. Pulse rate and respiration
The student is asked to breathe slowly but deeply in and out whilst the pulse rate and rhythm is observed.

D. Valsalva manoeuvre
The student is asked to make a forced expiration against a closed glottis, holding it for as long as possible. The pulse is recorded, and particular note should be taken of the pulse after the student takes a breath again.

E. Effects of exercise
Two experimenters are required for this experiment. The student's pulse and blood pressure are taken at rest. The student is then requested to run up and down stairs until he or she is exercising really hard. The blood pressure and pulse are recorded *simultaneously* by both experimenters immediately after exercise has finished. The blood pressure observations should include the systolic and diastolic differences before and after, and the proportionate changes. The pulse observation should include the time taken to return to pre-exercise level.

   Results can be compiled under the categories athlete/non-athlete and smoker/non-smoker, for comparison with other students.

motivation for revision. Motivation can be increased even further if the teams are selected from each teacher's personal tutees, as this may spur each team to do well on behalf on their own teacher. The rounds can be spread over the course of a week, with the final being played off on the last day, with a small prize for the winning team.

STRATEGIES FOR TEACHING PSYCHOLOGICAL CONCEPTS

Psychology, like biology, forms one of the major disciplines contributing to nursing and midwifery and plays a significant part in curricula at both pre-registration and post-registration levels. The question of whether or not a qualified psychologist should teach the subject is an interesting one;

many Colleges of Nursing and Midwifery have teaching staff who are also qualified psychologists, and it is obviously preferable if they are allocated to teach the area. If no qualified member of staff exists, then it may be appropriate to request a psychologist to service the course from another department within higher education. It is an important principle, I believe, that specialist subjects should be taught, wherever possible, by a teacher qualified in that area, since they can bring not only expertise in the subject, but a feel for the culture of the subject and its research.

Planning to teach psychology

When planning to teach psychology the teacher utilizes the general principles that apply to any subject, and which are dealt with at appropriate points in this book. However, there are one or two specific issues that need to be addressed with regard to teaching psychology to nurses and midwives. In my experience, these professional groups often find the subject frustrating because, unlike biology, there are few if any 'concrete' facts to get one's teeth into. It can seem vague and speculative as a discipline, and this runs counter to the professional training of nurses and midwives, who have tended to see things as 'black and white' in traditional nurse education.

What aspects of psychology should be taught to nurses and midwives?

One of the greatest problems facing curriculum planners is the acute shortage of time within curricula to include everything that is considered too important to be left out. In the case of psychology, it takes three years full-time study to become a psychology graduate, and even then it is considered to be only the starting point in a psychology career. How then is the teacher to approach a series of teaching sessions on psychology when it is only one component of a crowded course?

The first consideration, as always, is the level of the students and the course or pathway level and learning outcomes. It may be safe to assume that post-registration students already possess a good grounding in psychology, but in my experience this does not seem to be the case, except perhaps for those trained in mental illness nursing. In pre-registration programmes, psychology is usually taught early in the Common Foundation Programme along with the other contributory disciplines, and consists of teaching the fundamental concepts of psychology in much the same way as they appear in undergraduate textbooks. Whilst this is based upon a sound rationale, i.e. students must understand the basic concepts before they can apply them to patients/clients, students tend to find difficulty in relating it in any meaningful way to their everyday life and professional education. It is ironic that one of the canons of educational psychology is that the material must be relevant to the student if it is to be meaningful, yet starting a series of psychology lectures with child development is about as far removed from adult nurses and midwives as one can get. Of course, if the student happens to have children, then it may well be

The course team has utilized the principles of educational psychology in designing the sequence of topics for the unit, and these are as follows:

Relevance for you
Most introductory psychology courses commence with study of the infant and then progress through all the stages of development. We have chosen to begin with study of the adult, as this allows you to relate the material directly to yourself as an adult. In this way you can apply the material to your own psychological processes, making use of experiential learning.

Relevance to nursing
It is essential that this introductory unit should provide you with information that helps you understand nursing. The team has therefore made interpersonal communication a central theme for the first half of the unit, and this should help you to communicate more effectively with patients, staff and fellow students.
    The diagram below indicates the key topics for the unit and their relationship to each other:

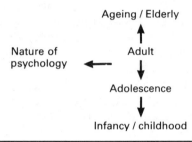

Fig. 17.6 Rationale and conceptual framework for a unit on the psychological basis of nursing and health.

perceived as relevant, but my argument is that much of fundamental psychology comes across as obscure and difficult for pre-registration students.

One way in which I have tackled this dilemma with Project 2000 students is to ignore completely the traditonal way of teaching psychology, i.e. in a linear progression from infancy to old-age, and to commence with a topic that has relevance and application to their immediate situation. This topic was Interpersonal Communication which involved aspects such as verbal and non-verbal communication, interpersonal relationships, etc. and which could be applied to every interaction they have with people, both socially and professionally. Thus, from the very outset, they encounter psychology that is immediate and relevant to them as people and nurses or midwives, with consequent benefits on motivation and understanding. Figure 17.6 shows an extract from the rationale and conceptual framework for a unit on The Psychological Basis of Nursing and Health for a Project 2000 course.

Another important aspect of pre-registration teaching is for the teacher to make sure that there are lots of references to patients, diseases etc, as students find this motivating also. In some cases, Project 2000 courses have gone overboard on the concept of health in the Common Foundation Programme, with the effect that students receive little or no information about illness or disease. I find that by including references to this during psychology lectures, students seem to become animated and interested. For example, in lectures on personality I include reference to Type A personality and its link with coronary heart disease, and this usually results in an enthusiastic group of students at the end who want to talk further about it.

When giving psychology lectures, it is important to involve the students in activities, and this can be done quite easily even in groups of 100 or more. For example, when teaching information-processing and memory, I get the students to form pairs with their neighbour, one acting as 'experimenter' and one as 'subject'. The 'subjects' are shown a list of names on the overhead projector for some twenty seconds (but not allowed to write any of them down), after which it is switched off. They then have to tell the 'experimenter' all the names they can remember, and when the results are calculated the teacher can discuss the experiment in the light of the limited capacity of short-term working memory. The activity only takes five minutes, but students become interested and are interacting with each other. Another strategy I use is Transcript Analysis of a brief audio-cassette extract when teaching non-verbal communication. Students are asked to listen carefully to the extract and to note any non-verbal aspects of the talking, such as prosodic, paralinguistic and indexical features. After three or four minutes of tape, the students are invited to comment on what they have observed, and this provides a motivating activity within a large lecture setting. Another useful strategy for small-groups is practical psychology work, and a useful reference is the British Psychological Society Manual of Psychology Practicals (McIlveen *et al.*, 1992) which gives fifteen practical exercises under the headings experimental method, observational method, and correlational method.

Health psychology

Health psychology is a relatively new branch of psychology that is concerned with the application of psychology to health promotion, prevention and treatment of illness, and the analysis and improvement of health care policies and systems. It has become an important topic in nursing and midwifery education at post-registration level, and there is much debate currently about the notion of a core curriculum for those working in the field of health psychology. Questions are being raised about whether training should be restricted to psychology graduates, or extended to include people from other backgrounds. Suggestions for a core curriculum are made by Rumsey *et al.*, (1994).

REFERENCES

Ausubel, D., Novak, J. and Hanesian, H. (1978) *Educational Psychology: a Cognitive View*, 2nd edn, Holt, Rinehart and Winston, New York.

Barnes, B. and Clawson, E. (1975) Do advance organisers facilitate learning? *Review of Educational Research*, **45**, 637–59.

Bruner, J., Olver, R. and Greenfield, P. (1966) *Studies in Cognitive Growth*, John Wiley, New York.

Dallas, D. (1981) *Teaching Biology Today*, Hutchinson, London.

Gagne, R. (1985) *The Conditions of Learning*, 4th edn, Holt, Rinehart and Winston, New York.

Klausmeier, H. (1985) *Educational Psychology*, 5th edn, Harper and Row, New York.

McIlveen, R., Higgins, L. and Wadeley, A. (1992) *BPS Manual of Psychology Practicals*, BPS, Leicester.

Quinn, F.M. (1984) Acquisition of content from a nursing lecture; role of advance organiser and mathemagenic activities. University of London Institute of Education. Unpublished MSc Dissertation.

Rumsey, N., Maguire, B., Marks, D. *et al.* (1994) Towards a core curriculum. *The Psychologist*, **7**(3), 129–31.

18 Facilitating interpersonal communication skills and teaching skills

The teaching of interpersonal skills is seen by many educationalists as being synonymous with experiential learning. Although experiential learning techniques are used extensively within interpersonal skills training, the concept of experiential learning has much wider implications for nurse education as a whole, as outlined in Chapter 7. This chapter explores two aspects of communication, interpersonal communication skills and teaching skills, both of which are closely intertwined in professional nursing and midwifery practice.

Nurses and midwives require a complex repertoire of professional skills in order to practise effectively and these include technical, managerial, interpersonal and teaching skills. Interpersonal communication skills are fundamental skills involved in relationships with other people, and are of particular relevance to nurses and midwives whose role involves them in constant and intimate contact with patients/clients and their relatives. The quality of this interaction is wholly dependent upon the practitioner's interpersonal communication and teaching skills, but there is evidence that nurses are not as effective as they might be. (Ashworth, 1980; Faulkner, 1980; McLeod Clarke, 1982).

A number of studies have been undertaken by Burnard and Morrison to determine students and trained staff perceptions of their interpersonal skills (Burnard and Morrison, 1988; Burnard and Morrison, 1991). Using Heron's six-category intervention analysis (Heron, 1986) they asked subjects to rank or rate the categories that they felt most skilled and least skilled in using, and found that the ranking of categories was identical in different samples of trained staff. Respondents felt most skilled in using the supportive category (offering general support), with the informative category (informing and teaching) and the prescriptive category (advising and suggesting) in second and third positions respectively. These three categories are termed 'authoritative' by Heron. The catalytic category (reflective) was fourth, the cathartic category (release of emotion) fifth, and the confronting (challenging) category last. These three categories are termed 'facilitative' by Heron. Trained staff perceived themselves to be less skilled in the other three categories. The authors suggest a number of factors that militate against a facilitative style of interpersonal relations between nurses and patients/clients, such as organizational culture, lack of time and a need to do the job, reluctance of nurses to make an emotional investment, and an emphasis on information-giving in nursing. The authors point out that some categories will be used more often than others. Catalytic, cathartic, and confrontational interventions will probably be used less in everyday contact with patients/clients, but the authors argue that these skills need to be available when required.

FUNDAMENTALS OF INTERPERSONAL COMMUNICATION

Communication is the transmitting or imparting of signals or information to a receiver. In the case of interpersonal communication, both transmitter and receiver are human beings, although they need not necessarily be in direct physical contact with each other. Intention to communicate is not a prerequisite; indeed, signals are often conveyed despite the transmitter's attempts to prevent this, as in non-verbal leakage of anxiety during an interview. Communication is usually classified into two broad categories – verbal communication and non-verbal communication, as illustrated in Figure 18.1.

Verbal communication

This involves the use of words as in speech and writing, but there is more than simply the meaning of the words themselves to be considered in a communication. There are three aspects of speech that need to be considered: prosodic, paralinguistic and indexical aspects.

Prosodic aspects   These are aspects closely related to the meaning of the spoken words and include stress placed on syllables and the intonation of the voice. A rise in intonation at the end of a sentence usually indicates a question, even though the sentence is not in the interrogative form.

Paralinguistic aspects   These reflect the attitude or emotions of the speaker; very rapid talking may indicate anxiety and loud volume usually signifies aggression, depending on the context.

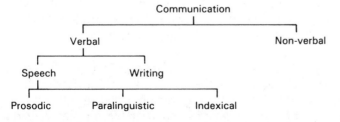

Figure 18.1   Classification of communication.

Indexical aspects   Regional accents and an individual's voice timbre are permanent features of the voice that convey information about the transmitter.

It is a good idea to use audiotaped voices when teaching these aspects of verbal communication; students can be asked to note down any particular aspects as outlined above and then compare with the rest of the group to see if common inferences were made.

Non-verbal communication

Non-verbal communication can be considered as a relationship language that conveys the correspondent's emotions, either consciously or otherwise. The main kinds of non-verbal signals used by man have been identified by Argyle (1983): facial expression, appearance, gestures, posture, proximity and orientation, bodily contact, and gaze. It is important to bear in mind that the meaning of any particular non-verbal signal will depend largely upon the context in which it is emitted, as well as the culture in which it occurs.

Facial expression   Probably the first thing we look at when we meet someone, facial expression is the main vehicle for signalling emotion. The mouth and eyebrows are capable of a wide range of variation in signals, as in surprise, smiling and anger.

Appearance   This conveys information about occupation, group affiliation and social class, although much is now dictated by fashion.

Gestures   These can be linked to a variety of emotions and social situations; clapping conveys appreciation to the recipient, a raised fist conveys solidarity or defiance. Many gestures are linked to speech, to give emphasis or describe spatial relationships.

Posture   This can convey passivity or assertiveness in social settings, according to the degree to which the body is held upright. A forward lean may indicate friendliness in some contexts and aggression in others.

Proximity and orientation   Proximity means the amount of distance between two persons during interaction and it seems that each of us has our own idea of personal space. If someone draws too close, we re-establish the space by moving backwards. Orientation is concerned with the angle between individuals, 90 degrees being the most common.

Bodily contact   This is the most intimate of non-verbal signals and involves such things as shaking hands, kissing and stroking. Many people are unhappy about being touched by persons other than their close friends and family, a point that comes out often when teaching interpersonal skills by experiential techniques.

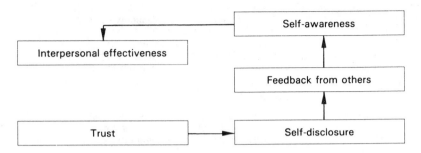

Figure 18.2 The components of interpersonal effectiveness.

Gaze A person looks at another person much more when listening than when talking. Eye contact is mutual gaze and becomes uncomfortable if held for any length of time. Eye contact has been traditionally held as a gesture of sincerity.

Non-verbal communication is best taught using video or film sequences for students to analyse. It is interesting to turn off the volume on a film and watch the non-verbal elements in action.

Interpersonal effectiveness

Relationships with other people depend upon our effectiveness in communicating with them; interpersonal effectiveness has been defined as 'the degree to which the consequences of your behaviour match your intentions' (Johnson, 1978). Interpersonal effectiveness is dependent upon a series of prerequisites as outlined in Figure 18.2.

One of these is self-awareness, which in turn is dependent upon feedback from other people; similarly, feedback is dependent upon a degree of self-disclosure that will only occur in an atmosphere of mutual trust.

Self-awareness

The notion of 'self' refers to all the thoughts, feelings and experiences relating to 'I' or 'me' and arises from both biological and environmental determinants. It comprises the way in which individuals see themselves – body image – and the way they feels about themselves – self-esteem. Our self-concept develops as a result of experiences and also by receiving feedback from other people. We tend to see ourselves in terms of a number of different roles, such as nurse, mother, athlete and so on, and during the course of development, the self-concept may be influenced by role models in real life or from the mass media. We are also influenced by what we think other people feel about us, the so-called 'looking-glass' self. Hence, we have a concept of what constitutes our 'self' and this concept is called self-awareness. Since the self is an entity that changes over time, we can never say that total self-awareness has been achieved. A useful device

	Known to self	Unknown to self
Known to others	Free self: open to self and others	Blind self: seen by others, but not by self
Unknown to others	Hidden self: seen by self, but not by others	Unknown self: Unseen by self and others

Figure 18.3 Self-awareness: the Johari window.

for conceptualizing self-awareness is the Luft Johari window (Luft, 1969), as illustrated in Figure 18.3.

The aim of self-awareness training is to extend the area of 'free self' and to reduce the other quadrants. There are two main ways in which we can become more self-aware: introspection and feedback from other people. Introspection involves looking within oneself and attempting to recognize and own our feelings and reactions. This needs considerable practice as well as a change in attitude, since socialization processes during childhood have tended to regard introspection as somewhat unhealthy. The ability to be able to recognize that one is feeling resentful during a conversation may well enable that person to guide the conversation in a more useful direction.

Burnard (1990) suggests a simple method of enhancing self-awareness through focusing on three hypothetical 'zones':

- Zone 1 involves outward focusing of attention on the outside world and our behaviour, and is synonymous with wakefulness;
- Zone 2 involves inward focusing attention with introspection of our thoughts and feelings; and
- Zone 3 involves fantasy such as day-dreaming and imagining.

Burnard suggests that it is important for nurses to be aware of their focus of attention and its shift between the three zones, since this will improve their abilities of observation and interpretation.

Meditation is a useful technique for getting in touch with one's emotions and the basic principle is that the person positions themselves in a relaxed, comfortable atmosphere and then concentrates on a single object or idea. Another interesting technique for self-awareness is the 'twenty statements test', in which the student is asked to write down twenty answers to the question 'who am I?' It is easy enough for the first ten, but much more difficult to think of another ten.

Feedback, self-disclosure and trust

Introspection alone is not sufficient for developing self-awareness; we need to be told by other people how they see us. Being able to give and receive constructive feedback is an important interpersonal skill, although one should avoid forcing feedback on someone else. When giving feedback to someone about a negative aspect of their behaviour, it is vital to avoid global condemnation of them as a person. By focusing on the specific behaviour and describing it clearly, one can provide constructive feedback without devaluing the person as a whole. It is more constructive to say 'It annoys me when you leave the treatment room untidy' than to say something like 'You are so unprofessional, leaving the treatment room in a mess like that'. Video recording provides the best way of seeing oneself as others see us and is often combined with role-play to provide feedback to students about their relationship skills.

PLANNING TO TEACH INTERPERSONAL COMMUNICATION SKILLS

In no other aspect of nurse education is detailed planning more important than in this very sensitive field. Table 13.1 shows a three-stage model for planning and implementing this area of the curriculum and each of these areas will be explored in this chapter.

Setting up the group

The introduction of training in interpersonal communication skills needs to be preceded by careful and detailed explanation to students about the purpose and goals of the topic. Students may be wary of the notion at first and require opportunities for free and frank discussion about the nature of the sessions. This can allay many anxieties if done in a sensitive manner by the teaching team. Topics such as self-awareness may engender considerable anxiety in students, particularly if they fear humiliation or exposure of 'weakness' in front of a group. It is a useful idea to introduce some of the research findings about communication skills in nursing, so that

Table 18.1 Planning model for teaching interpersonal communication skills

A. Setting up the group	1. Detailed explanation of purpose 2. Outline of current research 3. Negotiation of ground rules 4. Dealing with anxieties of members 5. Facilitating relationships
B. Choosing a conceptual framework for the course	6. Include all aspects of interpersonal communication, as in Figure 18.4
C. Implementing the programme	7. Consider the importance of warm-up 8. Emphasize the importance of briefing and debriefing after activities 9. Encourage the keeping of experiential diary throughout the course 10. Consider formative and summative evaluation

Table 18.2 Some ground rules for groups learning communication skills

1. Members must address other members by name.
2. Each member is responsible for himself/herself and must decide how far he or she wishes to go in any activity.
3. Members must not speak on behalf of other group members, but should refer to 'I' when making statements.
4. Members must treat the events that happen in the group as confidential, and not repeat incidents outside the group.
5. Members should try to react honestly to other members, but without 'put-downs'.
6. Members must try to accept other members' expressions of feelings rather than discounting them.

students have some idea about the importance of this area and are motivated to learn the skills themselves. One way of helping students to gain confidence with their peers is by negotiating ground rules for the conduct of the group; these ground rules identify the parameters of behaviour that the group agree upon and some common examples are given in Table 18.2.

Another useful way of lowering anxiety is to use an exercise called the 'worry box' in the very first session on interpersonal skills. This exercise is designed to allow each group member to voice an anxiety they may have about the topic, but in an anonymous setting. Each group member is invited to write down on a slip of paper one anxiety or concern they feel about the learning of interpersonal skills. This is done without using names, and then the group leader collects all the slips into a box; after shuffling the slips the leader goes around the group and invites each member to take a slip from the box and silently read it. Each student is required to formulate a response to the anxiety voiced on their slip and this response should offer some supportive comment to the rest of the group. In this way, each group member receives some positive supportive comment from another member of the group and the exercise serves to illustrate that most group members have similar anxieties or concerns about the topic. It has the added advantage that no student is identified by name, hence avoiding the threat of disclosure in the early stages of group formation. It is of crucial importance to start helping students to initiate relationships with other group members right from the outset of the programme and there are many ways in which this can be accomplished. One way, which is both enjoyable and non-threatening is to have the students work in pairs to exchange aspects of themselves; each can be given a couple of minutes to do this and then they are asked to change partners and do another exercise. This can be repeated several times so that each group member meets most or all of the group. An example is given in Table 18.3.

Choosing a conceptual framework

Many students find it difficult to see why the various activities used in interpersonal skills training are important, so it is vital that the nurse

Table 18.3   Exercise for initiating relationships in a group

This exercise consists of a number of pairings with group members. You are asked to choose partners whom you know LEAST WELL amongst the group. Please begin each partnership by INTRODUCING YOURSELF to your partner.

1. Choose a partner whom you know LEAST WELL. Each take a couple of minutes to DE-BAGGAGE, i.e. tell the other person of any frustrating incidents or 'hassles' you have experienced within the past week, e.g. difficult journeys, personal conflict, etc.
2. Choose another partner whom you know LEAST WELL. Each tell the other person about the following:

    If you were to imagine that you were a well-known book, which one would you be? Why did you choose this particular one?

3. Choose another partner whom you know LEAST WELL. Each take a couple of minutes to tell the other person about the following:

    If you were to imagine that you were a famous character from history, who would you choose, and why?

4. Remain with your present partner and join TWO OTHER PAIRS. In this group briefly discuss your feelings about the exercise.

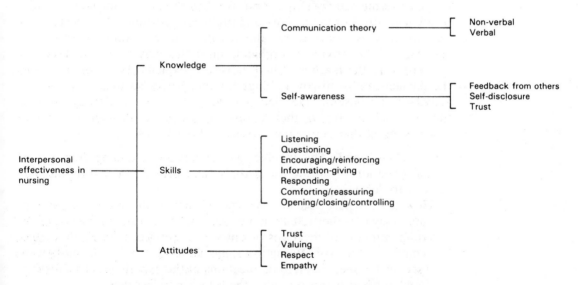

Figure 18.4   Systematic network-analysis of interpersonal effectiveness in nursing.

teacher spend time with the group explaining the overall framework for the programme of training in this field. Clearly, any programme of training must involve a selection from the enormous range of possible topics for inclusion, and a conceptual framework is useful to help delineate this selection. Figure 18.4 shows a systematic network-analysis of interpersonal effectiveness in nursing, and this can serve as a basis for the planning of the course content. It has been divided into the domains of knowledge, skills and attitudes, but obviously these are not separate categories, as each of the components is influenced by all three. However, it is useful for clarification, provided it is not seen as rigid or inflexible. An outline of the main components of this network is given later in the chapter.

Implementing the programme

Having decided upon a conceptual framework for the course and having carefully set up the group, the programme can then be followed according to the chosen sequence. This sequence should, in my opinion, be graded so that group trust and confidence can be built up gradually, and this implies the use of activities that are not highly threatening in the early phases of the programme. As confidence and trust develops, it will be possible to introduce activities that call for greater personal investment and disclosure.

Whether the student is pre-registration or post-registration, it is always very important for the teacher to plan carefully for briefing and debriefing. Briefing is carried out prior to any learning activity or experience and consists of a careful and detailed explanation of the aims, goals or purposes of the activity in question. Briefing should also include any rules or other features of the activity and provide opportunity for questions by the students. In some cases, the teacher will not want to reveal the purposes of an activity beforehand, since this may spoil the discovery element in it; the teacher should, however, explain that he or she wants the participants to discover things for themselves so that they feel the activity is purposeful. Debriefing is vital after every activity, as it is through such debriefing that learning takes place. Pearson and Smith (1985) suggest that debriefing consist of three stages:

1. What happened? This involves participants in describing their actions and experiences during the activity, and provides a non-threatening start to debriefing.
2. How did the participants feel? The teacher invites the main participants to say how they felt about the activity, then brings in the rest of the group. Emotional reactions or outbursts may occur during this stage.
3. What does it mean? During this stage the teacher helps the students to discover the meaning and implications of the experiences and feelings they have had by encouraging them to generalize these.

Another useful concept prior to group activities is the notion of warm-up activities or 'ice-breakers'; these are brief activities, usually of a physical nature, which are designed to facilitate the relaxation of students so that they enter the main activity in a state of readiness, similar to the way in which athletes warm-up before a big race. Table 18.4 gives examples of simple warm-up exercises.

One very useful strategy for use in learning interpersonal communication skills is the keeping of a 'reflective diary or record'. Students are encouraged to reflect on each experience and to enter this reflection into

Table 18.4 Examples of warm-up activities

1. 'SWAN LAKE': Members are asked to imagine they are ballet dancers performing in front of an audience. They are asked to dance around the room for about two minutes.
2. DE-BAGGAGING: Members are asked to form pairs and to spend two minutes each telling the other person about any problems or hassles they had that day, such as getting to work late.
3. NAME BALL-GAME: Members of the group form a circle and the leader gives a large sponge ball to one of the members. The object of the game is for each member to throw the ball at another member, whilst at the same time shouting out that member's name. If correct, the recipient throws the ball to someone else; if incorrect, the recipient throws the ball back to the thrower at the same time giving his or her correct name. The thrower then throws it at the same person again, this time saying the correct name.

their diary as soon as convenient. Over the course of the training programme, the student will build up a valuable record of his or her feelings and reactions to the experiences encountered and in this way can monitor progress.

STRATEGIES FOR TEACHING INTERPERSONAL COMMUNICATION SKILLS

Giving and receiving constructive feedback

A systematic way of giving feedback to students about their group skills is to use interaction-analysis techniques.

Group interaction analysis involves using a variety of observational techniques to record what is happening in a group and systems have been devised by many people (Bales, 1950; Turner, 1983). I prefer to use a simulated case study for the group discussion, with about eight students forming the discussion group. The remainder of the students are assigned different observational roles for recording what happens during the group discussion, as outlined in Table 18.5.

The eight students are asked to form a group and to discuss the material contained in the case study for about twenty minutes. This gives sufficient time for students to become really involved in the issues and also allows them to become accustomed to the video camera so that eventually they forget it is there. After the discussion, each type of observation is discussed by the total group, including the replay of the videotape. The data from the record sheets is used to show participants which kind of behaviours predominated in their interaction with other members of the group. Table 18.6 shows the record sheet for group behaviours and Table 18.7 the descriptions of each behaviour.

Self-disclosure

In order to encourage feedback from someone, it is necessary to disclose a little about oneself. Mutual self-disclosure results in increasing trust and

Table 18.5   Roles of observers for group interaction analysis

Data	Method of recording
1. Number of contributions per individual	Each group member is given a tally for every contribution made. These are totalled up at the end.
2. Length of individual contributions	Every five seconds a note is made of which group member is speaking.
3. Flow of interaction across group	A map of group members' positions is made on flipchart, and the direction of interaction drawn as arrows from person to person.
4. Group processes	Using a record sheet each group member is given a tally for specific behaviours such as questioning, etc.
5. Group processes	The whole discussion is videotaped.

Table 18.6   Record sheet for group interaction analysis

NAMES OF GROUP MEMBERS

Behaviours								
Initiating								
Inviting-in								
Controlling								
Obstructing								
Building								
Summarizing								
Supporting								
Tension-relieving								
Monopolizing								
Evaluating								
Requesting information								
Questioning								
Timekeeping								

development of a relationship, provided that the disclosure is appropriate to the stage that the relationship has reached. People may choose to disclose a wide range of details about themselves, such as interests, aspirations, family relationships and so on, which help the other person to

Table 18.7 Description of behaviours for group interaction analysis

Behaviour	Description
Initiating	Starting off discussion; starting a new line of discussion
Inviting-in	Inviting another group member to contribute
Controlling	Steering the course of discussion
Obstructing	Preventing another member from making a point
Building	Adding to a previous contribution from another member
Summarizing	Stating what the group has discussed so far
Supporting	Showing agreement with another member by verbal or non-verbal means
Tension-relieving	Making jokes or humorous comments when group is intense
Monopolizing	Dominating the discussion to the exclusion of other members
Evaluating	Giving opinions about the value of the discussion
Requesting information	Asking for facts or opinion
Questioning	Seeking further clarification from a specific member
Timekeeping	Monitoring the time available for discussion

get to know them. A useful way of assisting students to learn about self-disclosure is that of a 'self-disclosure inventory'. The student is asked to spend about 20 minutes completing the inventory on their own and then to join another student to discuss each other's responses to the questions. Finally, this pair of students joins with another pair and each person talks a little about their partner's inventory responses. Table 18.8 shows such an inventory; the questions can be answered at any depth, from the superficial to the profound, the students making the choice as to what they feel is right for them.

Trust

Underpinning all interpersonal skills is the concept of trust, which implies confidence that the other person will not let you down. In a trusting relationship, we can share thoughts and feelings without fear of the consequences and this is the hallmark of a meaningful relationship. Of course, it is not always appropriate to place one's trust in some other person, but it is an important concept when learning interpersonal skills in nursing. There are a number of trust exercises that can be useful for exploring this area, many of which involve physical trust. Students can be blindfolded and then led by another student around an obstacle course; two other examples of such trust exercises are shown in Table 18.9.

Effective listening skills

The ability to be able to listen to people is an important social skill in any setting, but in nursing it is particularly vital to the effectiveness of communication. Encouraging patients to talk about their worries and

Table 18.8 Self-disclosure inventory

Question 1. Please complete the following sentences:

         (a) I'm quite good at . . . .

         (b) I'm not very good at . . . .

Question 2. How would other people describe you?

Question 3. What are your present feelings about yourself?

Question 4. Over the next five years what is your greatest wish?

Question 5. Over the next five years what is your greatest fear?

Question 6. Over the past year what do you consider has been the most successful achievement in your life?

Question 7. Over the past year what has been the least successful achievement in your life?

Question 8. In the space below, draw a sketch or cartoon to illustrate where you see yourself at this stage of your life.

Table 18.9 Examples of trust exercises

1. *'Blade of Grass'*: One group member is asked to stand with feet anchored to the floor like a blade of grass, with eyes closed. She is surrounded by a circle of group members. She is instructed to act as if she were being blown by the wind, swaying over in any direction but always keeping her feet on the same spot. The role of group members is to stop her falling over by gently pushing her back towards the other side of the circle. This continues for three or four minutes and then a debriefing session is held to discuss feelings and reactions.

2. *'Lump of Clay'*: One member is asked to lie on the floor and six other members kneel beside her, three on each side. They work in pairs, lining up with each other at the shoulders, hips and legs of the recumbent student. They knead the student's body for two minutes, stroke it smooth for two minutes and then finish off by rapidly patting the body. De-briefing is carried out as before, with discussion of how it felt to trust other group members to handle your body.

anxieties is a key function of the nurse, but patients can be so easily discouraged by a listener who is plainly not paying attention. A distinction is often made between passive listening and active listening, the latter being preferred for effective communication. Active listening involves a high degree of concentration on the part of the listener with avoidance of interruption or judgement. The active listener is attending not only to the

Table 18.10 Guidelines on effective listening skills

1.	Convey attention to speaker	Give non-verbal signals by alert posture, gaze and eye-contact, nodding and smiling as appropriate.
2.	Focus on total content of message	Listen to what is said, but attend also to any paralinguistic aspects such as anxiety.
3.	Listen for cues from speaker	Cues are often indirect questions or key words that are repeated during a conversation, and signify concerns that are important to the speaker.
4.	Observe and listen for incongruence	The speaker's non-verbal signals may convey a very different message from the words being spoken.
5.	Make effective use of silences	Silences give the speaker opportunity to think about what to say next, or to reflect on what has been said. Avoid the temptation to fill these with questions or talk.
6.	Convey acceptance of what is being said	Show the speaker that you are accepting what is being said without judging it in any way.
7.	Make appropriate use of paraphrasing	It can be helpful to the speaker to have a paraphrase of what has been said, as a means of clarifying issues.
8.	Make appropriate use of summarizing	Summarizing can help the speaker by reviewing what has been said; it also serves as a check for the listener as to the accuracy of the listening.

words that are being conveyed, but all the other accompaniments of speech outlined earlier. The tone of voice of the patient, the volume or loudness, any signs of emotion, can all convey important data to the nurse and may not be congruent with the words that are being uttered. Effective listening utilizes silence to the patient's advantage, giving time for them to formulate ideas, and the effective listener encourages the speaker to carry on talking.

Triadic exercises are very useful ways of teaching effective listening skills. Students form groups of three and take the following roles: one speaker, one listener and one observer. The speaker can choose any topic to talk about, such as where they went on holiday and the listener is instructed to behave in a way that indicates they are not listening very attentively. After a few minutes, the triad discusses how it felt to talk to someone who is not interested and then the exercise is repeated using effective listening skills. Students change roles after each exercise so that everyone has a chance to try out the three roles. Table 18.10 gives guidelines on effective listening skills.

Effective questioning skills

As well as being a skilled listener, nurses need to be skilled in the art of conversing with patients and colleagues and Macleod Clark (1984) has identified a number of sub-skills of verbal communication. These involve encouraging patients to communicate, questioning, responding and giving information. Nurses can encourage patients to talk by active listening, as outlined previously, and by the use of reflecting, which involves saying what the patient has just said, or a paraphrase of it.

It needs to be borne in mind that questioning has a very different role in normal social interaction from that used in educational settings. In education, the person asking the question usually knows the answer already, whereas in normal social interactions, the questioner is seeking information or data.

- *Cognitive questions* require the respondent to answer from his or her knowledge base and can range from recall of specific information to the evaluation of courses of action
- *Affective questions* require the respondent to answer about his or her feelings and values.

These two major categories or domains of questions can be further subdivided in a variety of ways.

1. *Closed questions* involve a narrow range of response choices, such as 'yes' or 'no', or a specific factual answer such as name and address. They are useful for gathering data quickly.
2. *Open questions* allow the respondent to answer as they wish, without a framework imposed by the questioner.
3. *Leading questions* encourage the respondent to answer in a predetermined direction, e.g. 'You're not worried about your operation, are you?'
4. *Probing questions* follow-up previous questions, to try to glean more information from the respondent.

The questioning skills of nurses are extremely important when dealing with patients and clients and the literature suggests that they overuse closed questions and leading questions. Closed questions in themselves are not necessarily wrong, in fact they are very efficient in getting precise information and facts. However, if used to elicit feelings, they are much less appropriate than open questions; the latter are very important in following up cues emitted by the patient. There is some evidence that nurses tend to make few positive responses to cues emitted by patients, which means they are either unskilled in detecting such cues or else they are choosing not to respond to them.

Other conversational skills

As well as questioning skills, there are a range of other conversational skills that are important to develop. The nurse needs to be able to encourage patients and clients to discuss their problems by giving full attention to them, using verbal and non-verbal cues such as eye-contact, posture and orientation. The use of reinforcement in the form of smiles, head-nodding and touch can help the patient to continue talking and it is important to provide reassurance and comfort when the patient feels distressed or worried.

Student nurses may need much practice in the effective opening of conversations with patients and it is surprising to find that nurses often forget to do the normal social greetings before engaging in questioning or information giving. During the course of a conversation or patient interview, it is all too easy for the busy nurse to control the direction and content. In some instances this may be appropriate, particularly if the purpose is information-giving, but even here there is a danger in being too nurse-centred. Because nursing is a very busy and demanding profession, there is pressure to deal with issues quickly and efficiently and it is tempting to try to cut out any digressions during an encounter with a patient. However, it may well be that the patient has important things to discuss that he or she cannot easily raise directly and so they give hints or cues to these in an indirect manner. The experienced nurse will quickly spot such cues, particularly when they are repeated in the course of conversation and allow the patient to focus on them by the skilful use of open questioning.

There are many ways of teaching effective conversational skills, and one of the most useful ones is the technique of 'transcript analysis'. This technique involves the student in making an audio or video recording of an interaction with a patient or member of staff and then making a written transcript of the recording. The transcript can then be analysed in terms of the communication skills that the student displayed in the interaction and provides a powerful tool for individual or group development.

Transcript analysis is used in the following sequence.

1. The student is asked to make a recording of an interaction with a patient or member of staff, using either audio or video recording. The interaction can be real or simulated, the former being preferred if at all possible. The recording should be of fairly short duration, five to ten minutes maximum, so that the task of writing a transcript is not too burdensome.
2. A written transcript of the recording is then made by the student to include any non-verbal accompaniments such as pauses or laughter. An example of a page of transcript is given in Table 18.11.
3. The student then subjects the transcript to a detailed analysis, checking for the effectiveness of communication in all aspects of listening and conversation referred to above. The student is also required to evaluate his or her effectiveness overall and to identify any further skills development required.
4. The transcript is copied to other members of the interpersonal-skills training group and each group member's recording is played to the rest of the group for feedback and discussion.

The peer-group feedback can be extremely useful, as it gives the individual a range of opinions about the skills that were demonstrated and the things that require more training. If any group member feels they wish to criticize any aspect of an encounter, they must say what they would

Table 18.11 Example of an audiotape transcript

Interviewer	Well, Carol, thank you for agreeing to talk to me about something that concerns you in the field of health education. Would you like to tell me what the topic is?
Respondent	The topic is head lice in schools, which is rife at the moment.
Interviewer	Er, would you like to tell me what it is that concerns you about it?
Respondent	Yes – until a few years ago the school nurse always used to inspect children's heads to see they were free from lice or nits, but recently, because so many children have now got head lice and nits, the school nurse feels it is no longer her responsibility, but the responsibility of the mothers to pick up and consequently treat head lice, and I feel because there are *more* head lice in schools now that it *is* the school nurse's place to educate the mothers, even if she doesn't look in the actual children's heads, which is time consuming, she shouldn't just leave it and say that there are so many children with head lice – she should make more of an issue out of it and have groups of mothers and have actual health education classes concerning head lice.
Interviewer	You seem to feel very strongly about that.
Respondent	Yes, yes. Because lots of mothers, quite well motivated mothers, look at their children's head recently and pick up that they've got head lice and realize that this has to be treated, not just for their own children's sake but for the sake of the other children who can easily become infested from their children, but it is the less motivated mothers, who don't bother to think that there's anything abnormal about having head lice, who never treat their children, who in turn keep causing the children who are being treated to become re-infested with the lice, and I feel that the school nurses shouldn't just wash their hands of the problem because it's too vast a problem to cope with, but should have health education classes and therefore try to motivate the mothers who don't understand the problem. Don't you agree that this is now an issue, because something is common in schools, the school nurses shouldn't say that you shouldn't do anything about, there's nothing you can do?
Interviewer	Well now, you use the word 'issue' – do you think generally speaking people see that as being a major issue?
Respondent	Yes, I think that probably it's becoming more and more obvious that they do. It's causing great concern – and probably great concern to teachers as well, who themselves are quite at risk – and the mothers, of course, are at risk from also getting head lice.
Interviewer	Mm-mm. Mm-mm.
Respondent	Because it's well known that nits jump from child to child pretty quickly, but they also can live in brushes and combs just for a little while, obviously not for any length of time; and I think mothers need, really, to have it brought into the open that all kinds of children – dirty and clean children – can become infested with head lice or nits.
Interviewer	Mm-mm. Mm-mm.
Respondent	Lots of mothers don't know the difference between head lice and nits, and what they're actually looking for.
Interviewer	Mm-mm. Brought into the open? What were you thinking of.
Respondent	Because lots of mothers like to hide it, and they will probably find that their children become infested with nits and lice, rush off and treat it and don't like to tell anybody else their children have got it, and therefore the children that they have already been in contact with are at risk. Because the mothers probably feel ashamed. Though most mothers are aware of this problem now, still there's a stigma about nits.
Interviewer	Stigma. Mm-mm. What would you like to happen?
Respondent	I think that there should be more health education in schools regarding nits – not just an examination of the children's heads as there used to be, but more groups – groups of mothers with the school nurse, all talking properly about head lice. Having a film – even having real head lice, which are easily obtainable, to show the mothers what they actually do look like, and what they're looking for.
Interviewer	Mm-mm. So it seems to me you're saying that really it needs an intensive campaign to re-educate or educate . . .

Table 18.11 *continued*

Respondent	Yes. I think an intensive campaign is starting, apparently there was a programme on breakfast television, which not all mothers watch because breakfast television tends to be on at the time when mums are taking children to and from schools anyway. So that's the kind of programme they would miss, but probably . . . obviously the media are becoming aware that it is a problem, well then maybe it is coming more into the open – but then therefore some mothers will think it even more of a stigma. Don't you agree?
Interviewer	Have you thought of ways of how you could overcome that problem? In terms of publicity and so on, getting people to . . .
Respondent	Yes, as I've just said, I think the schools' nurses should not just wash their hands of the affair and say it's up to the mums and give them a vague little leaflet with a silly drawing of a creature with legs, of any kind of size, nothing relevant to the actual size of the lice . . .
Interviewer	Mm-mm.
Respondent	And I think that mothers should be encouraged to go to the school, if it's only just for a few minutes before the end of school, when they're actually there chatting about nothing much outside school anyway, they could be in the school for five minutes talking to the school nurse.
Interviewer	Mm. How do you see your own involvement progressing, and can a single health visitor do very much to . . .

have done to make it better, thus ensuring that all feedback is constructive rather than negative.

TRANSACTIONAL ANALYSIS (TA)

Since its invention by the late Dr Eric Berne in the early 1960s, transactional analysis has mushroomed into a major psychological movement. Berne was a practising psychiatrist and his system derives from the analysis of the basic structural unit of social intercourse, the transaction. Transactional analysis is a tool that anyone can use as a teaching or learning device for understanding behaviour in interpersonal interaction. It has its own language and this is the keystone of the system, since the language used is that of everyday life rather than the exclusive 'language of the priesthood' characteristic of psychiatry. The analysis of social transactions can enable people to understand what happens when they are involved in interaction so that they can exercise freedom of choice in what they do, rather than feeling that events simply take over. The basic concept in the method is that of the ego state, which Berne describes as 'a system of feelings accompanied by a related set of behaviour patterns' (Berne, 1966). Each person has three such ego states in his personality: parent, child and adult.

Parent

This is best explained using the analogy of Harris (1973). He describes this ego state as a kind of tape-recording of all the transactions which took place between the parents of an individual in the early formative years of his life. These data were recorded raw, without any modification such as interpretation of meaning and consist of all the rules, censures and 'do's and don'ts' of his first five years of life. Also recorded are the pleasure data from that period and all data are recorded as being true, even if this is not really the case.

Child

This consists of the recordings of the internal events that took place in the first five years, that is the feelings and emotional responses to the conflicts of these years. The recording can be said to have two sides, the first a negative one, in which the feelings are of frustration, rejection, aggression, etc. and the second that of the positive feelings. These include the wonder of the first discoveries, the exploration, creativity and all the other feelings of happiness in early childhood.

Adult

This stage commences at the age of about ten months, when the individual begins to exert some control over his world. The thinking process is used to work out life. 'Through the adult the little person can begin to tell the difference between life as it was taught and demonstrated to him (parent), life as he felt it or wished it or fantasized it (child), and life as he figures it out by himself (adult)' (Harris, 1973, p. 30).

The adult functions like a computer, examining both the parent and the child data against the reality of today, accepting or rejecting it as appropriate. Another function is that of estimating probabilities so that solutions can be devised if required. Creativity is also a major concern of the adult, and stems from curiosity.

The fundamental importance of these ego states lies in their influence on the individual during social interaction. At any point in a transaction one of these states will predominate, so that an individual may respond as a parent, adult or child. These states may vary during an interaction, and a person can be said to be 'in his or her child, adult or parent state'. Being in one's 'child' is not to be equated with being childish, since the child can be considered as the most valuable aspect of personality, contributing creativity and pleasure to life. The language of transactional analysis includes another important concept, namely that of 'OK-ness'. A person who feels OK experiences feelings of approval towards himself, feelings of being alright. 'Not OK' means the opposite of this, and the vocabulary of transactional analysis is used to describe the four possible life positions for a two-person transaction:

1. I'm not OK, you're OK.
2. I'm not OK, you're not OK.
3. I'm OK, you're not OK.
4. I'm OK, you're OK.

The first position is universal for the early years of infant life and stems from feelings of inferiority towards the adult. This position of OK-ness is either accepted by the child, or is replaced by positions (2) or (3) during the third year of life. The new position is then maintained throughout life unless a conscious decision is made to change it to position (4). The first three positions are related to 'stroking', which is another major concept in transactional analysis. A stroke is the unit of social action, an exchange of strokes being a transaction. Stroking is wider than just physical contact, implying any action that acknowledges the presence of the other person. Berne states than an individual seeks recognition in the form of strokes, and that this stems from the need for physical stroking during infancy in order for survival. Strokes may be positive or negative, but both can function as survival value, in that any form of stroking is better than none. In position (1) stroking is present from the parents, and the person who remains at this position tends to try to win approval and recognition from others, possibly by 'creeping'. The people from whom approval is sought tend to have a large parent, which forms the source of the strokes. Position (2) is the result of lack of stroking by the mother or father, leading to the viewpoint that no one is OK and an individual who remains at this position tends to reject all strokes that are offered and simply gives up, perhaps ending up in a psychiatric hospital.

Position (3) is described by Harris in terms of the child with non-accidental injury, who has concluded that his cruel parents are not OK. His source of stroking then becomes his feeling of peace when he is alone, and he rejects stroking from others. A person who is at this position tends to think that he is right, and that everything is the fault of other people. An example is the psychopathic personality, who displays no conscience about his behaviour. The fourth position, 'I'm OK, you're OK', is a position taken, a conscious, deliberate decision that is not controlled by past personal experiences, but by such things as values and philosophy. The most common position, however, is that of 'I'm not OK, you're OK', with most people falling into this category. Analysis of a transaction involves identifying the particular ego state that each of the transactors is in at any given time and this can be assessed by various clues, physical and verbal, which indicate the behaviour of parent, adult and child respectively. Transactions can be divided into two main types, complementary and crossed. Figure 18.5(a) shows the typical diagram used to illustrate

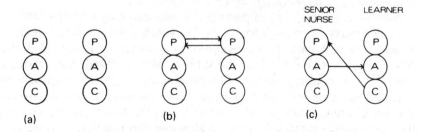

(a)　　　　　(b)　　　　　(c)

Fig. 18.5 (a) Typical transaction diagram: (b) complementary transaction; (c) crossed transaction.

transaction, and in Figure 18.5(b) we can see an example of a complementary transaction between parent and parent states. A complementary transaction is one where the lines of transaction are parallel; these complementary transactions are in agreement, and can continue indefinitely. Figure 18.5(c) shows an example of a crossed transaction indicated by the non-parallel lines on the diagram. Whenever a crossed transaction develops, communication comes to a standstill.

The kind of transaction illustrated in Figure 18.5(b) might take the following form:

Nurse teacher A: These Project 2000 nurses seem so superior, they need bringing down a peg or two.
Nurse teacher B: I quite agree, in my day we daren't say anything unless we were asked.

Both teachers are in their parent, using the sort of language that their parents used when they were small. Figure 18.5(c) might take the following form:

Senior nurse: Would you collect a sputum specimen for Mr Jones, please, nurse?
Student: Why do I always get the unpleasant jobs to do?

In this case, the senior nurse is addressing his or her adult to that of the student, but the student is responding from his or her child to the senior nurse's parent.

The aim of this analysis is to help people to make sure that their adult is in control of any transaction and this can be assisted by developing the ability to recognize one's parent and child and also to be aware of the child in other people. If the latter is achieved, then the other person's child can be cared for, stroked and allowed expression.

All transactions can be classified into one of six categories.

1. *Withdrawal* occurs when a person opts out mentally, whilst remaining physically present. For example, students in a group may allow their attention to drift to the events of the previous evening, rather than attending to the discussion.
2. A *ritual* is a series of socially defined actions, such as greetings, leave-taking and more formal things such as religious services.
3. An *activity* is a way of structuring time, usually in ways useful to the individual such as working, doing odd jobs, etc.
4. A *pastime* is a social way of passing the time and may take the form of chat at a party, with such topics as 'Do you know so-and-so?', etc.
5. A *game* is a very important concept in transactional analysis and Berne has devoted a whole book to the subject (Berne, 1966). He defines a game as 'an ongoing series of complementary ulterior transactions progressing to a well-defined predictable outcome'. Games always involve ulterior motives and a pay-off, and the following example of the best-known game will serve to illustrate the function of games.

Imagine the following transaction taking place in the office of a nurse teacher in the college or department of nursing.

Student: I can't stand living in the halls of residence any longer.

Teacher: Have you thought about taking a flat?

S: Yes, but I couldn't afford it.

T: What about sharing with some other students; that would save money.

S: Yes, but I don't know anyone who wants to move out.

T: Have you asked the residence manager if they have any addresses?

S: I don't get on with her; she doesn't like nurses.

T: Why don't you advertise on the student union notice board?

S: I don't fancy sharing with a stranger.

T: What about living back at home?

S: I couldn't go back home again, mum would drive me mad.

This game is called 'Why Don't You, Yes But,' and can be explained by reference to the child/parent interaction. The teacher here is in their parent state and the student in their child and the purpose is for the student to reject all the suggestions given until the teacher lapses into silence, defeated. This demonstrates to the student the inadequacy of the parent. In order for this game to be played, the teacher has to indulge in a game called 'I'm Only Trying To Help You'.

6. *Intimacy* is free of games, and occurs in the absence of fear. In this situation the transaction is conducted by the adult but allows the natural child to come through, with all its advantages.

ASSERTIVENESS TRAINING

I still have vivid memories of an incident that occurred on my first day in a new job. I had parked my car in the college car park and was walking away when a man bore down on me. 'You're not supposed to park here,' he said and I responded by saying, 'I'm sorry, I didn't know'. He then said, 'Well you know now', and walked away. I felt very angry about this incident, mainly because I was annoyed with myself for responding in the way I did. As I mulled over the encounter I began to imagine all the alternative responses that I could have made, which would have made me feel much better about myself. What I needed was an assertive response that would leave me feeling good even if I did not win the encounter. Assertiveness means defending your own rights without infringing on those of another individual. It involves open and direct expression of feelings and reactions without devaluing self or others. It is not a common response, since we tend to be conditioned from childhood to avoid causing fuss or embarrassment; this accounts for the tendency to put up with bad service, cold food and many other unsatisfactory aspects of life. It is sometimes suggested that nurses are lacking in assertiveness in their professional role and that this has left them in a much less favourable position in terms of power and financial rewards in comparison with medical staff and other professionals. Assertiveness can be a way of bringing an element of choice into social situations; our responses to others are often made as a result of habit rather than by careful choice according to the circumstances. Assertiveness training aims to give the individual another way of behaving that may leave them feeling more autonomous and satisfied within themselves, thereby increasing self-esteem. Assertiveness training involves not only changes in behaviour, but also changes in beliefs about the self. It is necessary to internalize a number of beliefs, such as the right to be treated with respect and the right to say 'No'. The following responses are commonly-seen behaviours in social settings, and contrast markedly with an assertive response.

Apologetic response

As the name implies, this form of behaviour uses apology as a way of obtaining satisfaction and is often preceded by phrases such as 'I'm very sorry to be a nuisance, nurse but . . .'

Aggressive response

A very common approach to unsatisfactory situations, this involves verbal aggression plus non-verbal cues to convey dissatisfaction. It usually contains global condemnation of the person concerned or the establishment. 'I've been waiting in this casualty department for two hours now and there's still no sign of anyone coming to attend to me. The NHS has gone completely to the dogs.'

Whining response

Usually made when there is more than one person involved with the respondent and consists of mutual complaining about a situation. The complaints, however, are never made to the cause of the difficulty, just to each other. A typical dialogue would occur as follows: 'This new GP is not as good as the last one . . . he doesn't listen to what you say. I certainly wouldn't recommend him to anyone.'

Assertive behaviour contrasts markedly with these three forms of behaviour in that the response is expressed directly and openly without devaluing the other person. The response is made with appropriate non-verbal cues such as upright posture and eye contact and the avoidance of incongruent cues such as smiling. 'I would prefer not to discuss this matter in front of the patient; can we go somewhere in private.'

Any of the three aforementioned forms of response may be quite successful in getting one's own way; indeed, the apologetic response can be extremely powerful in this respect. However, what really matters is how you feel after having made a response and it is here that assertiveness may offer something different. Even if an encounter results in 'failure', we may still feel good within ourselves if we chose an appropriate mode of responding. Selection interviewing is a good case in point. It is important that the applicant does not emerge from an interview feeling that he or she has 'sold my soul', particularly if they were unsuccessful anyway.

Teaching assertiveness is best done by triadic exercises and I usually begin by taking one or two common social situations where assertiveness may be an advantage.

Situation 1: Saying 'No'

I introduce this topic by emphasizing that two beliefs are important when saying no. The first is that everyone has a right to say no and the second is that by refusing the request you are not rejecting the whole person. There are four basic techniques about saying 'No' (Turner, 1983).

1. *Cracked record* This involves saying the same thing over and over again until the requester gives up, e.g. 'I don't want to discuss it at the moment.'
2. *Time-out* We often feel that we have to make an instant decision when meeting a request. Time-out means taking a few minutes to think about the request and then letting the person know the outcome.
3. *No excuses* There is no need to justify a refusal unless you want to, so it is better not to make excuses. Excuses often provide more ammunition for the requester to use in persuasion.
4. *No waiting* Having turned down a request, it is common for an individual to remain with the requester trying to off-load any guilt feelings about the refusal. The best thing is to leave the requester as soon as you have said no.

Having given some guidelines to the students I then ask them to act out a scenario such as being asked to go out in the evening with another student. It is a good idea to begin with non-threatening everyday situations such as this, and then gradually progress to professional ones. One student is the requester, one the respondent and one an observer, and the role of the requester is to try to persuade the respondent to agree to go out for the evening. The respondent tries out the various techniques of saying no and then the triad members discuss their feelings and reactions.

Situation 2: Facing devaluation by other people

It is a fact of life that most people encounter negative criticism or devaluating comments from others and the following techniques are designed to help cope with this.

1. *Fogging* As the name suggests, this involves putting up a 'fog' that absorbs all the comments that are directed against you. The first rule is to avoid denying the criticism or defending yourself and the second is never to counter-attack. It is virtually impossible to keep negative criticism going in the face of this 'fog', e.g. 'I can see that you must find my behaviour inexplicable.'

2. *Negative enquiry* Asking for more information about the behaviour at issue can be a useful way of defusing criticism, e.g. 'What is it about my approach that makes you unhappy?'

Situation 3: Facing aggressive attacks from others

There are two basic points to bear in mind when dealing with an angry outburst:

1. Do not accept that you are the cause of the anger; it may well lie completely elsewhere, but it is likely to lie within the angry person.
2. You have the right to walk away from anyone shouting at you.

A possible sequence for dealing with outbursts is as follows:

1. Gain attention by repeating a phrase such as 'Please listen to me.'
2. Establish eye contact and hold it.
3. Have ready a phrase consisting of:
    (a) recognition of the anger;
    (b) your own reactions;
    (c) willingness to co-operate.
4. Encourage them to sit down.
5. Listen to what they have to say.
6. Move to joint problem-solving.

These situations can be practised in triads, with each member taking turns to be the actor and the respondent. Having had some practise with these examples, the members should be asked to bring real-life nursing examples to act out, as this makes the exercises more realistic and useful.

TEACHING EFFECTIVE TEACHING SKILLS TO STUDENTS

Although teaching is generally acknowledged to be an important aspect of nursing and midwifery practice, it is ironic that so little attention is paid to this aspect during courses for initial registration. The post-registration provision for teaching skills is much better, with a variety of short courses available such as the ENB 997/998 courses for Teaching and Assessing in Clinical Practice, and the University of Greenwich/Nursing Times Open Learning (NTOL) unit Teaching and Learning in Practice, and the City and Guilds of London 7307 course. There are also recognized courses of initial teacher training leading to either a certificate, postgraduate certificate, or postgraduate diploma in education. However, it seems to me that in leaving teaching skills training until after the student has qualified we are missing an opportunity to build in teaching as a fundamental part of the education and training programmes for nursing and midwifery. It is so much easier, and more effective, for students to learn teaching skills alongside the other nursing or midwifery skills during their initial training, rather than having to accommodate them as new ideas once they have qualified. Patient education is an important part of the role of nurse or midwife, and students must be given the opportunity to undertake the

Table 18.12 Example of a students' guide to a unit on teaching and learning: the educational role of the nurse (Source: University of Greenwich)

Introduction: Teaching is one of the key roles which you will undertake as a nurse, and will involve patients, clients, families and other students. As well as helping people to learn, you need to be able to present information at meetings to colleagues or other professionals, and such presentations need to be of high quality for maximum impact.

This unit aims to give you the basic knowledge and skills to enable you to fulfil your teaching role with greater insight and effectiveness.

Sequence of topics for unit

Session	Type	Title
1	Workshop	Introduction to Unit 10
2	Lecture	Planning for teaching
3	Workshop	Planning exercise
4	Lecture	Verbal exposition
5	Workshop	Verbal exposition
6	Lecture	Questioning
7	Workshop	Questioning skills
8	Lecture	Explaining
9	Workshop	'Explaining' exercise
10	Lecture	Assessment of learning
11	Workshop	Audiovisual aids 1
12	Lecture	Theories of learning 1
13	Workshop	Audiovisual aids 2
14	Workshop	Student consultation
15	Lecture	Theories of learning 2
16–20	Workshop	Student micro-lesson presentations

Teaching and learning strategies: The unit consists of lectures and group work at Avery Hill Campus. The emphasis will be on the acquisition of planning and teaching skills, supported by theoretical perspectives. Lectures will provide key information, and group work will involve the production of teaching plans, audiovisual resources, and micro-teaching sessions.

Assessment: You are required to carry out a TEN-MINUTE TEACHING SESSION to your peer group according to the following criteria:

1. You must choose a HEALTH TOPIC that you would teach to a patient/client e.g. healthy eating; giving own insulin etc.
2. The session must be based on a PLAN containing details of aims/goals, sequence of development, content notes, learning aids used, and assessment of learning.
3. Following the presentation, the PLAN AND MATERIALS used must be HANDED IN as part of the assessment.
4. The plan must also be accompanied by a RATIONALE (1000 WORDS) consisting of the following:

   (a) An introduction that states why the topic you chose is relevant to the role of the nurse.
   (b) An explanation of the reasons underlying your choice of teaching method and approach. This explanation must make reference to educational theories.
   (c) A critical self-evaluation of how you felt the lesson went, and any changes you would make in the light of your own and your peers' evaluation of your lesson.

(Peer evaluation consists of brief written feedback by students and tutor following each student presentation.)

Please note: The actual presentation of your lesson, although compulsory, does not count towards your grade. You will be graded only on the written materials and accompanying rationale. This decision is to help reduce the stress that inevitably accompanies a student's first formal presentation to a large group.

teaching of patients whilst they are still students. Without adequate preparation this is unlikely to be effective, and raises serious questions about the adequacy of the curriculum. The lack of teaching skills training is also evident on the occasions when students are required to make presentations to their groups during their course. They may feel embarrassed about explaining things to their peers, and their timing and delivery are often poor. Even when students have taken the trouble to produce posters or overhead projection materials they are often badly designed or illegible.

A couple of years ago, an invitation to join a curriculum development group for a new Project 2000 course gave me the opportunity to raise the issue of teaching skills training at pre-registration level. I was fortunate enough to convince my colleagues that this was an important aspect to include in the curriculum, and as a result was asked to write a unit for the Project 2000 course. I called the unit 'Teaching and Learning: the Educational Role of the Nurse', and Table 18.12 shows the Unit Guide for Students. This unit has run several times on a Project 2000 programme in which I am involved, and students' evaluation provides evidence that it has been of considerable benefit to them.

REFERENCES

Argyle, M. (1983) *The Psychology of Interpersonal Behaviour*, 4th edn, Penguin, Harmondsworth.

Ashworth, P. (1980) *Care to Communicate*, RCN, London.

Bales, R. (1950) *Interaction Process Analysis: A Method for the Study of Small Groups*, Addison-Wesley, Cambridge, Mass.

Berne, E. (1966) *Games People Play*, Andre Deutsch, London.

Burnard, P. (1990) *Learning Human Skills. An Experiential Guide for Nurses*, 2nd edn, Heinemann, Oxford.

Burnard, P. and Morrison, P. (1988) Nurses' perceptions of their interpersonal skills: a descriptive study using six category intervention analysis. *Nurse Education Today*, **8**, 266–72.

Burnard, P. and Morrison, P. (1991) Nurses' interpersonal skills: a study of nurses' perceptions. *Nurse Education Today*, **11**, 24–9.

Faulkner, A. (1980) The Student nurse's role in giving information to patients. Unpublished M. Litt thesis, University of Aberdeen.

Harris, T. (1973) *I'm OK, You're OK*, Pan, London.

Heron, J. (1986) Six category intervention analysis, Human Potential Research Project, University of Surrey.

Johnson, D. (1978) *Reaching Out*, 2nd ed, Prentice-Hall, New Jersey.

Luft, J. (1969) *Of Human Interaction*, National Press, Palo Alto.

Macleod Clark, J. (1982) Nurse-patient verbal interaction: an analysis of recorded conversations from selected surgical wards. Unpublished PhD thesis. University of London.

Macleod Clark, J. (1984) Verbal communication in nursing, in *Communication*, (ed. A. Faulkner), Churchill Livingstone, Edinburgh.

Pearson, M. and Smith, D. (1985) Debriefing in experience-based learning, in *Reflection: Turning Experience into Learning*, (eds D. Boud, R. Keogh and D. Walker), Kogan Page, London.

Turner, C. (1983) *Developing Interpersonal Skills*, Further Education Staff College, Blagdon.

19 Teaching research and enquiry skills

Professional practice in nursing, midwifery, and health visiting takes place within a context of continuous change, which can be on a macro scale, such as the NHS reforms, or a local scale, such as the adoption of an alternative model of care within a practice setting. Regardless of the nature of the changes, it is axiomatic that both students and practitioners require access to education in order to help them to adapt appropriately, and thereby ensure the quality of patient/client care is maintained. However, educational programmes must also adapt to change if they are to remain relevant to practice, and this implies they should be planned on the basis of sound research findings. A number of terms are often used synonymously in relation to research, namely inquiry, investigation, and study, but these are viewed by some as being less rigorous than research.

INSTITUTIONAL RESEARCH CULTURE

The argument for a research-based approach to education is overwhelming, but the implementation of research-based education is not as easy as it sounds. One of the main stumbling-blocks is the lack of a research culture in Colleges of Nursing; this is not a criticism, since nurse education has evolved in response to different imperatives from those of HE. Institutions with a culture of research perceive teaching and research as being of equal importance and academic staff are required to undertake research as part of their role. However, research activities should not be so demanding that they adversely affect the quality of teaching that students receive. A culture of research and teaching within an institution is a potent formula for quality education, as academic staff are able to combine the two roles to ensure that their teaching is informed by research which is often their own. As well as generating research, academics also supervise research students who are undertaking research projects at undergraduate and postgraduate levels. In Colleges of Nursing and Midwifery the absence of a research culture may lead staff to believe that their only role is teaching, and whilst they willingly incorporate research findings into their sessions, they may resist the idea of becoming active researchers themselves. It is therefore of crucial importance that staff development is provided to help nurse teachers to appreciate the importance of research as a basis for teaching and practice, for supervising research students, and for generating income in the form of research grants and research consultancy. The latter can provide a significant source of external funding for the institution, but requires a well-established culture and track-record in research. The NHS and the Statutory Bodies have given impetus to the development of a research culture in nursing, midwifery and health visiting. For example, in its response to the Strategy for Research in Nursing, Midwifery and Health Visiting, the English National Board outlines its Research and Development position (ENB, 1993). A Research and Development (R&D) Group has been appointed to advise the Board, and three key issues are identified: R&D priorities, research education and training, and dissemination and implementation of research findings.

The R&D group has adopted six overlapping dimensions as part of its identification of R&D priorities:

1. Disease/practice-related, e.g. mental health, cancer, stroke
2. Management and organization, e.g. purchaser/provider contracting
3. Client groups, e.g. physical disabilities, elderly people
4. Consumer issues, e.g. user inputs to decision-making
5. Health technologies, e.g. assessment of new technologies
6. Methodologies, e.g. identification and development of methodologies to address NHS issues

The Board has already established mechanisms to ensure quality research education by means of conjoint validation events and educational audit, both of which ensure that research awareness and application of research to practice are included in educational programmes.

Research findings are disseminated in a variety of ways, including published materials such as executive summaries and research highlights, conferences, and regional workshops and seminars.

Staff development for teaching research

From the foregoing discussion it is apparent that research forms a crucial agenda item in the development of the nursing, midwifery and health visiting professions. Teachers of these professions will be key players in the design and delivery of education for research, but there is some question as to whether they have the appropriate knowledge and experience to do this effectively. In an exploratory study of nurse teachers' perceptions about research, Clifford (1993) found that over half the subjects felt inadequately prepared for research. Similar findings are reported by the National Board for Nursing, Midwifery and Health Visiting for Northern Ireland (1990), where 43% of nurse tutors in the sample had no research training. Teachers therefore need staff development if they are to teach research effectively, and to undertake research themselves. However, staff development will be of little use unless resources are made available to free the teacher from some of his or her other college commitments. Staff development for research requires pump-priming investment on the part of the college if the initiatives are to bear fruit. One of the key staff development strategies in Colleges of Nursing and Midwifery is to encourage and support teachers to undertake higher degree studies in which research forms a central component, especially M.Phil and PhD degrees. Other staff development activities include attendance at research conferences, local and regional exchange of research information, workshops on research methods and writing articles for journals, and specific staff appointments such as research assistants who can assist staff in undertaking research projects. One useful strategy is 'research-mentoring', in which a teacher with knowledge and experience of research acts as a mentor to a member of staff who lacks confidence in research.

STRATEGIES FOR TEACHING RESEARCH

Essentially, students can learn research by being told about it or by doing it, although the ideal strategy involves a combination of both. The experiential approach to teaching research is much more common now that nursing and midwifery programmes are offered at undergraduate and postgraduate level. In fact, a research project or investigation of some kind is a hallmark of CATS level 3 learning, and at postgraduate level takes the form of a research dissertation comprising a significant proportion of taught masters degrees. The inclusion of research projects in nursing and midwifery education may present problems if the teachers are not equipped to carry out effective supervision of research students.

SUPERVISING STUDENTS' RESEARCH PROJECTS

Christopherson (1992) suggest that there are two main aspects to supervision of students' research projects. The first and most important concerns the abilities of the supervisor to challenge and motivate the student with a steady stream of ideas. The second involves the mechanics of facilitating the progress of the student. He cites the following common reasons for non-completion of research projects.

1. *A slow start* The student needs to work hard in the initial stages to avoid slippage in the deadlines.
2. *Perfectionism* Some students are never satisfied with their results and are constantly trying to improve them. Taken to the extreme, this will prevent the project from ever being completed.
3. *Distraction* It is relatively easy for a student to be distracted by some aspect of the project, such as computer analysis of data, and as a result, spend too much time on this aspect to the detriment of the overall project.
4. *Inadequate collation of data* This may be detected during the writing up of the project, and results in a need for further analysis which then delays the writing stage of the project.

The supervisor/student relationship

The student/supervisor relationship is the most important factor in project supervision. Students tend to face similar problems when undertaking research, regardless of the level of the project. Once allocated a supervisor, the student must be supervised and not left entirely to his or her own devices.

The supervisor should provide appropriate support while ensuring that the progression of the project remains firmly the responsibility of the student. A probing, questioning approach by the supervisor can be helpful in making the student focus more clearly on the key issues, and to think more critically about the project. It is very difficult when a supervisor is presented with detailed materials at a meeting and asked to comment there and then, and a much more considered opinion is likely if the supervisor has had time to read and criticize material in advance of the meeting. It is very important that an agreed system for contacting the supervisor is negotiated; some supervisors are happy to give their home telephone numbers to students, but others may, understandably, be reluctant to do this. If home telephone numbers are given, the student should avoid contacting their supervisor during meal-times, bank holidays and other inconvenient times.

Scientific enquiry

Research is a rational process of scientific enquiry directed towards a question or problem and resulting in extension of the total sum of knowledge. It is a way of making sense of the world through explanation, but the definition makes clear that it is not just ordinary enquiry such as that of casual observation. Research is scientific and science is characterized by objectivity and the empirical nature of its explanations (Kerlinger, 1979). Empirical research is a term used to describe the systematic, controlled gathering of evidence that characterizes science, including behavioural sciences. Objectivity means that the explanations are independent of the experimenter's own bias and this is ensured by the detailed reporting of every step in the research so as to enable another scientist to replicate the study. The publication of research exposes it to the scrutiny of the scientific community and this provides a measure of quality assurance.

These criteria are the foundations of the scientific method of enquiry, a process of investigation consisting of a logical sequence of steps as follows:

1. defining the problem or question;
2. searching the literature;
3. formulating a hypothesis;
4. designing the study;
5. carrying out pilot study;
6. collecting the data;
7. analysing the data; and
8. drawing conclusions and making recommendations.

Research is classified into quantitative research, which is about collecting facts that are analysed using statistics, and qualitative research, which is more concerned with gaining insights, and data is analysed by qualitative methods.

SUPPORTING STUDENTS DURING THE STAGES OF THE PROJECT

The next sections use the steps of the scientific method to describe the role of the teacher in advising and supporting supervisees doing their research projects.

Defining the problem or question

The research process begins with an observation about some phenomenon, or perhaps a feeling about something, and from this germ of an idea a research project may develop. We need to distinguish scientific problems from two others kinds, engineering problems and value problems. An engineering problem is concerned with how to do certain things such as 'how to improve patient care', whereas a value problem asks about what is good and which is best. A scientific problem has an advantage over these other kinds of problem because it is formulated in such a way as to render it capable of being tested. Scientific problems are to do with relationships between variables, and there are three criteria for a scientific problem (Kerlinger, 1979) – it must:

1. be stated in interrogative form, i.e. as a question,
2. state a relationship between variables, and
3. imply empirical testing.

Students usually have difficulty in choosing a research topic and it is helpful to advise them to identify a broad area of interest, and then focus down to clearly defined questions to which answers can be found. These answers may be empirical or literary. They also need to consider why the topic is worth investigating and what the likely benefits will be. If the student wishes to attempt to solve a concrete, practical problem in the immediate work setting, then this is considered to be an example of action research, which is typified by a requirement for specific knowledge for a practical problem in a specific situation (Bell, 1993).

When the project idea has crystallized, the student completes a research project proposal form which is then signed by their supervisor and the course director once they are happy with the proposal. Within health care settings, research involving patients and clients has to be approved by an ethics committee, and this may take some time. Students must put their proposal in writing to the secretary of their local ethics committee. Students registered for an MPhil or PhD degree will also have to have their proposal approved by the university research committee.

Searching the literature

Before embarking upon a research study the student must search the literature in order to gain an understanding of the theoretical background. In addition, study of the literature will indicate whether previous work has been done in the same area. Even if this is the case, the student may wish to replicate previous study and compare the results. Another advantage is that there may be methods of measurement in other studies that could be used. A search of the literature is often done in two stages: a general overview of the secondary sources, such as textbooks, CD-ROM, etc., and a specific review of the primary source material in written research reports. This will result in a great deal of information, so it is imperative that an efficient system of recording is used.

Formulating a hypothesis

A hypothesis is a supposition or conjecture about the relationship between variables that is couched in declarative rather than interrogative form. The hypothesis must be testable and therefore requires to be stated in operational terms that specify which operations are necessary to measure the variables. A hypothesis is usually stated in the null form, which is a negative statement that uses the form 'will not'. The null hypothesis is preferred in practice because it is easier to test statistically and adds a measure of objectivity to the acceptance or rejection.

Designing the study

In designing the research study the student must consider the type of research design that best meets the aims of the project.

Experimental research design

This is a type of research in which the situation to be studied is artificially controlled by the experimenter. Some form of treatment is administered and the effects observed, whilst maintaining other variables at a constant level. By systematically altering the treatment and observing the results, the experimenter may come to the conclusion that a cause-and-effect relationship exists. The treatment may involve such things as administration of a drug, and is termed the independent variable because it is independent of the results of the experiment. The dependent variable is the observed changes in the subject's performance following treatment by the independent variable. The dependent variable is dependent upon the way in which the independent variable is manipulated, hence the independent variable is the antecedent and the dependent variable the consequence. This relationship is often stated as: 'If p, then q.' However, in the experimental situation, it is important to have a control group of matching individuals who are not given the treatment, but who are assessed on the same test as the experimental group. This has the effect of

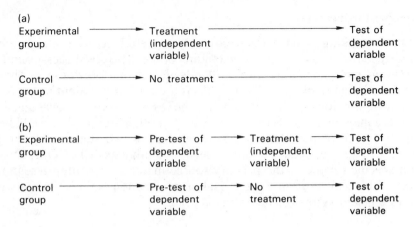

Fig. 19.1 One-way experimental design: (a) without pre-test; and (b) with pre-test.

dealing with irrelevant variables that might confuse the findings, and allows the experimenter to assume that any difference in the experimental group is due to the treatment rather than to other factors. There are, however, confounded variables that the experimenter needs to consider; it is possible that there is another, unknown, variable that is acting to produce the effect, rather than the independent variable.

There are two vital aspects to be considered when designing an experiment: internal and external validity. Internal validity is concerned with aspects of credibility within the design itself, including such things as changes due solely to the passage of time, the effects of a test being affected by prior tests, and changes due to other events occurring between the independent and dependent variables.

External validity refers to the generalizability of the results and can be affected by such things as pre-testing causing sensitization of subjects to the phenomenon in question and thereby affecting results. There is also a notion called ecological validity, which questions the applicability of laboratory-based research to the real world.

In experimental research there are two types of design – 'one-way' and 'two-way' – named according to the number of independent variables employed. A one-way design (as in Figure 19.1) uses only one independent variable and is often referred to as the 'classic design'; it consists of an experimental group and a control group, the experimental group is treated by the independent variable, whereas the control group receives no treatment. Both groups are subsequently tested for changes in the dependent variable (Figure 19.1 (a)). Additionally, a pre-test can be given prior to the treatment to establish the existing level of the variable under study (Figure 19.1 (b)). One of the limitations of one-way designs is the reliance on a single variable, which in the social sciences is rarely useful, since most behaviour is the result of many variables working together.

Two-way designs allow the use of more than one independent variable and are also termed factorial designs. Not only can the effect of each

Table 19.1 Advantages and disadvantages of experimental research

Advantages	Disadvantages
A high degree of control over potential confounded variables.	Independent variables used in laboratory may not be as strong as naturally occurring ones.
Situations are flexible enough to test a variety of aspects.	Laboratory setting may lead to loss of ecological validity.
They can be replicated by other experimenters.	There are ethical difficulties in some areas where experiment is not acceptable.
Hypothesis is used as a predictor for relationships between variables.	
Data is generated which is objective and can be subjected to statistical analysis.	By focusing on objectivity and control, the experiment may lose valuable subjective data.
Independent variables can be manipulated to demonstrate effects on dependent variable.	It is not always practically possible to use experiments.

variable be measured as a separate entity, but also the effects of any interaction between them; these are called the main effect and interaction effects respectively. Interaction effects can be described as: 'If p, then q, under condition r.'

The use of experiments, then, brings a degree of control that is important in determining the effects of the independent variable, but the student needs to be aware of the disadvantages in using them. Table 19.1 shows some of the pros and cons of this method.

Non-experimental research design

This is research in which the researcher is unable to manipulate variables or to randomly allocate subjects and conditions. It is also termed *ex post facto* because it is research after the event, i.e. after the variables have already affected the subjects. For example, a postgraduate student may wish to ascertain if a correlation exists between pre-operative visits by an anaesthetic nurse, and perceived post-operative anxiety in surgical patients. Both experimental and non-experimental research make the assumption 'if p, then q', but non-experimental research uses surveys as its means of enquiry. In this method, a population is sampled to determine aspects of certain variables such as distribution and relationships, the latter being referred to as correlation. Correlation means literally the co-relation between two sets of values, such as pre-operative visiting and perceived anxiety in surgical patients, and occurs in two dimensions, magnitude and direction. Magnitude is the strength of correlation on a scale of between -1 and $+1$, with 0 being no relationship, $+1$ meaning that a high score on one variable is accompanied by a high score on the other and -1 meaning that a high score on one variable is accompanied by a low score on the other. Magnitude is expressed as a 'coefficient of correlation' and direction is indicated by the plus or minus sign.

The simplest form of survey is the case study, which is a single study of an individual or organization. The main weakness from a research point of view is that the results cannot be generalized. Descriptive surveys are used to collect information from a representative sample of individuals in order to make generalizations. Opinion polls are examples, and this form of survey does not attempt to explain the information in any way, so if one wishes to know if there is any relationship between variables, then an explanatory survey is required.

Another form of non-experimental research is ethnographic research which utilizes the technique of participant observation. This involves the researcher in sharing the experiences of the subjects in order to gain insight into phenomena.

New paradigm research

The term 'new paradigm research' was coined by John Rowan and Peter Reason to describe a group of approaches that constitute a new paradigm in human research (Reason, 1988). According to the authors, traditional or normative research tends to alienate subjects from the work of the researcher, from other subjects, and from the products of the research. In new paradigm research no distinction is made between subject and researcher, the aim being to work with people rather than on people. It is an approach that emphasizes action rather than intellectual problems, and this is exemplified in a technique called 'co-operative inquiry' (Heron, 1985). This approach makes no distinction between researcher and subject, with each individual taking both roles. It is used in conjunction with experiential learning, emphasizing the importance of reflection in the validation of experience. A group of student nurses may wish to enquire into some aspect of nursing, and they begin as co-researchers reflecting and clarifying the purpose and methods they will use. The study is then undertaken co-operatively by members of the group, and then the experience of this is reflected upon in order to help them to understand the meaning and implications of the study with a view to further modification of the original idea.

Sampling

This is a crucial aspect of research design and students usually need much help sorting it out. Sampling is the term given to the selection of the subjects for research, and implies that they are taken from a 'whole'. Sampling is necessary in research, in order to be able to generalize the results beyond the group that was investigated. The term 'population' implies any group of people or observations that includes all possible members of that category. A sample taken from a population must be representative of the characteristics of the population that is being studied. Samples are used because it is not usually possible to study every member of a particular population, so it is important to remember that the results of any one sample cannot be generalized beyond the population from which it was drawn. Measures of characteristics of a population are termed parameters and of a sample, statistics. There are a number of designs of sampling, the simplest being random sampling.

Random sampling In this method, each member of the population has an equal chance of being selected, as in drawing names out of a hat. A more sophisticated method is to use computer-generated random numbers. Random samples allow results to be generalized to the rest of the population from which the sample was drawn, but it must be remembered that such generalization is never totally accurate, there being some sampling error always. This means that we must talk about inference and probability rather than certainty, and in simple random sampling the error diminishes as the sample size grows.

Systematic sampling This is another type, in which the sample is taken from some kind of list at fixed intervals, for example, every fifth one. In this type, some members of a population have no chance of being selected and the randomness will be affected by the frame from which the names were taken. If this was done by simple random sampling, then the systematic sample will be equivalent. However, if the list is in some form of rank order, this would affect the representativeness.

Stratified sampling This involves the researcher in dividing the population into layers or strata, on the basis of such characteristics as sex, social class, educational attainment, etc., according to the variables under study. A simple random sample is then taken from each stratum. If the sample is proportionate, i.e. reflects the proportion of subjects in the population, then this method is more representative than simple random sampling.

Cluster sampling This involves the selection of natural groups on a random basis, and can be used where the size and cost of sampling a population in a simple random manner would be too great.

The decisions that the researcher must make with regard to sampling design are affected by a number of factors and Fox (1969) has put forward this adage: 'No data are sounder than the representativeness of the sample from which they were obtained, no matter how large the sample.' There are constraints on availability of time, finance and the facilities and assistance required, and non-response may alter the representativeness. The design of the sampling should be within the scope of the researcher, and compromise may have to be reached between this need and the type of sampling employed.

Measuring instrument or tools

Selection of instruments is a crucial stage in the research process, and the student needs to consider such points as the validity and reliability, practicality and so on, and whether or not the instruments are already available, or have to be designed. The two most common instruments used in survey research are the questionnaire and the interview.

The questionnaire This consists of a sequence of questions that the respondent is required to answer: there are two main areas in which it can be used: opinions and attitudes. When designing a questionnaire it is important to produce a specification of the subject area that is to be measured, and also to consider the practical aspects such as:

- whether the questionnaire will be posted to the sample, or administered on a group or individual basis
- what the sequence of questions will be, and,
- will it use open or closed questions.

Open questions allow the respondent to answer in his own words, but are difficult to analyse, while closed questions give the respondent a limited number of choices from which to select his responses (Oppenheim, 1966). This makes analysis much easier and is recommended for most types of questionnaire. The sequence of questions is important, as the initial questions should put the respondent at ease so that some kind of rapport is developed. The more searching, personal questions can be left until later in the sequence, when the respondent is convinced of the seriousness of the questionnaire. Wording of the questions is crucial and every effort must be made to eliminate ambiguity and possibility of bias. Leading questions are those that contain an implicit value as to what the behaviour in question ought to be. Prestige bias is the term given to responses which reflect distortion of the facts due to a prestige element. Questions that contain two elements are best avoided and it is essential that the questions are subjected to a pilot study, so that any of these problems can be resolved before the main data collection commences.

The interview Interviews have a number of advantages over questionnaires, although questionnaires or schedules are used in an interview. The presence of an interviewer ensures that the respondent understands the purpose of the study and any misunderstood questions can be explained. The respondent's non-verbal communication can be noted, and the interviewer can be instructed to probe further into the responses to a question. However, there is a danger of bias when using an interview technique, because the interviewer may introduce his or her own attitude without being consciously aware of this. The interviewer's responses, manner and other non-verbal cues may influence the response of the individual being questioned. Research students need to be made aware of the practical constraints on the use of this technique, particularly the problems of finance, training in interviewing technique, and the time involved in collection of data. There is a spectrum of interview techniques, ranging from the totally structured to the totally unstructured interview.

Carrying out a pilot study

Students should be strongly encouraged to undertake a pilot study to check out their methodology, as this will pay dividends in the data collection phase. A pilot study is really the main study done on a smaller scale, the purpose being clarification of procedures and methodology. The questionnaire should be tried out on a sample of people representative of the population to be studied, and the size of the pilot will be influenced by the time available and the size of the sample to be studied in the actual survey, but 10% seems a reasonable number for groups larger than 50. This pilot trial-run must go through all the stages in the research design, so that no aspect is omitted that might turn out to be a problem in the real survey. The results of the pilot study must be carefully evaluated and any improvements introduced into the final version. In the case of question-naire design, the improvements made to questions mean that those questions need to be piloted again in the revised form.

Data collection

The actual collection of data will vary according to the instruments used, but some basic principles should be borne in mind. The research student should be encouraged to conduct the data collection with due considera-tion for other people. Access to a sample depends upon the goodwill of the people concerned and is not a question of the researcher's right to be there. The student must also bear in mind that other researchers may wish to approach an institution for access to a population and that the conduct on his or her research may well affect the kind of reception that subsequent inquiries receive. The approach must be made in ample time, so that arrangements can be fitted around the normal routine. Research students may forget that the prime purpose of an institution is not to provide a population for research, but to go about its business as efficiently as possible. In this sense, all research is at best an intrusion and at worst a nuisance. The sample must be put at their ease during the collection of data and the guarantee of anonymity assured. It is often necessary to take great pains to explain that results will not identify any individual, since many surveys may involve the statement of attitudes towards an authority or employer. At the end of the study, the student should send a written acknowledgement to the people involved in assisting the researcher, although it is not possible to thank individually the members of the sample.

Data analysis

Having obtained the data during the collection stage, the next step is to subject it to analysis. If the research has used a qualitative approach the data analysis is likely to be partially or entirely qualitative, whereas a quantitative approach would require quantitative analysis using statistics.

Qualitative analysis

Statistical methods of analysis are not ruled out totally when analysing qualitative data; for example, students commonly use percentages to illustrate aspects of subjects' responses. However, there are severe limitations to statistics when attempting to analyse a wide range of qualitative data such as textual transcripts and the like. Qualitative analysis utilizes techniques such as network analysis, textual analysis, conversational analysis, etc. to gain insight into phenomena. Grounded theory is a common approach in social science research and is one of many styles of qualitative analysis of data. It is designed specifically for generating and testing theory, and theory should be grounded in qualitative data (Strauss, 1987, p. 22):

> Grounded theory is a detailed grounding by systematically and intensively analysing data, often sentence by sentence, or phrase by phrase of the field note, interview or other document; by constant comparison, data are extensively collected and coded, thus producing a well-constructed theory.

Quantitative (statistical) analysis

Statistics is invariably an area that causes students to become anxious, since the formulae can appear intimidating if the student does not have a good mathematical background. Teaching statistics need not be the dry presentation of figures and sums that characterizes students' views of statistics. I use the very first session of a research unit to involve the students in a Carousel Exercise (see Chapter 7) that generates data for subsequent statistical analysis. This has the effect of motivating students because the self-generated data is relevant to them. Henshaw (1992) describes experiential methods of teaching statistics, utilizing existing quantitative and qualitative data that nurses are already familiar with, e.g. TPR charts, fluid charts, accident reports and the like.

However, statistical analysis need not be difficult and the amount required will depend on whether the research project is largely quantitative or qualitative. There is a danger that the raw data may be transcribed in error when being transferred, so it is essential to double-check the results. Accurate records must be kept and the original raw data should be kept until the study has been completed. The use of a computer for calculations can save considerable time, and there are statistics packages available such as Statistical Package for the Social Sciences. The term statistics is used in three main ways (Guilford and Fruchter, 1973).

1. Statistics is a branch of the science of mathematics which deals with numerical data such as amounts, relationships, etc., in a sample.
2. Statistics is commonly used to describe numerical details in reports or records, particularly vital statistics such as births, marriages and deaths.

3. A statistic is a particular value, for example the average of a group of data. (The correct term for average is arithmetic mean).

Research information is termed data which is the plural form of datum, a numerical detail or fact. The original data gathered during research are termed raw data, since they have not yet undergone any kind of processing following collection. Processing of data is important in providing clarification, although there is inevitably some loss of fine detail which is referred to as degradation of the data.

Percentage   Percentages provide a useful method of comparing data on an equal basis, the assumption being that data are considered in terms of so many out of 100, that is, so-and-so per cent. If we want to calculate, in terms of percentage, five cases out of ten then one can simply write 5 out of 10 as a fraction, and multiply by 100%:

$$\frac{5}{10} \times 100\% = 50\%$$

Percentages must be interpreted with caution when using a small number of cases. For example, in a group of 20 cases a change in one case would result in 5%, whereas in a group of five cases a change in one case would be equivalent to a 20% change. There are two further concepts that are closely related to the percentage – proportion and ratio.

Proportion   This is a part, or fraction of 1.0. For example, out of 60 student nurses commencing a course, 6 withdrew in the first year. The percentage of withdrawals is 10% and the proportion of withdrawals is 0.10.

Ratio   This is a statistic denoting a relationship between parts and is expressed as a fraction. The ratio a to b is the fraction a/b, and the baseline is 1.0. For example, out of 40 students, 35 passed their assessment and 5 failed. The ratio of successful students to unsuccessful students in 35/5, i.e. 7:1.

   These two latter concepts, ratio and proportion, are very closely related. In fact, a proportion is a particular kind of ratio that is limited to the relationship of a part to the total. A ratio on the other hand, involves the relationship between parts.

Measures of central value

Central value is commonly called the average, but there are really three different measures of this concept, namely the mean, the mode and the median.

Arithmetic mean   To obtain the mean or average of a group of scores, the scores are added together and then divided by the number of scores.

Mode   The mode is defined as the score that occurs with most frequency in a set of data.

Median   The median is the point in a set of ordered scores that divides it into halves, so that exactly half the scores are less than the median and exactly half are greater than the median value. Calculation of the median value involves the use of a frequency distribution, so we need to examine this concept before returning to the median.

Frequency distribution

A frequency distribution is a table that separates the data into certain classes and shows how many data fall into each class. Frequency distributions can be plotted for both un-grouped and grouped data, the latter conveying much more clearly the information it contains.

Table 19.2 shows a frequency distribution on a set of un-grouped data which consists of a list of each of the average scores followed by the number of times each one occurred in the results. Table 19.3 shows the same data plotted in a frequency distribution, but using grouped data, i.e. scores that have been classed into score intervals rather than individually.

This distribution shows much more clearly the arrangement of the scores and renders the data capable of being converted into a visual form of display. There are conventions for deciding upon the number of intervals and also the size of each interval, the former being from 10 to 20, and the latter being selected from 2, 3, 5, 10 and 20. When making calculations on an interval it is important to bear in mind that in statistics a

Table 19.2   Frequency distribution of un-grouped data

Score	Frequency	Cumulative frequency	Cumulative percentage
84	1	20	100
82	1	19	95
81	1	18	90
78	2	17	85
77	2	15	75
75	1	13	65
74	2	12	60
73	1	10	50
72	1	9	45
71	1	8	40
70	1	7	35
69	1	6	30
66	1	5	25
65	1	4	20
63	1	3	15
61	1	2	10
58	1	1	5

Table 19.3 Frequency distribution on grouped data

Score interval	Frequency	Cumulative frequency
82–84	2	20
79–81	1	18
76–78	4	17
73–75	4	13
70–72	3	9
67–69	1	6
64–66	2	5
61–63	2	3
58–60	1	1

score is never seen as an exact point on a scale, but as something occupying a whole interval, from half a unit below to half a unit above. Thus, with our data, the interval 58–60 really extends from 57.5 to 60.5, and a single score such as 84 really extends from 83.5 to 84.5.

Graphic display of frequency distribution

Figure 19.2 shows two methods of presenting the information contained in the frequency distribution. Figure 19.2(a) is called a histogram and Figure 19.2(b) a polygraph, both illustrating the information in a visual way, conveying maximum meaning.

Having discussed the concept of frequency distribution, we can now return to the calculation of the median. This was defined as the point that separates the top half of the ordered scores from the bottom half, so for the data in Table 19.3 we need to separate the top ten scores from the bottom ten scores, i.e. the half way point. If we examine the frequency distribution we can see that the third column is headed cumulative frequency and is derived by adding up the frequencies from the bottom to the top. We need the point below which ten cases fall, so we check up from the bottom of the cumulative frequency column until we reach the point we require. Unfortunately, in these data there are nine cases up to Interval 70–72, and the next interval contains four cases. Now we require only one more case to make up our ten, so this must be taken from the next interval, i.e. 73–75. As we have already seen, this interval contains four cases, so we need to extend one quarter of the way into the next interval to reach our extra case. The interval 73–75 really has as its exact limits from 72.5 to 75.5, i.e. a total of three units. We need to extend one quarter of three units, i.e. 0.75 of the way into the next interval. This 0.75 is thus added to the lower limit of the category, giving a median of

72.5 + 0.75 = 73.25.

This can be checked for accuracy by working down from the top in a similar fashion, but subtracting the figure from the upper limit of the interval that contains the median. If, when calculating the median, the

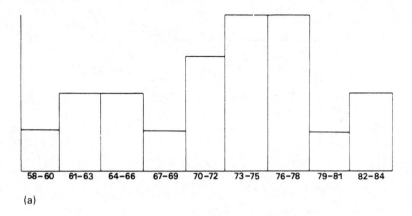

(a)

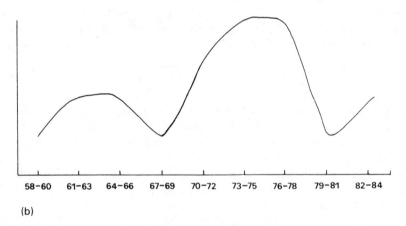

(b)

Fig. 19.2 Graphic displays of frequency distribution: (a) histogram; and (b) polygraph.

required number of cases works out exactly right in an interval, then the upper limit of that interval is taken as the median.

Percentiles

Another useful concept for processing data is that of percentiles. A percentile is the point below which a given percentage of scores fall. For instance, the 80th percentile is the point at which 80% of scores fall below and 20% fall above. The reader will see that the median is also the 50th percentile, as 50% of the scores fall above and 50% below. Percentiles allow a comparison to be made on two sets of data, by providing a common unit of measurement. The calculation of percentiles is quite straightforward, as is shown in Table 19.3. We must add a fourth column to the frequency distribution, namely the cumulative frequency percentage, which is obtained by taking each frequency in the second column and calculating what percentage of the total frequency it comprises. Now, the total frequency for all scores is 20, so commencing at the bottom of the column we can see that a frequency of one is equivalent to

$$\frac{1}{20} \times 100 = 5\%$$

The next frequency up is also one, so this 5% is added to the first 5%, giving a cumulative percentage of 10%. This is carried on for all the percentages in the list, until the final one arrives at 100%. Reading across the table, it is easy to see that a score of 69 is at the 30th percentile, as 30% of the scores fall below it and 70% fall above. Similarly, a score of 81 is at the 90th percentile. In addition to percentiles, the term quartiles is also employed. The first quartile contains the scores up to the 25th percentile, the second up to the 50th percentile, the third up to the 75th percentile and the fourth up to a hundredth.

Scales of measurement

So far we have seen how raw data can be converted into processed data by using such statistics as the percentage, measures of central value, and frequency distribution. However, we need to examine another important aspect of statistics, namely scales of measurement.

There are four of these used in statistics, and they form a hierarchy of levels, with the higher ones subsuming the lower.

Nominal scale   This consists merely of names or labels for the data it contains, with no further details of quantities. The only criterion is that the classes be mutually exclusive, i.e. no member of the data can belong to both classes, e.g. gender of patient (male/female), nationality (English, Scottish, Welsh, . . .).

Ordinal scale   This scale involves data in rank order but it does not assume that the distance between intervals is equal, e.g. satisfaction level (poor, satisfactory, good, excellent).

Interval scale   This scale does assume that the intervals between data are equal, and is thus termed the interval scale. The distance between scores 63 and 73 is the same as that between 74 and 84, namely ten. In the interval scale, e.g. when recording temperatures, however, a score of 80 is not twice that of a score of 40, because the zero point is arbitrarily defined rather than being an absolute zero.

Ratio scale   The highest form of measurement scales is the ratio scale, which does possess an absolute zero point. Most measures in the physical sciences possess an absolute zero point, so that one can safely assume that 10 litres is twice as much as 5 litres. In the behavioural sciences, however, the ratio scale is of little use, as it is very rare indeed to find a subject with zero characteristics.

Variability

The mean can be a useful measure, but is limited when dealing with more than one set of information. For example, two groups of subjects could obtain the same mean for a test, but the range of scores could be quite different. This could occur if the first group had a large number of high and low scores, with few in the middle, while the second had mostly middle-range scores. It is therefore useful to have a measure of the dispersion or variability of the scores. There are three main measures used to indicate variability: the total range, the semi-interquartile range and the standard deviation.

Total range   This is a very crude indicator of the dispersion of a set of scores, as it relies on the two extreme scores. It is calculated by subtracting the lowest score from the highest and in our data (Table 19.2), the range is 84 minus 58, i.e. 26.

Semi-interquartile range (Q)   This measure is closely related to the median and is one half of the range of the middle 50% of scores. The middle 50% of scores lie between the 25th and 75th percentiles and this range is referred to as the interquartile range, since these two percentiles separate the top and bottom quarters of the scores. The interquartile range is 77.5 minus 66.5, i.e. 10, and the semi-interquartile range is one half of this, namely, 5. This figure shows the average distance from the median to the 25th and 75th quartiles, and indicates the range of variability of the scores.

Standard deviation   This is the commonest and most reliable form of dispersion and is based upon the deviation of each score from the mean. The standard deviation is calculated using the following procedure:

1. Find the mean score for the group of data.
2. Calculate the amount by which each score 'deviates' from the mean, by substracting each score from the mean.
3. Square each of these deviations, by multiplying each one by itself. (NB. If a deviation in negative, its square will be positive.)
4. Find the sum of these by adding them all together.
5. Divide this total by the number of scores.
6. Extract the square root of this figure, which gives the standard deviation.

The standard deviation is probably best explained by referring to the concept of the normal distribution, which is a mathematical concept consisting of a bell-shaped distribution curve. Many human characteristics are distributed this way, such as height, weight and intelligence. Figure 19.3 shows the normal distribution curve and its relationship to the standard deviation.

It can be seen that 68.2% i.e. about two-thirds of all the scores fall between minus one and plus one standard deviations from the mean. Approximately 95% will fall between minus two and plus two, and

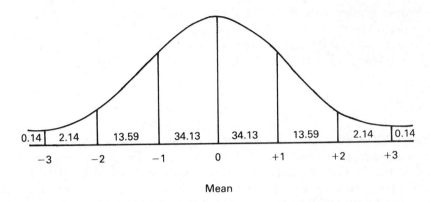

0.14 | 2.14 | 13.59 | 34.13 | 34.13 | 13.59 | 2.14 | 0.14

-3   -2   -1   0   +1   +2   +3

Mean

Fig. 19.3 Normal distribution curve and its relation to standard deviation.

virtually all cases will fall between minus three and plus three standard deviations. Thus, the full range of the normal distribution covers six standard deviations (99.72% of the scores) and this fact provides a simple test of the normality of the distribution. If we divide the total range of scores by the standard deviation then the result should be approximately six. If it is less, then the distribution is more compressed than normal, and if greater, then the distribution is elongated.

Correlation

Correlation concerns the extent to which one set of measurements is related to another and is the basis upon which causation is inferred in statistics. It is measured using the correlation coefficient (r), which is a single number indicating the extent to which two variables are related. This figure varies from plus one, which means perfect positive correlation, to minus one, which means perfect negative correlation. In the former, high scores on test A are always accompanied by high scores on test B, whereas in the latter high scores on A are always accompanied by low scores on B. The main requirement for computing a correlation is that the data must arise from the same source.

The actual calculation of a correlation coefficient can be done using a variety of formulae, the most common one being Pearson's product moment correlation coefficient. The formula for this is somewhat complex at first glance, but is fairly straightforward to calculate:

$$r_{XY} = \frac{\Sigma xy}{N\sigma_x\sigma_y}$$

r_{XY} is the correlation between a learner's score on test X and the score on test Y.

xy is obtained by first multiplying deviation x by deviation y for each learner.

All these products are then added up to give Σxy.
N is the number of scores in the test.
σ_x is the standard deviation of all the X scores.
σ_y is the standard deviation of all the Y scores.

Probability

Probability is an important concept in statistics, as it is used to estimate the odds against a result occuring by chance. If the probability value is higher than a certain figure, then the results are said to be statistically significant, which means that the odds are in favour of the result being true. Probability is defined by Guilford (Guilford and Fruchter, 1973) as 'the ratio of the number of ways in which that favoured event can occur to the total number of ways the event can occur'. By favoured event he means the event in which one is interested, for example the ratio

Ways in which a coin can land 'heads' up, i.e. one	: (TO)	Total number of ways the coin can land, i.e. two

The ratio is 1/2, or 0.5 and this comes midway on the range of probability, which extends from zero to 1.0. Zero implies that there is no chance whatever of the event happening, and 1.0 implies absolute certainty that it will occur. Another example is the probability of getting a six when throwing a dice, i.e. 1/6 or 0.17. Probability is also additive, so that chance of either a five or a six coming up is $1/6 + 1/6 = 1/3$ or 0.33. Probability levels are actually fixed in practice for statistical tests, at three levels:

	Odds against
(a) Probability of 0.05, or five chance occurrences in 100.	19–1
(b) Probability of 0.01, or one chance occurence in 100.	99–1
(c) Probability of 0.001, or one chance occurrence in 1000.	999–1

Generally, the lower the probability, the greater the confidence that can be placed on the result. Values higher than 0.05 are considered to be 'not statistically significant'.

Interpretation of data, conclusions and recommendations in the research report

It is important to advise students that their research project should be written up as they go along, and not all left until the research has been completed. For example, the literature search needs to be done early so as to influence the methodology of the study, so the student can begin to write this chapter quite early on in the project. Although it depends upon the exact nature of the research project, the following sequence of chapters might be suggested to the student:

1. *Abstract*   This is a short (300 word) summary of the research project, i.e. what it is about, what the student found out, and what the implications are.
2. *Introduction and context of the study*   This should include: the context in which the study is based, e.g. community nursing, midwifery practice; why the student chose the topic/issue; and what problem/issue the student is attempting to address.
3. *Review of the relevant literature*   This chapter should critically review the literature relevant to the project and should inform the design of the study.
4. *Design of the study*   This chapter should include methodology, sampling, data collection, and methods of analysis of the data.
5. *Analysis and results of the study*   This chapter presents the data collected, in the form of summary tables, pie-charts, etc.
6. *Discussion of findings*   This is the key chapter, in which the student demonstrates critical thinking, analytical and interpretive skills. Findings should be discussed in depth, and attempts made to explain them. The discussion should address any aspects that appear to conflict with the literature. The student has to take responsibility for what he or she writes by weighing the evidence and arguing the case.
7. *Conclusions and recommendations*   This chapter summarizes the arguments, and identifies the implications of the results for professional practice.
8. *References*   These are very important indeed as they indicate the range and depth of the student's reading.
9. *Appendices*   These are for material that, whilst being relevant to the study, is not necessary to include within the main body of the text, e.g. examples of raw data, specimen materials etc

REFERENCES

Bell, J. (1993) *Doing Your Research Project*, 2nd edn, Open University Press, Buckingham.

Clifford, C. (1993) The role of nurse teachers in the empowerment of nurses through research. *Nurse Education Today*, **13**, 47–54.

Christopherson, Sir D. (1992) *Research Student and Supervisor: An Approach to Good Supervisory Practice*, Magdalene College, Cambridge.

English National Board for Nursing, Midwifery and Health Visiting (1993) The Board's Response to the Strategy For Research in Nursing, Midwifery and Health Visiting: The Report of the Taskforce, ENB, London.

Fox, D. (1969) *The Research Process in Education*, Holt, Rinehart and Winston, New York.

Guilford, J. and Fruchter, B. (1973) *Fundamental Statistics in Psychology and Education*, McGraw Hill, Tokyo.

Henshaw, A. (1992) Statistics: a painless injection. *Nurse Education Today*, **12**, 142–7.

Heron, J. (1985) The role of reflection in a co-operative enquiry, in *Reflection: Turning Experience into Learning*, (eds D. Boud, R. Keogh and D. Walker), Kogan Page, London.

Kerlinger, F. (1979) *Behavioural Research: A Conceptual Approach*, Holt, Rinehart and Winston, New York.

National Board for Nursing, Midwifery and Health Visiting for Northern Ireland (1990) Attitudes Towards Research: Report of a Survey of Views of Nursing Service and Nursing Educational Staff in Northern Ireland, Occasional Paper No. 1, NBNI.

Oppenheim, A. (1966) *Questionnaire Design and Attitude Measurement*, Heinemann, London.

Reason, P. (1988) *Human Inquiry in Action*, Sage, London.

Strauss, A. (1987) *Qualitative Analysis for Social Scientists*, Cambridge University Press, Cambridge.

Author index

Subject index